AF560823

HEALTH PSYCHOLOGY AND COUNSELLING

HEALTH PSYCHOLOGY AND COUNSELLING

Edited by
Dr. M.V.R. Raju, *Ph.D.*
Professor & Head
Department of Psychology
&
Director
Centre for Psychological Assessment & Counseling
Andhra University
Visakhapatnam

DISCOVERY PUBLISHING HOUSE PVT. LTD.
NEW DELHI-110 002

First Published - 2009

Reprinted - 2017

ISBN: 978-81-8356-373-4

Health Psychology and Counselling

Published by:

DISCOVERY PUBLISHING HOUSE PVT. LTD.

4383/4B, Ansari Road, Darya Ganj

New Delhi-110 002 (India)

Phone: +91-11-23279245, 43596064-65

Fax: +91-11-23253475

E-mail: discoverypublishinghouse@gmail.com

sales@discoverypublishinggroup.com

web: www.discoverypublishinggroup.com

Printed at:

Infinity Imaging Systems

Delhi

DEDICATED TO

Dr. B.L. MUNGEKAR

Member, Planning Commission

New Delhi

Foreword

The present volume is the result of the proceedings of the International Conference on 'Health Psychology and Counseling' organized by Prof M.V.R Raju in Andhra University.

The deliberations of the conference gave a new insight in to the problems of professionals working in positive mental health and Psychology.

I was fortunate to participate in the seminar and the quality of the papers and the deliberations that took place indeed stimulated the interest of professionals working in health psychology.

This volume consists of four sections dealing with various aspects of health psychology and its applications. Section 1 on Stress, Adjustment and Coping consists of 16 presentations made by psychologists working in the area.

Section 2 deals with Health and Life style and 10 papers broadly cover this area of research.

Section 3 on Applied Organizational and Educational aspects is on the impact of the socio-cultural environment and health psychology. Five presentations discuss various aspects. Section 4 is exclusively on disability with four research papers presented.

Educational and health psychology is well accepted and recognized as helping profession in our country and the recent contribution from psychologists made a positive impact in the area of health. Significant contributions and research findings are great help to the allied fields like medicine social work and organizational development.

I am sure this volume will definitely make a positive & valuable contribution to the developing area of health psychology as a profession in India.

Prof. K. Kunhikrishnan
Pro Vice Chancellor
Kannur University

Preface

This book in its present form is expected to adequately meet the basic objective of providing research oriented aspects of stress, health, organizational and educational for the benefit of mental health professionals, psychologists, teachers, counselors and researchers. And recognize to meet the need for an Indian and cross cultural perspectives of Health Psychology and Counseling related issues.

This book defines Health Psychology and Counseling and has incorporated the mixture of empirical and theoretical research. Starting with topics, they are categorized under four sections as stress, adjustment and coping, stress and health educational and organizational health and disability.

All in all, this text sets the standard for the field; it is exemplary in coverage, organization, and perspective. It is a wonderful throwback to the vanished texts of yesteryear in making a scholarly contribution as well as educating its readers.

The text discusses specific topics on stress, health in different areas and its prevention through counseling and other psychological interventions.

I would like to acknowledge my senior faculty members for their support and cooperation in this regard. I am especially grateful to Prof.V.S.Pramila, Prof. Shanti V.Prasad, Prof. P.Nirmala Devi, who read drafts of the original text and provided helpful criticism and suggestions. I would like to thank Dr. N.D.S.Naga Seema for her valuable assistance, support and cooperation in the preparation of the book.

My sincere thanks go to all these people and to my family and colleagues, each of whom helped in bringing this book fruition.

M.V.R.RAJU

Contents

SECTION—1
STRESS, ADJUSTMENT AND COPING

1

Mental Health Problems of Adolescents

The Case of Students in Addis Ababa City, Ethiopia

Abdinasir Ahmed*, M.V.R. Raju**

ABSTRACT

The aim of this study is to investigate the mental health problems of adolescent students in Addis Ababa City by examining emotional problems in relation to such factors as age, gender, and socioeconomic status of the subjects. A sample of 702 subjects (357 males and 345 females) was randomly selected from sample schools. The data were collected through the Youth Self-Report and a demographic questionnaire. The results were analyzed using both descriptive and inferential statistical techniques. The results indicated the middle adolescent students have significantly higher emotional problems than early adolescents ($p < 0.01$). Female adolescents were found to have significantly higher ($p < 0.01$) emotional problems than males. The study revealed that subjects from lower socioeconomic status (SES) group has significantly higher emotional problems than middle and upper SES groups at $p < 0.05$ and $p < 0.01$, respectively. These findings were duly discussed and suggestions forwarded for practical intervention.

* **Abdinasir Ahmed (Ph.D), Assistant Professor, Jijiga University, Ethiopia. P.O. Box 1020, Jijiga University, Email:** *abdinasir786@yahoo.com*

** **Professor and Head, Department of Psychology, Andhra University.**

Psychologists and other experts involved in dealing with mental health problems of adolescents classify adolescents' psychological problems into two: emotional and behavioral problems. This study focuses on emotional (internalizing) problems. Emotional problems are those problems in which the adolescents turn their problems inwardly and exhibit the problems in emotional symptoms: anxiety, depression, withdrawal, and psychosomatic disorders.

Various cultures view adolescence as a time of intense moodiness and emotionality. Young people are thought to experience higher emotional feelings compared to adults (Verma, and Larson, 1999). Adolescence period is universally known as a period of fundamental biological, cognitive, and social changes (Hill, 1983). Authorities in the area stress that adolescents are more emotional than adults and exhibit also more emotional extremes than adults. (Bradburn, 1969; Campbell, 1981; Diener et al., 1985; and Verma, and Larson, 1999).

Different researchers identified a number of determinants of adolescent emotional problems. These determinants, among others, are age, gender, and socioeconomic status (SES) indices. The timing of pubertal development has been found to have an impact on the adolescents' mental health (Graber et al 1997). Twice as many adolescent girls as boy were reported to have emotional problems (Achenbach and Edelbrock, 1979; and McGee et al., 1990). Adolescent girls were also found to have more psychological problems of clinical range than boys (Lawlor and James, 2000). It was also found that girls have a tendency towards internalizing symptoms such as depression and anxiety.

In the same vein there is substantial number of research findings reporting that family attributes contribute to emotional problems. For example, social and economical disadvantage of parents and consequences that attend these disadvantages have implications for the adolescent mental health (Dekovic, 1999). Conditions like poverty, life stressors, and disruption of family processes have link to the development of emotional problems in adolescents (Stern et al., 1999).

There are different studies conducted about various aspects of Ethiopian adolescents. Although there are relatively sizable research works conducted on Ethiopian adolescent problems, most of them focus on different aspects of adolescent problems other than the emotional problems. The few studies on emotional problems of adolescents were carried out in other settings than schools (e.g. Abdinasir, 1995; Zenebe, 1996; Cox, 1967; Renner, 1974; and Yusuf, 1996). The available research evidences conducted in different countries pointed out that emotional problems negatively influence adolescent students in school. However, the emotional problems of Ethiopian adolescent students in school were not studied in a comprehensive manner. Therefore, it is paramount to investigate the emotional problems of adolescent students in school. The present study, specifically attempts to identify the degree of severity of emotional problems of adolescent students in relation to age, gender, and socioeconomic status of their parents.

OBJECTIVES OF THE STUDY

The general objective of this study is to examine the emotional problems of adolescent students. Towards this end, the specific objectives of this study are to identify:

- differences between male and female adolescent students in emotional problems.
- age differences between early, middle, and late adolescent groups in emotional problems.
- relationship between emotional problems of adolescent students and their parents' socioeconomic status group as measured by items available in their household.

METHODS AND MATERIALS

Sample: The data for this study were collected from a sample of 702 adolescent students (357 boys and 345 girls). The subjects were selected from upper primary (Grade 7&8), secondary (Grade 9&10), and preparatory (Grade 11&12) of the schools in Addis Ababa City. Equal number of students from Government and non-government schools was included in the sample. The sample was selected using simple random sampling technique.

Independent variables: In this study three independent variables were considered: age, gender, and socioeconomic status. The randomly selected subjects were grouped into male and female. Similarly, the subjects were assigned to three age groups: early adolescents (12 to 14 year old), middle adolescents (15 to 16 year old), and late adolescents (17 to 18 years old). Regarding the socioeconomic status (SES), the subjects were grouped into lower SES, middle SES, and upper SES groups based on the availability of household items and other appliances.

Tools: The Youth Self-Report Questionnaire (YSR; Achenbach, 2001) was adapted. In this study the first three subscales of the YSR were used. These subscales measure the mental health problems in the areas of anxious/depressed, withdrawn/depressed, and somatic complaints. The combined scores of these subscales form emotional problems scale. The YSR was translated into Amharic - the official language of Ethiopia. The translation was rated by judges using five-point scale. The ratings yielded high mean ratings with $\bar{X}$ = 4.58 and s = 0.51. The reliability analysis of a pilot test showed a coefficient alpha of 0.92.

A demographic questionnaire with 20 open and close-ended items was used to collect background information of the subjects and information pertaining to parents' material possessions.

Statistical Analysis

Descriptive statistics such as mean and standard deviation were employed. ANOVA was used to find out whether differences between groups of subjects in emotional problems are statistically significant. All the data were analyzed using SPSS (version 10.0 for windows) statistical package.

RESULTS

The age of the respondents ranges from 12 to 18 years. The mean age of the respondents was 15.76 year with a standard deviation of 1.65 year. The median and the mode of the age of the respondents were 16 years and 17 years respectively. Table 1 presents the percentage of the respondents by age group and gender.

Table 1

Frequency distribution by gender and age group

Age Group	*Male*		*Female*		*Total*	
	No.	*%*	*No.*	*%*	*No.*	*%*
Early Adolescent	94	13.39	74	10.54	168	23.93
Middle Adolescent	124	17.66	140	19.94	264	37.61
Late Adolescent	139	19.80	131	18.66	270	38.46
Total	357	50.85	345	49.14	702	100.0

The frequency distribution of the respondents showed that there were less early adolescents than either middle or late adolescents. The proportions of genders in age group showed that male respondents were slightly more in number in early and late adolescent groups compared to female respondents. Females were slightly more represented in the middle adolescent group.

Table 2 presents the summary results of one way ANOVA.

Table 2

Summary of ANOVA of emotional problem scores by age group

Source	*Sum of Squares*	*df*	*Mean Square*	*F*
Between Groups	947.60	2	473.80	6.47**
Within Groups	51199.78	699	73.25	
Total	52147.38	701		

** $p < 0.01$.

The results (Table 2), indicated that the mean differences between the adolescent age groups in emotional problems are statistically significant, $F(2,699) = 6.468$, $p < 0.01$. Further analyses of Post Hoc Tests revealed that middle adolescent group has significantly higher mean score compared to early adolescent group ($p < 0.01$). Whereas the mean differences observed between early and late adolescents and that between middle adolescents and late adolescents are not statistically significant ($p > 0.05$).

The scores of the respondents on emotional problems were examined in relation to gender. Table 3 presents the results of one-way ANOVA of emotional problems by gender.

Table 3

Summary of ANOVA of emotional problems by gender

Source	*Sum of Squares*	*df*	*Mean Square*	*F*
Between Groups	875.815	1	875.815	11.957**
Within Groups	51271.559	700	73.245	
Total	52147.375	701		

** $p < 0.01$.

The results (Table 3) showed that the difference between male and female respondents in emotional problem scores is significant, $F_{(1,700)} = 11.96$, $p < 0.01$. That is, female respondents reported more emotional problems compared to their male counterparts.

Table 4 depicts the results of the univariate analysis of variance of emotional problems scores by gender and age group.

Table 4

Summary of univariate analysis of variance of emotional problems by gender and age group

Source	*Sum of Squares*	*Df*	*Mean Square*	*F*
Gender	488.69	1	488.69	6.82**
Age Group	926.61	2	463.30	6.46**
Gender * Age Group	556.73	2	278.36	3.88*
Error	49884.93	696	71.67	
Total	339991.00	702		

* $p < 0.05$

** $p < 0.01$

The results (Table 4) indicated that there are statistically significant differences between the mean scores of female and male respondents in emotional problems, $F_{(1,696)} = 6.82$, $p < 0.01$, and age group $F_{(2, 696)} = 6.46, p < 0.01$. The interaction effect of gender and age group is also significant, $F_{(2,696)} = 3.88, p < 0.05$. That is, being in a given age and belonging to a given gender are important for emotional problems.

The scores of the respondents in emotional problems were investigated by parental socioeconomic status (SES). Table 5 presents the results of one-way ANOVA of emotional problems by socioeconomic status.

Table 5

Summary of ANOVA of emotional problems by socio-economic status group

Type of Problem	*Source*	*Sum of Squares*	*df*	*Mean Square*	*F*
Emotional	Between Groups	944.37	2	472.18	6.45**
	Within Groups	51203.01	699	73.25	
	Total	52147.38	701		

** p< 0.01.

The results (Table 5) showed that there are significance differences in emotional problems between the respondents from different SES groups, $F_{(2,699)} = 6.45, p < 0.01$. The results of post hoc tests also revealed that the mean score in emotional problems of lower SES group is significantly higher from that of the middle and upper SES groups at $p < 0.05$ and at $p < 0.01$, respectively.

DISCUSSION

The findings of this study showed that middle adolescent students reported significantly more emotional problems than the early adolescents. Adolescent students who are in different stage of development have different concerns and worries. According to the categorization used in this study, the middle adolescents are those who are 15-16 years old. Research evidence showed that, Ethiopian female adolescents experience menarche, on average, at 14.53 years (Tirussew, 1990), and male adolescents, though data is not available for Ethiopian boys, in general boys are one year behind girls in reaching puberty (Hurlock, 1988). Given these developmental changes adolescents in middle adolescence may face more social and psychological pressure in their life than their counterpart who are in early adolescence group and these in turn may lead them to exhibit emotional problems. Another possible explanation could be that most of middle adolescents are in first cycle of secondary education (grade 9 and 10 in Ethiopian education system) where there are more academic requirements and national examinations that determine their future life.

The findings of the present study on emotional problems are in agreement with the findings of other studies. Doepfner, et al (1997) found that occurrence of internalizing problems reported by parents for children and adolescents increases with the adolescents' age. Liu, et al., (2001) also found that emotional problems tend to increase with age. The results of the present study, however, are inconsistent with the study by Allgood-Merten, et al., (1990) which reported that no age effects in adolescent depression. It has to be mentioned here that the latter study focused on one component of emotional problems-depression and this could be a possible reason for the discrepancy with other studies including the present one.

The results of the present study indicated that there is gender difference in emotional problems. Female students have significantly higher scores in emotional problems than male students. Although there are no hard data that explain why girls have elevated emotional problems than boys, one explanation of these phenomena could be that of socialization. In most Ethiopian cultures female adolescents are expected and encouraged not to express their anger and frustration in aggressive manner and as a result they tend to resort to emotional outlets. In the case of male adolescents, it seems that there is a tacit rule that tolerate and even expect them to be aggressive. Other conditions being equal, the fact that these societal pressures occur at the decisive period of adolescence and provide differential opportunities for expression may have led the female adolescent students to incline to exhibit more emotional problems than male adolescent students.

Different studies have reported findings that agree with the finding of the present study. For instance, girls were reported to have higher emotional (internalizing) scores than boys (Liu, et al., 2001); similar results were reported for girls (Verhulst, et al., 2003;

Doepfner, et al., 1997; Lawlor and James (2000)). Furthermore, more depressive symptoms were found for female adolescents (Allgood-Merten, et al., 1990; Schraedley, Gotlib, & Hayward 1999).

The finding also indicated that students from the lower socioeconomic status (SES) group have significantly higher scores in emotional problems than students from middle and upper SES groups. This finding implies that socioeconomic status of the parents is a decisive factor in the emotional problems of adolescent students. The socioeconomic conditions of the family, especially the economic aspect of the family has impact on the emotional state of adolescent students. Adolescent students from the lower SES group, in addition to the emotional changes that come with their age, are more susceptible to emotional problems than their counterparts in middle and upper SES groups.

There are a number of studies that lend support to the findings of the present study in terms of socioeconomic status group. For instance, study by Larsson and Frisk (1999) found that youngsters from the lower SES group have elevated emotional/behavioral problem scores compared to youngsters from middle SES group. Similarly, Achenbach, et al., (1991), found that there are more problems and fewer competences for lower SES children compared to upper SES children.

There are findings of other studies that are in accord with some aspects of the present study's findings. For instance, among other things, depressive symptoms were found to differ by socioeconomic status (Schraedley, Gotlib, and Hayward, 1999). The family economic pressure was reported to eventually lead to elevated emotional distress in adolescents (Conger, et al., 1999).

CONCLUSION

In light of the findings of the present study, some conclusions can be drawn concerning the emotional problems of adolescent students in Addis Ababa City.

The study found that adolescent students have emotional problems that warrant due attention. The emotional problems are so serious and pervasive. Students in middle adolescence and female adolescent students are the most affected segments of adolescents by emotional problems. Students from lower socioeconomic status group suffer more from emotional problems than students from middle and upper socioeconomic status groups.

The level of emotional problems of the students is high to require professional intervention. Given the present low level of counseling services in Ethiopian schools, the emotional problems of adolescent students assume more weight. Concerned efforts of all concerned and professional interventions are needed to curb the current problems and lay ground for the prevention of these mental health problems in the future.

The present study, although it disclosed important findings in this less trodden area of research in the case of Ethiopian adolescent students, by no means can be regarded as all encompassing and final. This study used adolescent students as the sole source of the data on emotional problems. In the future researches, due attention be given to parents and teachers as the source of data.

RECOMMENDATIONS

The findings of the study disclosed that the adolescent students suffer from emotional problems of serious proportion. Based on the findings the following recommendations are suggested.

- Mental health professionals especially school counselors should be empowered through professional training to deliver their duties professionally so as to alleviate the emotional problems of adolescent students.
- The education policy makers should acknowledge the importance of mental health problems in schools and incorporate this to all relevant policy documents.
- Schools should establish link with mental health professionals and institutions outside the school system to provide professional services to the adolescent students.
- Efforts should be made to reach parents to raise awareness about the importance of mental health of adolescent students in schools to encourage preventive measures to minimize mental health problems.

REFERENCES

Abdinasir Ahmed (1995). *A study of behavioral problems of children in residential* Institutions: A case of children in Ethiopian Children's Amba at Zeway Unpublished M.A. Thesis, School of Graduate Studies. Addis Ababa University.

Achenbach, T. M. (1991). *Manual for the Youth Self-Report and 1991 Profile.* Burlingon, VT: University of Vermont, Department of Psychiatry.

Achenbach, T.M. (2001). *Youth Self-Report for Ages 11-18,* ASEBA, University of Vermont.

Achenbach, T.M. &Edelbrock, C.S. (1979). The child behavioral profile II: Boys aged 12-16 and girls aged 6-16. *Journal of Consulting and Clinical* Psychology, 47, 223-233.

Allgood-Merten, B., and Lewinsohn, P.M. (1990). Sex differences and adolescent depression. *Journal of Abnormal Psychology Vol. 99, 55-63.*

Bradburn, N. (1999). *The structure of psychological well-being.* Chicago: Aldine.

Campbell, A. (1981). *The sense of well-being in America.* New York: McGraw-Hill.

Conger, Rand D., Jewsbury Conger, Katherine; Mathews, Lisa S.; & Elder, Glen H. Jr. (1999). Pathways of economic influence on adolescent adjustment. American Journal of Community Psychology. Aug. Vol. 27(4) 519-541.

Cox, David R. (1967). Problems of Ethiopian Adolescents. *Ethiopian Journal of* Education, 1 (1) 50-56.

Dekovic, Maja (1999). Risk and protective factors in the development of problem behavior during adolescence. Journal of Youth & Adolescence. Vol. 28(6) 667-685.

Diener, E. Sanfred, E. & Larson, R.J. (1985). Age and sex effects for emotional intensity. *Developmental Psychology, 21, 542-546.*

Doepfner, Manfred et al., (1997). Psychic disturbances of children and adolescents in Germany: Results of representative survey: Methode, age, gender, and rater effects. *Zeitschrift fuer Kinder-und Jugendpsychiatrie. Vol. 25* (4) 218-233. Retrieved (April 17, 2003) http://www.apa.org/psychoinfo.

Graber, Julia A. et al. (1997). Is psychopathology associated with the timing of pubertal development? *Journal of the American Academy of Child & Adolescent Psychiatry. Vol. 36(12) 1768-1776.*

Hill, J. (1983). Early adolescence. A framework. *Journal of Early Adolescence,* 3, 1-12.

Hurlock, E., (1988). *Developmental Psychology (5th ed.).* New York: McGraw-Hill, Inc.

Larsson, B. and Frisk, M. (1999). Social competence and emotional/behavioural problems in 6-16 year-old Swedish school children. *European Child and* Adolescent Pscyhiatry. 81(1) 24-33.

Lawlor, M. and D. James (2001). Prevalence of psychological problems in Irish school going adolescents. *Irish Journal of Psychological Medicine. Vol.* 17(4) 117-122.

Liu X. et al., (2001). Behavioral and emotional problems in Chinese adolescents: parent and teacher reports. *Journal of American Academy of Child and* Adolescent Psychiatry. 40 (7) 828-36.

McGee, R., Feehan, M., Williams, S., Partrige, F., Silva, P., & Kelley, J. (1990). DSM-III disorders in a large sample of adolescents. *Journal of the American Academy of Child and Adolescent Psychology, 29, 611-619.*

Renner, Maria Theresa (1974). Adolescence in Retrospective. *Ethiopian Journal* of Education, 6 (2).

Schraedley, P.K., Gotlib, I. H.; Hayward, C. (1999). Gender differences in correlates of depressive symptoms in adolescents. *Journal of Adolescent* Health. Vol. 25(2) 98-108.

Stern, Susan B., Smith, Carolyn A., Joon Jang, Sung (1999). Urban families and Adolescent mental health. *Social Work Research. Vol. 23(1) 15-27.*

Tirussew Teferra (1990). Onset, bodily reactions and psycho-social consequences of Menarche among a group of Ethiopian girls. *Ethiopian Journal of Education. Vol. XI, no. 2: 1-27.*

Verhulst, F.C. et al. (2003). Comparisons of problems reported by youth s from seven countries. *American Journal of Psychiatry. 160(8) 1479-85.*

Verma, S. and Larson, R. (1999). Are adolescents more emotional? A study of the daily emotions of middle class Indian adolescents. *Psychology and Developing Societies,* 11, 2.

Yusuf Omer Abdi (1998). *Gender sensitive counseling: A Handbook for Ethiopian high school counseling*. Department of Psychology. Addis Ababa University.

Zenebe Mamo (1996). *Street children: Nature and magnitude of the problem and methods of intervention*. Conference on the situation of children and adolescents in Ethiopia, Addis Ababa.

2

Impact of Cartoon on Adolescents' Mental Health

Swaha Bhattacharya*

ABSTRACT

Now-a-days cartoon is one of the best audio-visual lucrative TV programme among the other TV programmes as accepted by the adolescents. It not only gives entertainment but also produces fun to the viewers. The aim of the present investigation is to study the impact of cartoon on adolescents' mental health and parental perception in this regard. Accordingly, a group of 100 adolescents (50 male and 50 female) and 100 parents (50 father and 50 mother) were randomly selected from different areas of Kolkata City. Three questionnaires, viz., General Information Schedule, Perceived Impact of Cartoon Questionnaire and Need Fulfillment Questionnaire were administered to them by giving proper instruction. The findings reveal that adolescents have strong and favourable attitude towards cartoon and they prefer to watch it than any other TV programmes, on the contrary, parents have unfavourable attitude towards it. According to them it creates violence , aggressive attitude, destructive tendencies which has a negative impact on their mental health. Besides this, reasons for need fulfillment as expressed by adolescents and parents also vary significantly. Adequate measures may be taken to create a congenial

* **Professor, Department of Applied Psychology, University of Calcutta, Calcutta.**

and healthy atmosphere for the viewers so that watching TV should actually give pleasure, recreation and keep the viewers good and healthy both physically and mentally.

INTRODUCTION

Now-a-days TV is considered as one of the best audio-visual media for all and that media is the best barometer of transformation taking place in our society. People are watching more television than ever before. People's dependence upon TV for recreation have increased. Among the different types of TV Programmes, Cartoon is one of the favourite show on television. Cartoon show just comes from animated picture. It is popular among children and adolescents. They watch an average of three or four hours of TV cartoons daily. Although cartoons are more entertaining, still it is difficult to consider that it is harmless and innocent way to keep the child, because now-a-days instead of indoor and outdoor games children spend much more time in front of the TV and they like to watch cartoons rather than other activities. It not only gives entertainment but also produce great fun to the viewers. Through the way of fun some cartoons increase knowledge among the viewers. Cartoon on TV is a clear incentive to the students and encourage to develop the notion of TV Literacy (Javier and Jose, 2002). TV cartoons are successful in broadening young children's knowledge, affecting their attitudes and increasing their imaginations (Indian Television.Com,Team,2006). After showing cartoon programme on television children and adolescents acquire more foreign language when it is in the sound track (Geryd and Marjke, 2004). Animated films, cartoons, comic books can address sensitive social and behavioural issues in an effective way if the audience is fully involved in creative process (Mckee and Aghi, 2004). Though cartoons are apparently more entertaining but it sometimes adversely induces the unhealthy behaviour and seriously affect the reading and writing skills of students. Preschool aged emotionally disturbed children's non-physical aggression increased from both aggressive and control cartoons (Kenneth, et.al, 1987). TV cartoons on sex-role stereotyping in young girls indicate that girls who viewed the low stereotyped programme received significantly lower sex-role stereotype scores than did girls in the high (Davidson, et. al. 1979). Media violence can encourage children to learn aggressive behaviour and attitude, cultivate fearful or pessimistic attitudes and desensitize children and adolescents to real world and fantasy violence.

Cartoon increases aggressive behaviour. In two separate studies, a class of younger and a class of older emotionally disturbed children were exposed to both high and low aggressive cartoons. Older class exhibited a significant increase in physical aggression. The younger group showed a somewhat different pattern of reactivity (Joyce, et.al,1987).Cartoon violence is a salient dimension which create discrepancies of behaviour among the viewers (Lambert, et.al.,1986). Another study reveals that violent cartoons increase physical aggressiveness among children and adolescents (David,1995). Watching cartoon for long hours adversely affect the daily routine of the students.

Besides this, it can be said that cartoon has an impact on reading and other academic skills which depends not only on the amount of television watching but also on what is being watched as well as age of the adolescents (Reinhing, 1990). Viewing violence in the television makes children and adolescents more violent. The most direct and obvious way in which viewing violence contributes to violent behaviour is through imitation and social learning. Children imitate televised words and actions from an early age. It increases aggression, desensitization and interpersonal hostility (Cantor,2002). Sometimes both children and adolescents do not understand reality and cartoon. It creates problems in their life. Sometimes the nature of cartoons causing confusion between fantasy and reality (Daniel,1997). Besides this, relationship between amount of television viewing and academic achievement shows that increased amount of TV viewing has increased good achievement among viewers (Razel, 2001). Television viewing increased young children's attentional abilities (Haward and Robers,2002). There are also some positive side of TV watching on children's social interaction (Mares, and Woodhan, 2005). It serves as a powerful socializing agent for easy understanding about values, beliefs and norms which is associated with health, illness and medicine. It has also great influence on both physical and mental health of the individual and society at large (Kline and Kimberly, 2003). Considering the above the present investigation has been designed to study the impact of cartoon on adolescents' mental health who belong to Kolkata City.

OBJECTIVES

1. To study the impact of cartoon as expressed by the adolescent viewers.
2. To study the impact of cartoon as expressed by the parents of adolescent viewers.
3. To study the need fulfillment by watching cartoon as expressed by the adolescent viewers.
4. To study the need fulfillment by watching cartoon as expressed by the parents of adolescent viewers.

HYPOTHESES

Hypothesis-I: Adolescents of male viewers perceive the TV Programme Cartoon more strong and favourable in comparison to the female viewers..

Hypothesis-II: Fathers perceive the TV Programme Cartoon more strong and favourable in comparison to the mothers.

Hypothesis-III: Adolescents of male viewers differ significantly with the female viewers in terms of perceived need fulfillment by watching Cartoon.

Hypothesis-IV: Fathers differ significantly with mothers in terms of perceived need fulfillment by watching Cartoon.

STUDY AREA AND SAMPLE

A group of adolescents (50 male and 50 female) and parents of them (50 father and 50 mother) were selected from different areas of Kolkata City following the stratified random sample technique.

The pertinent characteristics of the subjects are as follows:

Adolescent group :	**Parent group :**
Age: 13 to 18 years	Age: 35 to 50 years
Education: From Class VII to Class XII.	Education: At least Graduate

Both adolescents and their parents are willing to give data and they are aware about the TV Programme Cartoon..

TOOLS USED

1. *General Information Schedule*: It consists of name, address, age, gender, education etc. of both adolescents viewers and their parents.
2. *Perceived Impact of TV Programme Cartoon Questionnaire*: It consists of 20 statements answerable in a five-point scale where high score indicates good or favourable attitude towards the TV Programme Cartoon and vice-versa. Odd-even Split-half reliability is 0.81.

Item No.	*Discrimination Index*
1.	16.78
2.	14.55
3.	12.69
4.	17.11
5.	14.24
6.	15.78
7.	18.91
8.	11.79
9.	17.08
10.	15.88
11.	16.77
12.	17.95
13.	14.37
14.	12.45
15.	18.06
16.	17.64
17.	13.85
18.	16.43
19.	19.11
20.	15.82

3. **Perceived Need Fulfillment Questionnaire :** It consists of five statements by which an individual may fulfill his or her need by watching the TV Programme Cartoon. The subjects were asked to rank the items according to their perception.

ADMINISTRATION, SCORING AND STATISTICAL TREATMENT

General Information Schedule, Perceived Impact of TV Programme Cartoon Questionnaire and Need Fulfillment questionnaire were administered to a group of 100 adolescents and 100 parents by giving proper instruction. Data were collected and properly scrutinized. Scoring was done with the help of standard scoring key. Tabulation was done for male and female viewers of adolescents and also for father and mother separately for perceived impact of TV Programme Cartoon and for need fulfillment. questionnaire. Statistical treatment was done by applying t-test and chi-square.

Results and Interpretation

The general characteristic data inserted in Table-I reveals the characteristic features of the subjects, under study.

Adolescent	*Group*		*Parent*	*Group*	
Age	*Male*	*Female*	*Age*	*Father*	*Mother*
13-14 yrs.	16 (32%)	17 (34%)	35-40 yrs.	14 (28%)	19 (38%)
15-16 yrs.	19 (38%)	18 (36%)	40-45 yrs.	17 (34%)	18 (36%)
17-18 yrs.	15 (30%)	15 (30%)	45-50 yrs.	19 (38%)	13 (26%)
Education			Education		
VII-VIII	17 (34%)	18 (36%)	Graduate	18 (36%)	25 (50%)
IX-X	19 (38%)	16 (32%)	Postgraduate	16 (32%)	18 (36%)
XI-XII	14 (28%)	16 (32%)	Others (Engg, Law, MBA)	16 (32%)	7 (14%)

Data inserted in Table 2 reveals the impact of TV Programme -Cartoon as expressed by the male and female adolescents viewers belonging to different areas of Kolkata City. It can be said from the findings that both male and female viewers have strong and favourable attitude towards the TV Programme cartoon but male viewers have more favourable attitude in comparison to the female viewers. According to them, cartoon gives pleasure, entertainment, good break and many funny things. They also opined that in between the tight schedule of their study they get pleasure from it and they like it very much. Female viewers also expressed that they pass their leisure time by watching cartoon. But sometimes they feel tired due to long hours watching in case of interesting cartoons. Although both viewers have strong and favourable attitude towards cartoon still male viewers have more strong and favourable attitude in comparison to the female viewers. When comparison was made between the two groups, significant difference was observed. Thus the **Hypothesis-I** which postulates, **'Adolescents of male viewers perceive the TV Programme Cartoon more strong and favourable in comparison to the female viewers." – is accepted in this investigation.**

Table 2

Comparison between the male and female viewers in terms of Perceived impact of TV Programme Cartoon

Category	*Mean*	*S.D.*	*t-value*
Male viewers	80.50	9.43	4.84*
Female viewers	71.64	8.87	

Score range: 20-100, * $p<0.01$.

Comparison was also made between the fathers and mothers (parents of adolescents) in terms of perceived impact of TV Programme-Cartoon. Here, reverse picture has been observed as expressed by the parents. According to them, cartoon creates violence, aggressive and destructive attitude, different types of behavioural problem among the adolescents. Although there are some carton programmes which are entertaining and gives pleasure. and sometimes helps to pass the leisure time still it is not good at all. Overall picture reveals the unfavourable attitude towards it. Analysis of data also reveals that mother has more unfavourable attitude in comparison to the father. Thus, the **Hypothesis-II** which postulates, **"Fathers perceive the TV Programme Cartoon more strong and favourable in comparison to the mothers." – is accepted, but overall picture reveals unfavourable attitude towards cartoon as expressed by parents in this investigation.**

Table 3

Comparison between the fathers and mothers of adolescents in terms of perceived impact of TV Programme Cartoon

Category	*Mean*	*S.D.*	*t-value*
Father	55.67	6.74	7.25*
Mother	45.32	7.51	

Score range: 20-100, * p<0.01

Comparison was also made between the male and female viewers of Kolkata city in terms of need fulfillment by watching the TV Programme-Cartoon. Five important criteria were considered in this investigation, viz., opportunity for entertainment(A), opportunity for rest (B), opportunity for increasing knowledge (C), opportunity to increase imaginative power (D)and opportunity for good break (E). Analysis of data reveals that the male viewers gave top priority to the opportunity for entertainment and then opportunity to increase imaginative power, on the contrary, female viewers expressed that they fulfill their need by watching cartoon mainly because of opportunity for rest and opportunity for good break. When comparison was made between the two groups significant difference was observed. Thus the **Hypothesis-III** which postulates, **Adolescents of male viewers differ significantly with the female viewers in terms of perceived need fulfillment by watching Cartoon." – is accepted in this investigation.**

Table 4

Comparison between the male and female viewers of adolescents in terms need fulfillment by watching the TV Programme-Cartoon

Category	*A*	*B*	*C*	*D*	*E*
Male	35	6	21	24	14
Female	21	33	11	10	25

Chi-square : 34.16, df =4, Difference is significant

Comparison was also made between the fathers and mothers of the adolescents in terms of perceived need fulfillment by watching the TV Programme –Cartoon as expressed by them. Although opinion varies in connection with the five significant factors but overall picture reveals no significant difference between the two groups. Analysis of data reveals that fathers expressed top priority to the opportunity for entertainment, on the contrary, mothers expressed top priority to the opportunity for rest .Comparative picture reveals no significant difference between the two groups. Thus the **Hypothesis-IV** which postulates,

"Fathers differ significantly with mothers in terms of perceived need fulfillment by watching Cartoon."—is rejected in this investigation.

Table 5

Comparison between the fathers and mothers of adolescents in terms need fulfillment by watching the TV Programme-Cartoon

Category	*A*	*B*	*C*	*D*	*E*
Father	30	13	22	21	14
Mother	25	26	15	14	20

Chi-square : 8.55, df =4, Difference is insignificant.

CONCLUDING REMAKES

Cartoon is one of the favourite show on television. It not only gives entertainment but also produces great fun to the viewers. The major findings of this study are as follows :

1. Adolescents of both male and female viewers have strong and favourable attitude towards cartoon.
2. The reasons are mainly due to that it gives pleasure, entertainment, many funny things and good break specially in connection with the tight study schedule.
3. Male viewers have more favourable attitude than that of the female viewers.
4. Parents have unfavourable attitude towards cartoon.
5. The reasons are mainly due to that it creates violence, aggressive and destructive attitude and sometimes creates behavioural problems.
6. Mothers have more unfavourable attitude in comparison to the fathers.

7. Need fulfillment by watching cartoon differs between the adolescent male and female viewers.
8. Top priority in connection with the need fulfillment as expressed by male viewers is the opportunity for entertainment, on the contrary, need fulfillment as expressed by girls is the opportunity for rest.
9. Comparative picture reveals the significant difference between the male and female viewers in terms of perceived need fulfillment by watching cartoon.
10. Comparative picture reveals no significant difference between the fathers and mothers in terms of perceived need fulfillment by watching cartoon.

Considering the above findings it can be concluded that measures should be taken to create a congenial, good and healthy environment for all so that watching cartoon can't create any major problem to the adolescent viewers in the near future. Time management, counseling and engagement in other recreational activities is necessary to get rid of this problem. Parents have to take an important role in this regard. A friendly discussion is needed in this context. Not only parents, but also other family members, neighbours and programme setters should stretch forward their hands to create a healthy atmosphere in the society and to control the destructive and aggressive part of the programme. Adolescents also have to keep in mind that addiction for watching cartoon is not good at all and they have to control themselves for their future.

REFERENCES

Cantor, J. (2002) The psychological effects of media violence on children and adolescents, *Journal of Broadcasting and Electronic Media*, Vol. 45, 143-147.

Daniel,C. (1997) Children's understanding of what is real on television: A Review of Literature, *Journal of Educational Media*, Vol.23(1),67-82.

David, B.K. (1995) Massaging the medium : Analysing and responding to media violence without harming the first amendment, *Journal of Law and Public Policy*, Vol.14, 17

Davidson, S. Yasuna, A. and Tower, A.(1979). The effects of television cartoons on sex-role stereotyping in young girls. *Child Development*, Vol.50, 597-600.

Geryd,Y. and Marjke,V. (2004). Incidental foreign language acquisition by children watching subtitled television programmes, *Journal of Psycholinguistic Research*, Vol. 28, 3, 227-244.

Haward,S.M. and Robers,S. (2002). Winning hearts and minds : Television and the very young audience, *Contemporary Issues in Early Childhood*,Vol.3, 315-337

Indian Television.Com.Team (2006) Educational TV has positive effects on toddlers, preschoolers, *Indian Television. Com's Ideology.*

Javier, F. and Jose, M. (2002). Teaching physics by means of cartoons : A qualitative study in secondary education, *Physics Education*, Vol. 37, 400-406.

Joyce, S. and Kenneth, D.G. (1987). Effects of viewing high versus low aggression cartoons on emotionally disturbed children, *Journal of Pediatric Psychology*, Vol. 12 (3), 413-427.

Kenneth, D.W. Joyce, S. Thomas, J.F. and Springer ,N. (1987). Effects of viewing aggression-laden cartoons on preschool aged emotionally disturbed children, *Children Psychiatry and Human Development*, Vol.17, 257-274.

Kline, K.N. (2003). Popular media and health,: Images, effects, and institutions, *Handbook of Health Communication*, Mahwah, NJ, Vol. XII, 753.

Lambert, D. Dianne, E. Carr, K. (1986). Cartoons varying in low-level pain ratings not aggression ratings, correlates positively with funnies ratings, *Motivation and Emotion*, Vol.10, 207-216.

Mares, L.M. and Woodand, E. (2005). Positive effects of television on children's social interactions : A meta- analysis, *Media Psychology*, Vol.7,3, 301-322.

McKee, N. and Aghi, M. (2004). Cartoons and Comic Books for changing social norms : Meena, the South Asian Girl, Entertainment, Education and Social Change : History, Research and Practice, *LEA's Communication Series*, Mahwah NJ,Vol.XXII,458.

Razel, M. (2001). The complex model of television viewing and educational achievement, *Journal of Educational Research*, Vol.94, 371-379.

Reinhing, H. (1990). Television effects on reading and academic achievement, *Media and Family*, Vol. 70, 65-69.

3

Stress Among Women Teachers Working with Normal and Special Children

T. Santhanam*

ABSTRACT

The present study was conducted to assess the level of stress among women teachers working with normal and special children. The study was conducted on a sample of 100 women teachers, 30 teachers were from government schools, 35 were government aided schools and remaining 35 teachers were drawn from private schools. They were administered stress questionnaire by Latha. The results indicated significant difference in the level of stress among the women teachers handling normal and special children and also there was significant differences observed in the level of stress among teachers working under schools of different management.

Education is an enterprising activity, carving the society from the ancient times. It attempts to develop the personality of an individual and then prepares him for membership in a society. Education is the modification of behaviour of an individual for a healthy social adjustment in the society. It has grown complex and complicated due to the modern day technological development, problems of life and society. The teacher plays a vital role in spreading education and building up a healthy society. Teacher

* **Psychologist & Deputy Director, Government of India, Ministry of Labour Vocational Rehabilitation Centre for Handicapped, Guindy, Chennai – 600 032.**

plays an important role in the cognitive, social, intellectual and emotional development of children.

Among children some need special efforts focused on them. Thus, special educators are the teachers, who concentrate on the needs and development of these children. The special education teachers work with children with specific learning disabilities, mental retardation, speech, hearing or visual impairment, serious emotional disturbance etc. They are involved in a student's behavioral as well as academic development.

STRESS

Stress is a complex phenomenon. It is a very subjective experience. The term **"stress"** refers to an internal state, which results from demanding, frustrating or unsatisfying conditions. A certain level of stress is unavoidable. In fact, an acceptable level of stress can serve as a stimulus to enhance an individual's performance. However, when the level of stress is such that the individual is incapable of satisfactory dealing with it, then the effect on performance may be negative. Thus, extreme stress conditions are said to be detrimental to human health, but in moderation stress is normal and, in many cases, proves useful.

Selye (1956), an endocrinologist, perceived stress to be a neural physiological phenomenon. More specifically he defined it as a general adaptive syndrome or non-specific response to demands placed upon the human body. These demands could either stimulate or threaten the individual.

The term has been further defined by Gold and Roth (1993), "a condition of disequilibria within the intellectual, emotional and physical state of the individual; it is generated by one's perceptions of a situation, which result in physical and emotional reactions. It can be either positive or negative, depending upon one's interpretation.

In modern usage, however stress has come to imply the subjection of a person to force or compulsion, especially mental pressure or by overwork, which leads to strain or mental fatigue. In medical parlance, 'stress' is defined as a perturbation of the body's homeostasis. This demand on mind- body occurs when it tries to cope up with incessant changes in life.

There are unquestionably a number of causal factors for teacher stress. The most important factor is job satisfaction, good attitude towards the teaching profession. These factors lead to a healthy professional and personal life. When their job satisfaction gets lessened, their attitude towards their profession decreases and causes stress in their profession and thus affecting their physical, health and personal aspects.

METHODOLOGY

Aim

- To study the stress level of the women teachers handling normal and special children.
- To study the level of stress of women teachers working under different management of schools.

Hypotheses

- There would be significant difference in the level of stress among the women teachers handling normal and special children.
- There would be significant difference in the level of stress among teachers working under schools of different management.

Sample

The study was conducted on a sample of 100 women teachers dealing with normal and special children. The total sample of the study consisted of 100 women teachers among them 30 women teachers working in government schools, 35 were working in government aided schools and 35 teachers were working in private schools. The mean age of the total teachers is 19.6 years.

Scales

Keeping in view the objectives of the study and the nature of the research, questionnaire seems to be an ideal choice. Stress questionnaire is used to suit the specific needs of the study as well as the sample to be investigated. The general information regarding the women teachers, namely, their name and address and type of school was obtained.

Stress Questionnaire

Stress questionnaire was developed by Latha (1997). This test was administered to adults, as it was suitable to measure their level of stress. As it was standardized on Indian population it was more meaningful to use the scale for the present study. The scale consists of 52 statements arranged from mild stress (least affecting the everyday affairs), moderate to severe (which affects the adjustments and efficiency of an individual It has a control index, where the subject has to record whether he or she have complete, partial or no control over the experienced stressful situation.

Procedure

The present study was conducted to assess the level of stress among women teachers dealing normal and special children. The study was conducted on a sample of 100 women teachers, who are working in normal and special schools. The investigator approached the management of the school and got permission to conduct the study and requested the women teachers to participate in this study. The teachers were made to feel at ease and an initial rapport was established. The questionnaire was given to teachers and they were asked to fill it as per the instructions. There was no time limit given. They took approximately fifteen to twenty minutes to complete the questionnaire.

Data Analysis

The data obtained from the sample of 100 teachers was scored and analyzed. The analysis involved Mean, Standard Deviation and Analysis of Variance.

RESULTS AND DISCUSSION

Stress among women teachers working with normal and special children was examined by studying the level of stress and different types of management. Table 1 provides the results regarding the level of stress among women teachers handling different type children. The results regarding each variable are presented and discussed separately.

Table 1
The table shows that the level of stress among women teachers handling different type of children (Normal and special children)

Groups	*N*	*Mean*	*Standard Deviation*	*F-value*
Teachers handling normal children	25	20	4.13	3.314*
Teachers handling visually impaired children	25	20.24	3.74	
Teachers handling hearing impaired children	25	17.76	2.52	
Teachers handling mentally retarded children	25	20.40	2.96	

* p = 0.05

Level of Stress in Women Teachers

The table 1 shows that there is a significant difference in the level of stress among the teachers handling different special group of children and normal children. As per the selected stress questionnaire the score of 17 and above indicates a moderate level of stress. The above mean scores of all the teachers handling different special children and normal children fall within this category. Hence it can be interpreted as these women teachers are having moderate level of stress.

This result supports the findings of Boe et al. (1999), who showed that the special educators are significantly more likely than the general educators to transfer to other teaching assignments. This result may be due to excessive paper work challenging behavior of children they handle and inadequate support from administration, other professionals and colleagues (Ax. M & Stephens., 1998). Some of other reasons may be poor working conditions and facilities, poor salary, long hours of work, and heavy work load. Thus the level of stress of teachers handling special children is slightly more than that of the general teachers.

Table 2

Table shows the level of stress among women teachers working in schools under different management.

Groups	*N*	*Mean*	*Standard Deviation*	*F-value*
Teachers working in Government Schools	30	19.53	3.94	4.428*
Teachers working in Government Aided Schools	35	18.57	3.08	
Teachers working in Private Schools	35	20.97	3.19	

* p = 0.05.

Different Types of Management

The Table 2 indicates that there is a significant difference in the level of stress among the teachers working in schools of different managements. It is possible to say from this finding the level of stress is different among teachers working different managements. As per the selected stress questionnaire the score of 17 and above indicates a moderate level of stress. The above mean scores of the teachers working under different management fall within this category. Hence, it can be interpreted as these women teachers working under different management are having moderate level of stress.

This result may be due to more administrative jobs given, long working hours even after the normal school time, frequent and regular reporting to the school head and the parents, and inadequate support from the colleagues. Low status of esteem about the profession in the society due to the salary paid is also reported to cause stress in teachers. Pressure from parents and the administration about the children's academic and social improvement, extra-curricular activities, etc are also some of the cited reasons for stress.

Conclusion

This study revealed that the level of stress is moderately high in teachers handling mentally challenged children and as a whole among young and less experienced teachers mostly working in private schools. The reasons for stress by the teachers were workload, challenging behaviors of the children, inadequate administrative support, different degrees of disabled children in a class, student – teacher ratio and time constraint.

Moreover, the stress being an important psychological variable, experienced in day to day life, by everyone, causing psychological and physical health problems, is an additional cause for the teachers due to their professional requirements.

REFERENCES

Ax, M., Conderman , G., Stephens, and Todd. (1998). Principal support essential for retaining special educators. National Association of Secondary School Principals, NASSP bulletin.

Boe. E. E., Bobbit. S. A., Cook. L. and Weber. A. L., (1995). Retention, Transfer and Attrition of Special and General Education Teachers in National Perspective. Retention and Attribution, Washington. D.C.

Gold, Y. and Roth, R. A. (1993). Teachers Managing Stress and Preventing Burnout: The Professional Health Solution. Washington, D. C, Falmer Press.

Latha (1997). Development of stressful life events questionnaire. Journal of psychometry, 1997, Vol. 10, No. 2.

Selye, Hans. (1956). The Stress of Life. New York, McGraw—Hill.

Vimala, T.D., Prasad Babu. B. and Bhaskara Rao, D. (2007). Stress, Coping and Management. Sonali Publications, New Delhi.

4

Mental Health and Involvement of Working and Non-working Women

Explorng the Linkages

Sangeeta Rath* Fakir Mohan Sahoo**

ABSTRACT

More recently, the concept of mental health has received added significance because of changing societal complexity and global problems. Traditionally, the absence of negative mental states such as depression and anxiety present a picture of mental health. With the emergence of health psychology, psychologists have indicated presence of positive aspects like achievement, personal competence, autonomy etc as more important criteria of mental health. Involvement is a central life interest. It results in a commitment to a particular thing in which successful performance is regarded as an end itself. Involvement must enrich life experience. It can be conjectured that involvement and mental health criteria are related in a predictable pattern. In view of this rationale, the present investigation is geared to examine the role of involvement in determining the mental health of working and non working women.

The study adopted a 2 (working and non-working) x 2 (involved and less-involved) factorial design. Two hundred forty

* **Faculty PG Department of Psychology, Ravenshaw University, Cuttakc.**

** **Professor, Center for Advanced Study in Psychology, Utkal University, Bhubaneswar.**

married women (120 working and 120 non working) participated in the study. The non-working women were categorized into involved and less involved sub-groups on the basis of the median split of their scores on family involvement. Working women were also categorized into similar sub-groups on the basis of their combined scores on family involvement and work involvement. The participants of all the four groups were compared with respect to their mental health.

The result indicated involved women showed better mental health compared to less-involved women on almost all dimensions of mental health. Involved women have demonstrated better mental health in the areas of competence, achievement, trust, social support, autonomy, social contact, physical health, feeling of happiness with the family, satisfaction in work and person moral. Working women indicated greater personal competence, autonomy, coping effectiveness and achievement compared to non working women.

Most of the time, involved people exert greater effort because they are likely to see in their job / family a chance to satisfy their self-esteem. Hard work and effort always lead to success. Many empirical findings report positive relationship between involvement and success. It seems logical to assume that a successful person will be happy, competent, confident and all these factors will lead to better mental health. Married women's employment, however appears to have an effect. The independent financial base provided by the employment offers women an increased sense of competence, gives women more power within the marriage. The financial resource contributed by women's job enhances their social status, power, position and perceived self-efficacy.

More recently, the concept of Mental health has received greater research attention. Traditionally, the absence of negative mental states such as depression and anxiety present a picture of mental health. But with the emergence of health psychology, psychologists have indicated presence of positive aspects as more efficacious criteria of mental health. The critical examination of the literature in the field of mental health documents multi-dimensionality of the concept. The criteria are achievement, social contact, control, feeling of happiness with family, work satisfaction, personal competence, social support, autonomy, coping, etc. It is noted that both the absence of negative conditions and presence of positive conditions are considered important to define the construct.

Involvement is a central life interest. Involvement results in a commitment to a particular thing in which successful performance is regarded as an end itself. Psychologists are of the opinion that involvement denotes one's psychological identification with a particular thing (work or family) and perception of the same as contributory to his self-esteem. According to Kanungo (1982a) involvement (in work or family) may be defined as an uni-dimensional cognitive or belief state of psychological identification with work or family context. It is posited that the extent of involvement is determined by past cultural conditioning and socialization influences on one's beliefs about its potentiality.

The involvement must enrich life experiences. It can be conjectured that involvement and mental health criteria are related in a predicatable pattern. Traditionally, work and family are viewed as separate worlds, with males occupying the work world and females responsible for the family. Presently structural changes in the society encourage dual career life style. Today, women try to do the multiple roles or wife, mother and employee and they feel a need to justify their roles.

Employment provides either self-esteem boost or stress for women. Most studies indicate a high level of satisfaction among the employed mothers but stress can result when demands of the dual roles are excessive. There are two seemingly conflicting views. One is that employment can enrich a woman's life providing stimulation, adult contacts, and escape from repetitive routines of household and childcare. So, the mental health of the working women is likely to be better. The other approach, working women experience role conflict and role overload which produce stress and strain. Thus, the complexity of work and family linkage presents a challenge.

Ramu (1989) holds that in India, research on working women has been sparse and uneven. Working class does not get adequate attention in spite of being highly susceptible to the adverse effect of work on family. The most glaring deficiency is shortage of effort for

understanding the critical factors that connect work and family has tended to focus only on the potentials for disruption and overlook the possibilities of positive spill-over. The positive effect of each domain on the other also needs to be examined.

In view of this rationale, the present investigation is geared to examine the role of involvement of working and non-working women in determining their mental health.

METHOD

In this investigation, a series of activities were carried out to test the relationship between involvement and mental health of the subjects.

Subjects

In the present study, 240 women (120 working and 120 non-working were incidentally sampled from urban areas of Orissa. All the participants were married and had children. Working women were highly educated. So, the minimum qualification for the other half of the sample (non-working) was fixed at graduation level. All participants had middle socio-economic status and the age ranged from 30 to 45 and their average age was 36.41 years (SD=4.94).

Measures

In the present study, measure of work and family involvement and measure of mental health were applied.

Measure of Work and Family Involvement. Kanungo and Mishra (1988) developed a multipart questionnaire to measure both work and family involvement. This is a cross-culturally validated and standardized measure. The scale has been found to possess internal consistency, uni dimensionality and construct validity in bi national studies using both Indian and Canadian samples (Mishra, Ghosh & Kanungo, 1990).

A total of eight items each were used as measures of work involvement and family involvement respectively. Involvement in work context was measured by the use of the work involvement questionnaire and graphic scales developed by Kanungo(1982 b). Six involvement items are in the form of questionnaire and two are graphic items. The six questionnaire items of the work involvement include: (a) the most important thing that happens in life involves the work; (b) people should get involved in the work; (c) work should be a large part of one's life; (d) work should be considered central to life; (e) an individual's life goals should be mainly work oriented; (f) life is worth living when people get totally absorbed in work . The graphic scale had two items. In one graphic item, two circles representing work and self respectively are presented with varying degrees of overlap(no overlap representing total alienation to complete overlap representing total involvement).In other graphic item, work context was portrayed with a human figure(representing self) and a house (representing work) with varying distances between them. In this item, the degree of proximity represented the degree of involvement.

Involvement in the family context is measured by another set of eight items(six questionnaire items and two graphic items). This questionnaire scale included six items as listed above with the word "family" replacing the word "work" . In graphic item, where two overlapping circles are used, the two circles represented "family" and "self" respectively. The other graphic item portrayed a human figure(representing self) and a house(representing family) with varying distances between them.

All the involvement items for both work and family contexts used a seven-point response format. A rating of 1 indicates very little involvement and rating of 7 indicates high involvement .The score of questionnaire items and graphic items are added separately and the average score was calculated. The involvement score is obtained by summing up the average score of the questionnaire and graphic measures.

Measure of Mental health Sahoo (1990) has developed a Health Behaviour Questionnaire (HBQ) that includes both multi criteria features and cultural relevance. It has a grater degree of indigenous element compared to traditional inventories. Health Behaviour Questionnaire(HBQ) involves a number of techniques to measure mental health. Since the techniques are highly inter-correlated, the present investigation used only the semantic differential technique with a view to economizing on test administration time. The psychometric efficiency of the scale is represented elsewhere (Sahoo, 1990).

Semantic differential technique of Health Behaviour Questionnaire comprises of fifteen criteria related to health. The criteria include achievement, social contact ,control, feeling of happiness with family, good physical health, work satisfaction, value of spiritual quality, personal competence, social support, freedom from depression, autonomous activities, inter personal trust, effective coping, integrated personality, and freedom from anxiety. Bipolar adjectives are presented to denote each of fifteen criteria . Numerals from 1 to 7 between each set of descriptions are used. The individual is asked to think of her present life conditions or characteristics and evaluate it using each of the seven points by encircling a number for each set to depict her mental health.

While scoring, the direction of keying is considered. The closer and individual's rating to a desired criterion, higher the score. Score for each criterion was computed and the overall mental health score was calculated by summing up each criterion score of the individual.

The study involved 2 (working versus non-working) X 2 (involved versus less-involved) factorial design. Working women were given both work and family involvement questionnaires and they were categorized into involved and less-involved groups on the basis of the median split of their combined score on work and family involvement whereas non-working women were given only the family involvement questionnaire. They were also categorized into involved and less-involved subgroups on the basis of the median split of the scores on family involvement. However, the participants of these four groups were compared with respect to their mental health.

RESULTS

The summary of the analysis of variances of working versus non-working and involved versus less-involved on different mental health dimensions are presented in Table-1.

Table 1

Summary of the analysis of variance performed on mental health dimensions.

Mental Health Dimensions	*Sources*	*df*	*F*
Competence	Status	1	5.37 *
	Orientation	1	10.09 **
	Status x Orientation	1	0.02
	Error	236	
Physical health	Status	1	0.08
	Orientation	1	7.28 * *
	Status x Orientation	1	0.70
	Error	236	
Freedom from anxiety	Status	1	0.01
	Orientation	1	2.21
	Status x Orientation	1	0.30
	Error	236	
Personal morale	Status	1	0.05
	Orientation	1	5.59
	Status x Orientation	1	0.36
	Error	236	
Freedom from depression	Status	1	0.86
	Orientation	1	2.73
	Status x Orientation	1	0.38
	Error	236	
Autonomy	Status	1	6.75 **
	Orientation	1	6.28
	Status x Orientation	1	6.75 **
	Error	236	
Trust	Status	1	1.50
	Orientation	1	4.77 *
	Status x Orientation	1	2.48
	Error	236	
Social support	Status	1	3.32
	Orientation	1	8.36**
	Status x Orientation	1	0.44
	Error	236	

(Contd...)

Mental Health Dimensions	*Sources*	*df*	*F*
Control	Status	1	0.02
	Orientation	1	6.96**
	Status x Orientation	1	0.72
	Error	236	
Feeling of happiness in family	Status	1	0.45
	Orientation	1	8.59**
	Status x Orientation	1	16.51**
	Error	236	
Effective coping	Status	1	4.05*
	Orientation	1	9.75**
	Status x Orientation	1	7.94**
	Error	236	
Mental Health Dimensions	Sources	df	F
Feeling of satisfaction in work	Status	1	0.07
	Orientation	1	5.51*
	Status x Orientation	1	0.37
	Error	236	
Social contact	Status	1	1.02
	Orientation	1	10.37**
	Status x Orientation	1	0.30
	Error	236	
Achievement	Status	1	4.64*
	Orientation	1	11.37**
	Status x Orientation	1	0.04
	Error	236	
Spiritual quality	Status	1	0.51
	Orientation	1	1.34
	Status x Orientation	1	6.23*
	Error	236	
Overall mental health	Status	1	2.64
	Orientation	1	24.34**
	Status x Orientation	1	4.22*
	Error	236	

* P <.05.

** P <.01.

The summary of the mean ratings and standard deviations of the participants on different mental health dimensions are presented in Table-2.

Table 2

Summary of the mean ratings on different mental health dimensions

Mental health Dimensions	*Groups*	*Working Women*		*Non-working Women*		*Combined*
		M	*SD*	*M*	*SD*	*M*
Competence	Involved	5.85	1.37	5.37	1.55	5.61
	Less-involved	5.27	1.26	4.95	1.14	5.11
	Combined	5.56	-	5.16	-	-
Physical health	Involved	5.35	1.50	5.45	1.43	5.40
	Less-involved	5.01	1.54	4.82	1.22	4.92
	Combined	5.18	-	5.14	-	-
Freedom from anxiety	Involved	4.45	1.72	4.32	1.73	4.38
	Less-involved	4.02	1.54	4.12	1.64	4.07
	Combined	4.23	-	4.22	-	-
Personal morale	Involved	5.22	1.39	5.37	1.33	5.29
	Less-involved	4.90	1.47	4.83	1.33	4.87
	Combined	5.06	-	5.10	-	-
Freedom from depression	Involved	5.20	1.21	5.15	1.23	5.18
	Less-involved	5.03	1.40	4.78	1.18	4.91
	Combined	5.12	-	4.97	-	-
Autonomy	Involved	4.92	1.40	4.92	1.47	4.92
	Less-involved	4.93	1.39	4.00	1.26	4.47
	Combined	4.93	-	4.46	-	-
Trust	Involved	5.27	1.53	5.33	1.29	5.30
	Less-involved	5.15	1.38	4.62	1.64	4.86
	Combined	5.21	-	4.98	-	-
Social support	Involved	5.60	1.42	5.13	1.49	5.37
	Less-involved	4.93	1.53	4.72	1.32	4.83
	Combined	5.27	-	4.93	-	-
Control	Involved	5.43	1.26	5.60	1.27	5.52
	Less-involved	5.13	1.40	5.02	1.32	5.08
	Combined	5.28	-	5.31	-	-

(Contd...)

Mental health Dimensions	*Groups*	*Working Women*		*Non-working Women*		*Com-bined*
		M	*SD*	*M*	*SD*	*M*
Feeling of happiness In family	Involved	5.37	1.51	6.13	1.01	5.75
	Less-involved	5.55	1.18	5.00	1.24	5.28
	Combined	5.46	-	5.57	-	-
Effective coping	Involved	5.35	1.34	5.48	1.34	5.42
	Less-involved	5.30	1.19	4.50	1.23	4.90
	Combined	5.33	-	4.99	-	-
Feeling of satisfaction In work	Involved	4.95	1.55	5.12	1.35	5.03
	Less-involved	4.62	1.65	4.55	1.35	4.58
	Combined	4.78	-	4.83	-	-
Social contact	Involved	5.23	1.26	5.15	1.44	5.19
	Less-involved	4.75	1.39	4.47	1.48	4.61
	Combined	4.00	-	4.01	-	-
Achivement	Involved	5.55	1.35	5.20	1.54	5.38
	Less-involved	4.98	1.26	4.57	1.24	4.78
	Combined	5.27	-	4.89	-	-
Spiritual Quality	Involved	4.58	1.71	5.18	1.60	4.88
	Less-involved	4.83	1.19	4.50	1.18	4.67
	Combined	4.71	-	4.84	-	-
Overall mental health	Involved	78.32	11.46	78.90	10.63	78.61
	Less-involved	74.42	9.74	69.43	9.81	71.93
	Combined	76.37	-	74.17	-	-

The Analysis of Variance (ANOVA) performed on different dimensions of mental health measured by semantic Differential Technique indicates significant main effect for status in personal competence, autonomy, coping effectiveness and achievement, $F(1,236) = 5.37$, $P < .05$, $F(1,236) = 6.75$, $P < 0.01$, $F(1,236) = 4.05$, $P < 0.5$, $F(1,236) = 4.64$, $P < .05$ respectively (see Table 1). As shown by Table 2, working women report greater personal competence, autonomy, coping abilities and achievement compared to non-working women (M=5.56 & 5.16, M=4.93 & 4.46 personal competence, physical health, personal morale, autonomy, trust, social support, control, feeling of happiness with family, effective coping, work satisfaction, social contact and achievement, indicates significant effect for orientation. $F(1,236) = 10.09$, $P < .01$, $F(1,2136)$

= 7.28, P < .01, F(1,236) = 5.59, P < 0.05, F(1,236)=6.28, P < .05 F(1.236)=4.77, P < .05, F(1,236) = 8.36, P < .01, F(1,236) = 6.96, P < .01, F(1,236)=8.59, P < .01, F(1,236)=9.74, P < .01, F(1,236) = 5.51, P < .05, F(1,236) = 10.37, P < .01 and F(1,236) = 11.37, P < .01. It indicated involved women show greater personal competence, better physical health, personal morale, more autonomy, trust, social support, control, feeling of happiness with family, coping, work satisfaction, social contact and achievement than less involved women (M=5.61 & 5.11), (M=5.40 & 4.92), (M=5.29 & 4.87), (M=4.92 & 4.47), (M=5.30 & 4.86), (M=5.37 & 4.83), (M=5.52 & 5.08), (M=5.75 & 5.28), (M=5.42 & 4.90), (M=5.03 & 4.98), (M=5.19 & 4.61) and (M=5.38 & 4.78 respectively). On overall mental health also the ANOVA shows significant effect for orientation, F(1,236)=24.34, P < .01. The mean scores of overall mental health indicate that the involved participants experience greater mental health than do less-involved participants (M=78.61 & 71.93 respectively).

DISCUSSION

Findings regarding working versus non-working women reveal certain interesting features. Working women indicate higher personal competence, more autonomy, achievement and coping effectiveness than do non-working women. With respect to overall mental health also, they tend too show better mental health than do non-working women even though the result does not reach the level of statistical significane.

Married women's employment, however appears to have an effect. The independent financial base provided by the employment offers women an increased sense of competence, gives women more power within the marriage and increases their influence in decision making (Blood & Wolfe, 1960; Blood, 1965). In addition, the financial resource contributed by wife's job enhances family's social status, wife's power, position and perceived self-efficacy.

In general, employment, marriage and parenthood are associated with good physical and mental health in both men and women. Verbrugge (1983) found that employed married parents tend to be the most healthy ones whereas persons with none of these roles tend to have the poorest health. Studies of relationship between multiple role involvement and mental health typically show positive effects for both women and men. Thoits (1983) for example found that regardless of gender, occupancy of up to seven roles was positively associated with mental health. Similarly, other studies have shown higher level of life satisfaction (Stewart & Salt, 1981) among women who occupy the three roles of wife, mother and paid worker effectively compared with women who occupy fewer roles. In a study by Pietromonaco, Manis and Frohardt-Lane (1984), for example, there is no increase in reported stress associated with a greater number of roles and more roles a woman occupied, the more source of pleasure she reported in her life. Kessler and McRae (1982) found that paid employment is associated with improved mental health among married women.

A wide variety of well-controlled studies show significant mental and physical health differences that favours working over non-working women (Verbrugge, 1983; Waldron & Herold, 1984; Merikangas, 1985). Moreover, contrary to the belief that the more high powered a woman's career, the more dangerous it is to her well-being, the advantages are greater for women in occupations with higher status (Baruch, 1985). Although being employed is beneficial even to women in low-level jobs (Ferree, 1976; Belle, 1982), viewing one's work as a career rather than a job is associated with greater work satisfaction and less role conflict. Merikangas (1985) has noted that the lack of employment is a risk factor for depression in women. He further commented that perhaps "a job is to a woman as a wife is to a man".

Another interesting feature of this investigation is that the involved women indicate better mental health than less-involved women. Involved women have demonstrated better mental health in the areas of competence, achievement, trust, social support, social contact, autonomy, physical health, feeling of happiness with family, satisfaction in work and person morale. Since the mental health of involved women has been indicated in a number of domains, it is obvious that involved women experience greater overall mental health compared to less-involved women.

Involved ones attach greater importance to the satisfaction of esteem, achievement, autonomy, power, control and growth needs. Since most psychological literature suggests that involved people demonstrate greater degree of goal specificity and persistence than the less-involved, it is expected that achievement and feeling of competence should co-vary with Involvement (Steers, 1975; Saal, 1978) shared greater consistency in demonstrating a positive relationship between these two variables.

Past empirical literature has shown that the sense of control enhances one's mental health. Moreover, pertinent literature on control has also indicated that involved persons have more control than less-involved persons. The present study indicates similar affirmative results. Since the investigation indicates that involved women show more happiness in family and satisfaction in work, it is plausible that they remain happy because they are satisfied with their family and work. It has been argued in the literature that though satisfaction and involvement are conceptually distinct, they share many common determinants. Hence it is logical to except them to be related to each other. The theoretical model developed by Hall (1971) also seems to affirm the above reasoning. Finally, the empirical findings support such a position (Wood, 1971; Newman, 1975; Baba & Jamal, 1976).

Most of the time, the involved ones exert greater effort because they are likely to see in their job a chance to satisfy their self-esteem. Hard work and effort always lead to success. It is also suggested in literature that experience of success enhances involvement (Hall, 1971). Many empirical findings reported positive relationship between involvement and success. It seems logical to assume that a successful person will be hapy, competent, confident and all these factors will lead to better mental helath and feeling of happiness in family. Involved women have also indicated greater person morale compared to less-involved women. Person morale denotes the integrity of the individual i.e. integrity of words, deeds, thoughts and feelings of the individual. It is indicative of the harmonious relationship amongst different functions and sub-functions within the individual. Since involved women have indicated a higher level of personal accomplishment in the areas of achievement, competence, trust and autonomy, it appears plausible that these persons are capable of coordinating their thoughts, words and deeds in an effective manner. This is reflected in their higher morale.

Less-involved women indicate less-competence, achievement, success and ultimately enjoy less happiness in family and lower satisfaction in work. It can be conjectured that less-involved individuals with a low degree of confidence are likely to engage in social interactions less effectively so that they are not in a position to derive desirable outcomes. Perhaps for that reason, less involved women do not enjoy social contacts and social support to the extent the involved women do. However, it appears that involvement as a positive life process generates wellness as its outcome.

REFERENCES

Baba, V.V., & Jamal, M. (1976). On the nature of company satisfaction, company commitment and work involvement : An empirical examination of blue-collar workers *Relations Industrielle, 31, 434-47.*

Baruch, G.K. (1985). Women's involvement in multiple roles and psychological distress. *Journal of Personality and Social Psychology*, 49, 135-145.

Belle, D.(Ed.) (1982). *Lives in stress : Women and depression*. Beverly Hills, C.A.: Sage.

Blood, R.O. Jr. (1965). Long range causes and consequences of the employed married women. *Journal of the Marriage and the Family, 27(1), 43-47.*

Blood, R.O., &Wolfe, D.M. (1960). *Husband and wives : The dynamics of married living. Glencoe, IL : The Free Press.*

Ferree, M. (1976). House work and paid work as source of satisfaction : *Social Problems*, 23, 431-441.

Haal, D.T. (1971). Theoretical model of career sub-identity development in organizational settings. *Organisaitonal Behaviour and Human performance. 6, 50-76.*

Kanungo, R.N. (1982a). *Work alienation*. New York. Praeger.

Kanungo, R.N. (1982b). Measurement of job and work involvement, *Journal of Applied Psychology*, 67, 341-349.

Kanungo, R.N., & Mishra, S. (1984). An uneasy look at work, non-work and leisure. In M.D. Lee and R.N. Kanungo (Eds.). *Management of work and personal life*. New York. Pracger.

Kanungo, R.N., & Mishra, S. (1988). The bases of involvement in work and family contexts. *International Journal of Psychology. 23, 267-282.*

Kessler, R.C. McRae, J.A., Jr (1982). The effects of wives employment on the mental health of married men and women. *American Psychological Review*, 47, 216-227.

Merikangas, K. (1985). *Sex differences in depression*. Paper presented at the Murray center (Radeliffe College) Conference : Mental health in social context; Cambridge, MA, USA.

Mishra, S, Ghosh R., & Kanungo, R.N. (1990). The definition and measurement of family involvement. *Journal of Cross-Cultural Psychology*, 21, 232-248.

Newman, J.E. (1975). Understanding Organizaitonal Structure : Job attitude relationship through peceptions of the work environment. *Organizational Behaviour and Human Performance,* 13; 371-79.

Pietromonaco, P.R., Manis, J., & Frohardt-Lane, K. (1984). *Psychological consequences of multiple social roles.* Paper presented at the meeting of American Psychological Association, Toronto.

Ramu, G.N. (1989). *Women, work and marriage in urban India : A study of dual and single earner couples.* New Delhi : Sage.

Saal, F.E. (1978). Job involvement : A multivariate approach. *Journal of Applied Psychology,* 63, 53-61.

Sahoo, F.M. (1990). *Health Behaviour Questionnaire.* Unpublished report, Utkal University, Bhubaneswar, India.

Steers, R.M. (1975). Effects of need for achievement on job performance : Job attitude relationship. *Journal of Applied Psychology,* 60, : 678-82.

Stewart, A.S. & Salt, P. (1981). Life stress, life styles, depression and illness in adult women. *Journal of Personality and Social Psychology.* 40, 1063-69.

Thoits, P.A. (1983). Multiple identities and psychological well-beibng. *American Sociological Review.* 48, 174-187.

Verbrugge, L. (1983). Multiple roles and physical health or women and men. *Journal of Health and Social Behaviour, 24, 16-30.*

Waldron, I., & Herold, J. (1984). *Employment attitudes towards employment and women's health.* Paper presented at the meeting of the society of behavioural medicine, Philadelphia.

Wood, D.A. (1971). Enhancing attitude performance relationships by degree of job involvement. *Proceedings of the American Psychological Association,* Annual convention.

5

Stress and Erectile Dysfunction
The Effect of Psychological Interventions

M.V.R.Raju*, N.D.S. Naga Seema, T.S.Rao*****

ABSTRACT

The present study is intended to examine erectile function of males having sexual problems. The erectile factors are associated with anxiety and stress factors. The stress factors include situational stress, stress in body and stress in mind. The major objectives of the study are to examine (1) the impact of individual factors on erectile function and stress, (2) the effect of interventions on erectile function and stress. The tools used for the study were International Index of Erectile Function Questionnaire (IIEF, 1997) by R. C. Rosen, and a Seven Minute stress test (1989) developed by Ronald G. Nathan. The study was conducted on a sample of 322 males having sexual problems. They were selected from the Vasavya Nursing Home, Vijayawada, which is a private hospital and one of the famous hospitals in Andhra Pradesh for sexual problems. The data were analyzed and significant results were obtained. Erectile function appears to be high for sample aged above 35 years. Situational stress and stress in the body seem to increase with age. Stress in the body and mind decrease with higher educational qualification. It was found that interventions such as Counseling, Psychotherapy

* **Professor and Head, Department of Psychology, Andhra University.**

** **Research Scholar, Department of Psychology, Andhra University.**

*** **Research Scholar, Department of Psychology, Andhra University.**

and Jacobson's Progressive Muscle Relaxation had significantly improved erectile functioning, and reduced stress.

The term "Erectile Dysfunction" was coined by Kaplan in 1974. According to a National Institutes of Health (NIH) consensus panel convened in 1993 erectile dysfunction (ED) is defined as the inability to achieve and/or maintain an erection sufficiently for satisfactory sexual activity. Although never life threatening in the usual sense of being fatal, ED may yet juxtapose many effects on the quality of life by causing considerable loss of self-esteem and often putting important life relationships in jeopardy. It is difficult to assess the precise effect of ED on quality of life because the dysfunction may be partly a result of a pre-existing psychological problem, which complicates interpretation. Nevertheless, ED often results in anxiety, depression and lack of self-esteem and self-confidence, which in themselves can perpetuate the disorder. This, in itself, often compounds the physical problem, which at the nadir ends up in loss of self-esteem, and fear of humiliation associated with inadequate sexual performance.

Erectile dysfunction is the repeated inability to get or keep an erection firm enough for sexual intercourse. The word "impotence" may also be used to describe other problems that interfere with sexual intercourse and reproduction, such as lack of sexual desire and problems with ejaculation or orgasm. Using the term erectile dysfunction makes it clear that those other problems are not involved.

Erectile dysfunction can be a total inability to achieve erection, an inconsistent ability to do so, or a tendency to sustain only brief erection. These variations make defining ED and estimating its incidence difficult. According to the National Ambulatory Medical Care Survey (NAMCS), for every 1,000 men in the United States, 7.7 physician office visits were made for ED in 1985. By 1999, that rate had nearly tripled to 22.3. The increase happened gradually, presumably as treatments such as vacuum devices and injectable drugs became more widely available and discussing erectile function became accepted. Perhaps the most publicized advance was the introduction of the oral drug sildenafil citrate (Viagra) in March 1998. NAMCS data on new drugs show an estimated 2.6 million mentions of Viagra at physician office visits in 1999, and one-third of those mentions occurred during visits for a diagnosis other than ED.

The causes of ED are frequently multifactorial, with psychological, neurological, endocrinological, vascular, traumatic and iatrogenic components described. Erectile dysfunction is usually divided into organic and psychogenic, according to the main contributors to the dysfunction. Organic ED is the result of an acute or chronic physiological condition, including endocrinologic, neurologic, or vascular etiologies. Unless related to trauma or surgery, organic ED is associated with a gradual progressive decline in sexual, masturbated, and nocturnal erectile rigidity. Approximately 80% of cases are secondary to organic disease, 70% of those to arterial or venous abnormalities.

Also, surgery (especially radical prostate and bladder surgery for cancer) can injure nerves and arteries near the penis, causing ED. Injury to the penis, spinal cord, prostate, bladder, and pelvis can lead to ED by harming nerves, smooth muscles, arteries, and fibrous tissues of the corpora cavernosa. In addition, many common medicines—blood pressure drugs, antihistamines, antidepressants, tranquilizers, appetite suppressants, and cimetidine (an ulcer drugs,) —can produce ED as a side effect.

On the other hand, historical indicators of psychogenic ED include acute onset, often related to a specific event, and usually associated with normal nocturnal or masturbatory erections. The most common causes of psychogenic impotence are: performance anxiety, relationship conflict, sexual inhibition, conflicts over sexual preference, and fear of pregnancy or sexually transmitted diseases.

Psychological or relationship factors frequently coexist with organic causes. Even minimal organic disease may result in performance anxiety; stress, with heightened sympathetic tone; and secondary psychogenic sexual dysfunction. Psychogenic ED may also occur in patients with clear-cut organic problems, such as diabetes or post radical prostatectomy.

Experts believe that psychological factors such as stress, anxiety, guilty, depression, low self-esteem, and fear of sexual failure cause 10 to 20 percent of ED cases. Men with a physical cause for

ED frequently experience the same sort of psychological reactions (stress, anxiety, guilt, and depression). Other possible causes are smoking, which affects blood flow in veins and arteries, and hormonal abnormalities, such as not enough testosterone.

HOW IS ED DIAGNOSED?

Patient History

Medical and sexual histories help to define the degree and nature of ED. A medical history can diseases that lead to ED, while a simple recounting of sexual activity might distinguish among problems with sexual desire, erection, ejaculation, or orgasm.

Physical Examination

Physical examinations can give clues to systemic problems. For example, if the penis is not sensitive to touching, a problem in the nervous system may be the cause. Abnormal secondary sex characteristics, such as hair pattern or breast enlargement, can point to hormonal problems, which would mean that the endocrine system is involved.

Laboratory Tests

Several laboratory tests can help diagnose ED. Tests for systemic diseases include blood counts, urinalysis, lipid profile, and measurements of creatinine and liver enzymes.

Other Tests

Monitoring erections that occur during sleep (nocturnal penile tumescence) can help rule out certain psychological causes of ED. Healthy men have involuntary erections during sleep.

Psychosocial Examination

A psychosocial examination, using an interview and a questionnaire, reveals psychological factors. A man's sexual partner may also be interviewed to determine expectations and perceptions during sexual intercourse.

Discussing the relationship between psychological, social, and physiological factors in sexual difficulties and dysfunctions, particularly male erectile dysfunction Ducharme (2004) identified numerous psychological issues that impact on an individual's satisfaction and ability to satisfy a partner. According to the author, the most typical include: low self-esteem, body image issues, past sexual abuse or trauma, relationships difficulties, poor communication and stresses of daily living.

Schiavi et al. (1990) examined the effect of age on sexual function and behavior (as determined in psychosexual interviews) and on nocturnal penile tumescence (NPT) in 65 healthy married men (aged 45-74 yrs). There was a significant negative relation between age and sexual desire, arousal, and activity. Clerici et al (1994) suggested that a patient in his forties and with an acute onset of impotence should be assessed from a psychological point of view.

According to Moore et al (2003), the prevalence of ED increases with age. However, it may emerge at any time during the adult years, and may bear a close relationship to ongoing psychosocial issues affecting the patient and his partner.Urban and Bela (2003) examined that age, residence, psychological stress and two or three chronic diseases formed significant risk factors to ED. Fahrner (1987) investigated sexual dysfunction in male alcohol addicts, Tengs and Osgood (2001) studied the link between smoking and impotence. Wylie et al. (2002) found that high proportions of individuals with general psychiatric disorders or with substance misuse may also have psychosexual dysfunction.

Derogatis, Meyer, and Kourlesis (1986) that males with erectile sexual dysfunction reveal disproportionate levels of psychological symptoms and psychopathology. Goldstein (2004) examined that suppression and expression of anger were correlated with higher probabilities of moderate and complete impotence.

McCarthy, (1986) presented a cognitive behavioral approach to the treatment of couples affected by erectile dysfunction as an alternative to medical approaches. McCarthy (1992) described a cognitive-behavioral strategy for dealing with sexual dysfunctions of secondary erectile dysfunction that may be accompanied by male secondary inhibited desire and female primary or secondary inhibited sexual desire. Therapy is a multifocused intervention that attends to individual, couple, and sexual dimensions. Shrivastava, Kumaraiah, and Mishra (1993) conducted a study in India to match varied behavioral strategies to individual cases of male sexual dysfunction and to assess the clinical significance of such interventions in the Indian set-up. Five adult clients completed the therapy program; 3 of the subjects treated had male erectile disorder and 2 had premature ejaculation with secondary impotence. The procedures were based on anxiety reduction, positive feedback, and operant conditioning principles. Avasthi et al. (1994) studied short-term (1 yr or less) and long-term (7 yrs) outcome of 66 male, Indian patients (aged 15-44 yrs) with psychosexual dysfunction in the context of patients' sociodemographic and clinical characteristics. A combination of erectile dysfunction and premature ejaculation was the most common diagnosis. used treatment that included behavioral therapy and the use of psychotherapy and drugs. Improvement in the short-term indicated favorable long-term outcome.

The present study attempts to examine the role of individual variables (age, education, income, occupation) and habits (smoking and alcohol consumption) on psychogenic ED. The study also examines the role of counseling, psychotherapy and relaxation in alleviating the problem of ED.

Method

The study was conducted to examine erectile function, and stress among the males having sexual problems and to examine the outcome of counseling on these problems.

Objectives of the Study

1. To examine the erectile function of males
2. To examine the stress (situation, body and mind)
3. To examine the effect of counseling on erectile function, and stress.

Sample

The study was conducted in Vasavya nursing home, Viziawada, which is a private hospital and one of the famous hospitals in Andhra Pradesh for treating sexual problems. The sample included 322 males having sexual problems. The sample consisted of 266 married men and 56 unmarried men.

Tools

1. The International Index of Erectile Function Questionnaire (IIEF, 1997) developed by Rosen RC, Riley A, Wagner G, Osterloh IH, Kirkpatrick J, Mishra.
2. The Seven Minute Stress Test (1989) is a self-administered scale developed by Ronald G. Nathan, Thomas E. Staats and Paul J. Rosch.

Counseling Sample

The total sample size was 322 males and out of this the sexologist recommended 19 cases for psychological counseling. These subjects were suffering from erectile dysfunction, which was primarily psychogenic in nature. These 19 cases divided into four groups according to the reported psychological reason for dysfunction. These 19 cases were provided psychotherapy and counseling sessions. The specific techniques used which included eight sessions each are described below.

1. Counseling

The counseling is that interaction, which occurs between two individuals called counselor and client, takes place in a professional setting and is initiated and maintained to facilitate changes in the behavior of a climate. The relationship between people that lead healing, growth and change to be autonomous and caring in living with oneself and others. Counseling is to help individuals become self sufficient, self-dependent, and self directed. Counseling is to adjust among them selves efficiently for a better and meaningful life.

2. Sex Education

Sex education, which is sometimes called sexuality education or sex and relationships education, is the process of acquiring information and forming attitudes and beliefs about sex, sexual identity, relationships and intimacy. Sex education seeks both to reduce the risks of potentially negative outcomes from sexual behavior like unwanted or unplanned pregnancies and infection with sexually transmitted diseases, and to enhance the quality of relationships.

3. Behaviour Therapy

Behavior therapy systems from the work of Pavlov and is based on the assumption that maladaptive behavior results from (a) deficient conditioned reactions-the failure of the individual to acquire need adaptive responses, as consequence of either defective conditioning powers or lack of opportunity to learn, or (b) surplus conditioned reactions-maladaptive anxiety reactions which have been learned under certain conditions and have generalized to other situations. Therapy, in turn, becomes an attempt to provide corrective conditioning experiences in which missing responses will be learned and adaptive responses will be substituted for maladaptive ones. The techniques used are many, including simple classical conditioning, operant conditioning aversive conditioning, and reciprocal conditioning inhibition.

4. Self-hypnosis

Self-hypnosis is a powerful technique that one can quickly and easily learn to counteract stress and stress-related illness. In addition one can relax, use it to introduce and reinforce positive changes in your life. Hypnosis is very relaxing. But unlike sleep, you never completely loose awareness during hypnosis. When hypnotized, you are able to respond if necessary to things going on around you. While hypnosis is usually done with eyes closed to facilitate concentration and imagination, it can be done with eyes opened.

5. JPMR Technique

Progressive relaxation of your muscles reduces pulse rate and blood pressure as well as decreasing perspiration and respiration rates. Deep muscle relaxation, when successfully mastered, can be used as an anti-anxiety pill.

Progressive relaxation provides a way of identifying particular muscles and muscle groups and distinguishing between sensations of tension and deep relaxation. Four major muscle groups will be covered:

(a) Hands, forearms, and biceps.

(b) Head, face, throat and shoulders, including concentration on fore-head, cheeks, nose, eyes, jaws, tongue, lips and neck.

Considerable attention is devoted to your head, because from the emotional point of view the most important muscles in your body are situated in and around this region.

(c) Chest, stomach, and lower back.

(d) Thighs, buttocks, calves and feet.

6. Visualization

One can significantly reduce stress with something enormously powerful: through imagination. The practice of positive thinking in the treatment of physical symptoms was popularized by Emil Coue, a French pharmacist, around the turn of this century. He believed that the power of the imagination far exceeds that of the will. It is hard to will yourself into a relaxed state, but you can imagine relaxation spreading through your body, and you can visualize yourself in a safe and beautiful retreat.

Carl Jung in his work in the early part of century used a technique for healing which he referred to as "active imagination." He instructed his patients to meditate without having any goal or program in mind. Images would come to consciousness, which the patient was to observe and experience without interference. Later, if he or she wanted, the patient could actually communicate with the images by asking them questions or talking to them. Jung used active imagination to help the individual appreciate his or her own rich inner life and learn to draw on its healing power in times of stress. Jungian and gestalt therapists have since devised several stress-reduction techniques using the intuitive, imaginative part of the mind.

7. Auto Suggestions

Let's take an example of a person getting angry when someone does not agree with them or does something to them. The surface cause of the anger may be the specific act that of other person that triggered the anger in the seeker. In this case, the seeker can give the autosuggestion-"whenever someone does I begin to get angry, I will become aware of the anger and I will become calm and I will immediately say a prayer to god to over come my anger and start to repeat the lord's name." When basic root is quite apparent, then one can give immediate suggestions.

Analysis of Data

The main objective of the study was to examine the Erectile function. To achieve this objective the sample of 322 males has to be categorized in to various factors like age, education, occupation, income, marital status, smoking habit and alcoholic habit.

The results are discussed in the following sections

Section-A: Erectile Function and Independent Variables

Section-B: Stress and Independent Variables

Section-C: The Effect of Psychological Counseling on Erectile Function and Stress among the Males.

A. Erectile Function and Independent Variables

The influence of the individual variables on erectile functioning is presented in the following pages. Higher scores on the erectile function scale dimensions indicated greater satisfaction with the particular function.

Table 1

Age and Erectile function

Dimensions	*Mean/ S.D.*	*G-1 (n=24)*	*G-2 (n=90)*	*G-3 (n=116)*	*G-4 (n=55)*	*G-5 (n=37)*	*F*
Erectile Function	Mean	9.75	10.76	13.02	13.84	13.43	8.84**
	S.D.	6.13	4.95	3.70	3.06	2.99	
Orgasmic Function	Mean	3.33	3.84	4.73	5.27	4.51	9.16**
	S.D.	2.10	2.12	1.52	1.52	1.26	
Sexual Desire	Mean	6.33	5.36	5.95	6.33	5.97	3.84**
	S.D.	1.95	1.90	1.55	1.48	1.19	
Intercourse Satisfaction	Mean	4.42	5.09	6.53	6.73	6.70	10.84**
	S.D.	2.90	2.92	1.90	1.35	1.61	
Overall Satisfaction	Mean	2.96	3.80	4.93	5.20	4.84	11.94**
	S.D.	2.03	1.88	1.81	1.75	1.38	

* $p < .05$; ** $p < .01$

G-1 = 20 to 25 years, G-2 = 26 to 30 years, G-3 = 31 to 35 years

G-4 = 36 to 40 years, G-5 = 41 and above

One-way analysis of variance (ANOVA) tests were conducted for the five age groups i.e. 20 to 25 years, 26 to 30 years, 31 to 35 years, 36 to 40 years and 41 and above on scores of dimensions erectile function. The mean scores of the erectile function dimensions in comparison across the age groups are tabulated in table-1.The table indicates statistically significant differences in the dimensions of erectile function across the different age groups. The table shows that the subjects in the age group of 36 and 40 years had the highest mean scores on all the dimensions. These findings indicate that age of the patients has a significant influence on ED. Similar results have been reported by Schiavi et al (1990), Clerici et al (1994), Panser et al (1995), Lendorf et al (1998), Mulligan et al (1988), Hinchcliff and Gott (2003), Urban and Bela (2003), Carson (2004) and Moore et al (2003),

Table 2

Education and Erectile function

Dimensions	*Mean/ S.D.*	*G-1 (n=86)*	*G-2 (n=71)*	*G-3 (n=144)*	*G-4 (n=21)*	*F*
Erectile Function	Mean	11.70	11.73	12.90	13.00	2.07
	S.D.	4.72	4.73	3.89	3.95	
Orgasmic Function	Mean	4.46	3.93	4.81	4.90	5.13**
	S.D.	1.64	1.97	1.74	2.00	
Sexual Desire	Mean	5.86	5.42	6.03	6.43	2.99*
	S.D.	1.73	1.64	1.68	1.16	
Intercourse Satisfaction	Mean	5.70	5.70	6.29	6.57	2.00
	S.D.	2.49	2.67	1.99	2.49	
Overall Satisfaction	Mean	4.10	4.27	4.81	4.81	3.09*
	S.D.	1.76	1.96	1.91	2.09	

* $p < .05$; ** $p < .01$

G-1 = Below 10th, G-2 = Intermediate, G-3 = Graduation

G-4 = Post Graduation

One-way analysis of variance (ANOVA) tests were conducted for the scores of erectile function dimensions in comparison across education i.e. below 10th, intermediate, graduation and post graduation (see table 2). The mean scores are statistically significant across the groups in the case of the orgasmic function, sexual desire and overall satisfaction. In all the cases it is the subjects with postgraduate qualification that have the highest mean scores. This observation suggests that subjects with postgraduate qualifications tend to have lesser ED problems. The higher the educations the higher will be the awarness towards a problem and its solutions.This result is supported by the results of Aytac et al (2000) who have noticed that men with low education are more likely to develop ED.

Table 3

Occupation and Erectile function

Dimensions	*Mean/ S.D.*	*G-1 (n=141)*	*G-2 (n=96)*	*G-3 (n=43)*	*G-4 (n=42)*	*F*
Erectile Function	Mean	12.95	11.56	12.02	12.31	2.05
	S.D.	3.72	4.72	4.75	4.79	
Orgasmic Function	Mean	4.84	4.16	4.02	4.24	4.07**
	S.D.	1.68	1.88	1.83	1.90	
Sexual Desire	Mean	5.94	5.78	5.93	5.86	0.17
	S.D.	1.46	1.86	1.72	1.86	
Intercourse Satisfaction	Mean	6.32	5.77	6.16	5.45	2.00
	S.D.	2.08	2.58	2.33	2.62	
Overall Satisfaction	Mean	4.73	4.32	4.12	4.55	1.55
	S.D.	1.76	1.99	1.76	2.31	

** $p < .01$

G-1 = Employees, G-2 = Business, G-3 = Farmers, G-4 = Labor

Table 3 provides results regarding the influence of occupation on erectile function. It can be observed that significant differences are observed across the groups on the orgasmic function, with the employee groups obtaining the highest mean score. Cogen and Steinner (1990) and Aytac et al (2000) have also noted that ED is more common among the blue collar employees.

Table 4

Income and Erectile function

Dimensions	*Mean/ S.D.*	*G-1 (n=168)*	*G-2 (n=116)*	*G-3 (n=38)*	*F*
Erectile Function	Mean	11.85	12.72	13.26	2.37
	S.D.	4.85	3.74	3.40	
Orgasmic Function	Mean	4.25	4.40	5.47	7.39**
	S.D.	1.79	1.85	1.52	
Sexual Desire	Mean	5.74	6.06	5.92	1.24
	S.D.	1.71	1.75	1.22	
Intercourse Satisfaction	Mean	5.64	6.05	7.61	11.48**
	S.D.	2.47	2.11	1.84	
Overall Satisfaction	Mean	4.33	4.50	5.26	3.72*
	S.D.	1.92	1.90	1.80	

* $p < .05$;

** $p < .01$

G-1 = Below Rs. 3,000 per month

G-2 = Between Rs. 3,000 to 5,000 per month

G-3= Rs. 5,000 and above per month

The influence of income on erectile function was examined by comparing the differences across the income groups on the dimensions of erectile function and the results are presented in table 4. The three income groups considered were those with an income below 3,000 per month, between 3,000 to 5,000 per month and 5,000 and above per month. The table indicates that orgasmic function, intercourse satisfaction and overall satisfaction are the dimensions where the differences are statistically significant. Subjects with an income above 5000 per month report higher erectile function as their mean scores are the highest on the three dimensions. Subjects with higher income reported lesser ED problems. This is possible as they are very satisfied with their salary and work life, free from tensions and are easy going.

Table 5

Marital status and Erectile function

Dimensions	*Mean/ S.D.*	*Married (n=266)*	*Unmarried (n=56)*	*t*
Erectile	Mean	12.21	12.89	0.98
Function	S.D.	4.24	4.81	
Orgasmic	Mean	4.48	4.30	0.64
Function	S.D.	1.81	1.83	
Sexual	Mean	5.91	5.75	0.56
Desire	S.D.	1.62	1.92	
Intercourse	Mean	6.02	6.05	0.09
Satisfaction	S.D.	2.28	2.71	
Overall	Mean	4.51	4.46	0.16
Satisfaction	S.D.	1.91	1.96	

Differences in erectile function between the married and unmarried subjects were examined and the results are presented in table 5. The table indicates no significant differences between the two groups on the dimensions of erectile function were found.

Table 6

Smoking habit and Erectile function

Dimensions	*Mean/ S.D.*	*Smokers (n=189)*	*Non smokers (n=133)*	*t*
Erectile	Mean	12.48	12.11	0.73
Function	S.D.	4.09	4.68	
Orgasmic	Mean	4.59	4.25	1.61
Function	S.D.	1.70	1.96	
Sexual	Mean	5.88	5.87	.05
Desire	S.D.	1.58	1.81	
Intercourse	Mean	6.24	5.71	1.97*
Satisfaction	S.D.	2.05	2.71	
Overall	Mean	4.66	4.28	1.72
Satisfaction	S.D.	1.78	2.08	

* $p < .05$.

Table 6 provides results regarding the influence of smoking on erectile function. It can be observed from the table that the group of smokers has a significantly higher mean score on intercourse satisfaction than the group of non-smokers. This finding indicates that smokers tend to report more ED problems than the non-smokers. This is because smoking contributes a high range of impotency among males. Tengs and Osgood (2001) have also found higher prevalence of smoking among persons having problems of ED.

Table 7

Alcoholic habit and Erectile function

Dimensions	*Mean/ S.D.*	*Alcoholics (n=153)*	*Non Alcoholics (n=169)*	*t*
Erectile Function	Mean	12.63	12.06	1.18
	S.D.	3.84	4.75	
Orgasmic Function	Mean	4.63	4.28	1.71
	S.D.	1.68	1.92	
Sexual Desire	Mean	6.05	5.73	1.72
	S.D.	1.51	1.80	
Intercourse Satisfaction	Mean	6.19	5.87	1.22
	S.D.	2.15	2.52	
Overall Satisfaction	Mean	4.68	4.34	1.58
	S.D.	1.87	1.94	

The influence of alcohol consumption on erectile function was examined and the differences are presented in table 7. As none of the differences are statistically significant it can be said that the habit of alcohol in this sample has no influence on erectile function.

B. Stress and Independent Variables

The interaction between the individual variables and stress dimensions has been examined and the findings are discussed.

The influence of age on stress was examined by comparing means, stress scores of the various age groups are presented in table 8. Significant differences are observed among the age groups on the dimensions of situational stress, the age group of 36-40 years with mean 98.89 ($F=3.28$, $p<.05$) and stress in body is experienced by age group 41 years and above with mean score 39.41 ($F=6.47$, p<.01). The findings suggest that situational stress and stress in the body seem to increase with the age of the subjects. This is possible as they either experience a feeling dissatisfaction with their appearance or dissatisfied with their spouse/lover appearance. There is a strong feeling of inadequacy. The situational stress includes feeling pressures at work from one or more superiors. The stress in the body includes ulcers, heart burn, headaches and back pain for males with age 41 and above.

Table 8

Age and Stress

Dimensions	*Mean/ S.D.*	*G-1 (n=24)*	*G-2 (n=90)*	*G-3 (n=116)*	*G-4 (n=55)*	*G-5 (n=37)*	*F*
Situational Stress	Mean	84.17	98.04	94.75	98.89	98.76	3.28*
	S.D.	21.88	19.8	18.91	18.51	13.83	
Stress in Body	Mean	27.96	31.78	34.53	36.42	39.41	6.47**
	S.D.	10.1	10.81	10.44	10.63	7.92	
Stress in Mind	Mean	28.08	30.79	28.57	30.47	29.73	1.897
	S.D.	8.57	7.44	6.1	6.74	5.79	

* $p < .05$;

** $p < .01$

G-1 = 20 to 25 years,G-2 = 26 to 30 years,G-3 = 31 to 35 years,G-4 = 36 to 40 years,G-5 = 41 and above

Table 9

Education and Stress

Dimensions	*Mean/ S.D.*	*G-1 (n=86)*	*G-2 (n=71)*	*G-3 (n=144)*	*G-4 (n=21)*	*F*
Situational Stress	Mean	92.56	97.86	98.10	90.14	2.42
	S.D.	18.13	18.80	19.56	18.78	
Stress in Body	Mean	34.36	31.56	35.78	30.95	3.22*
	S.D.	8.80	11.18	10.72	13.26	
Stress in Mind	Mean	31.65	29.38	28.95	26.57	4.59**
	S.D.	6.28	6.67	6.88	7.22	

* $p < .05$;

** $p < .01$

G-1 = Below 10th, G-2 = Intermediate, G-3 = Graduation, G-4 = Post Graduation.

The various education groups were compared for differences in stress and the results are presented in table 9. The table indicates significant differences across the groups on the dimension of stress in body is significant among graduates with mean 35.78, (F=3.22, p<.05) and stress in mind is significant among those with below 10th class with mean 31.65, (F=4.59, p<.01). The findings suggest that stress in the body is experienced by graduates with regard to ulcers, headaches, tensions, muscle aches. Stress in the body is experienced by below 10th class. They reported a high level of heartburns, headaches, ulcers and back pain. This is due to their nature of work they are involved.

Table 10

Occupation and Stress

Dimensions	*Mean/ S.D.*	*G-1 (n=141)*	*G-2 (n=96)*	*G-3 (n=43)*	*G-4 (n=42)*	*F*
Situational Stress	Mean	100.68	94.54	88.84	91.33	6.14**
	S.D.	18.40	18.03	20.26	19.22	
Stress in Body	Mean	35.13	33.90	30.28	35.45	2.55
	S.D.	10.83	9.46	11.64	10.95	
Stress in Mind	Mean	29.06	30.03	29.86	30.26	0.57
	S.D.	6.44	6.05	8.65	7.65	

** p < .01

G-1 = Employees, G-2 = Business, G-3 = Farmers, G-4 = Labor

The results regarding the influence of occupation on the mean scores of the stress dimensions are tabulated in table-10. The differences are significant with regard to the dimension of situational stress among employees with mean value 100.68, (F=6.14, p<.01) only. The results indicate that situational stress is highest among the employees followed by the businessmen, labor and farmers. The employees were having pressures at work from one or more superiors, pressure to produce beyond reasonable limits, uneasy about an impending promotion or job change, feelings of underpaid, they hardly get any time for their own self.

Table 11

Income and Stress

Dimensions	*Mean/ S.D.*	*G-1 (n=168)*	*G-2 (n=116)*	*G-3 (n=38)*	*F*
Situational Stress	Mean	96.18	95.69	96.55	0.03
	S.D.	18.94	19.18	20.04	
Stress in Body	Mean	33.42	34.54	36.24	1.20
	S.D.	10.10	10.69	12.66	
Stress in Mind	Mean	30.36	28.73	29.00	2.13
	S.D.	6.58	7.08	6.79	

G-1 = Below Rs. 3,000 per month, G-2 = Between Rs. 3,000 to 5,000 per month, G-3 = Rs 5,000 and above per month

Table- 11 provides findings regarding the influence of income on stress. The table indicates that none of the stress dimensions are statistically different.

Table 12

Marital status and Stress

Dimensions	*Mean/ S.D.*	*Married (n=266)*	*Unmarried (n=56)*	*t*
Situational Stress	Mean	95.16	100.27	1.82
	S.D.	19.02	19.07	
Stress in Body	Mean	35.23	29.07	4.21**
	S.D.	10.52	9.8	
Stress in Mind	Mean	29.59	29.73	0.15
	S.D.	6.97	6.06	

** $p < .01$.

The married and unmarried subjects were compared for difference in stress dimensions and the results are presented in table 12. The comparison of the scores indicates that the married and unmarried are differing significantly on the dimension relating to stress in the body (t=4.21, p<.01). Stress in the body is higher among the married subjects. The married subjects were experiencing gastric problems, muscle aches, tension headaches, back pain and rashes.

Table 13

Smoking habit and Stress

Dimensions	*Mean/ S.D.*	*Smokers (n=189)*	*Non smokers (n=133)*	*t*
Situational Stress	Mean	97.46	94.05	1.52
	S.D.	17.03	21.61	
Stress in Body	Mean	36.39	30.98	4.51**
	S.D.	9.74	11.10	
Stress in Mind	Mean	30.06	28.97	1.36
	S.D.	6.14	7.65	

** $p < .01$.

The differences in mean scores of stress dimensions across smokers and non-smokers are presented in table-13. The table indicates that the stress in body (t=4.51, p<.01) dimension is statistically significant with the smokers reporting more stress in body. The findings indicate that smokers reported significantly higher body stress than the non-smokers. Smoking is injurious to health. The smokers were suffering with muscle aches, tension headaches and skin rashes.

Table 14

Alcoholic habit and Stress

Dimensions	*Mean/ S.D.*	*Alcoholics (n=153)*	*Non Alcoholics (n=169)*	*t*
Situational Stress	Mean	97.06	95.14	0.91
	S.D.	17.75	20.25	
Stress in Body	Mean	36.92	31.65	4.58**
	S.D.	9.95	10.66	
Stress in Mind	Mean	29.89	29.36	0.69
	S.D.	6.59	7.02	

** $p < .01$.

The mean scores and t-values of the stress dimensions in comparison across the habit of alcohol i.e., alcoholics and non-alcoholic are computed and tabulated in table-14. Significant differences are observed on the dimension of stress in body. The findings indicate that alcoholics reported significantly higher body stress than the non- alcoholics. Excess intake of alcohol leads to health related illness. The alcoholics were suffering with bodily stress. They were having ulcers, gastric problems, tension headaches, back pain and diarrhea.

C. The Effect of Psychological Counseling on Erectile Function and Stress are presented in the following tables-15 and table-16.

Table 15

Effect of Psychological Counseling on Erectile function (n=19)

Dimensions	*Mean/ S.D.*	*Before Counseling*	*After Counseling*	*t*
Erectile Function	Mean	12.16	17.05	4.59**
	S.D.	3.40	3.15	
Orgasmic Function	Mean	3.95	5.89	4.78**
	S.D.	1.35	1.15	
Sexual Desire	Mean	5.95	7.05	2.59*
	S.D.	1.65	0.85	
Intercourse Satisfaction	Mean	5.31	7.32	4.61**
	S.D.	1.53	1.11	
Overall Satisfaction	Mean	4.11	7.11	4.87**
	S.D.	1.63	2.13	

* $p < .05$;

** $p < .01$.

The tables 15 and 16 provide results regarding the influence of counseling on erectile functioning, and stress. It can be observed from the tables that counseling had significantly improved erectile functioning (high scores indicate better erectile functioning) and reduced stress. These findings indicate that counseling had helped the clients alleviate the ED. Each of these cases were provided counseling and other specific techniques and other specific techniques which continued over a minimum of 4 sessions to 8 sessions. Granero (1990) in his study on 8 subjects with secondary

ED had noticed that all his subjects were successfully treated to regain erection starting with the second session. Further, all subjects were successfully treated by the 6th session.

Table 16

Effect of Psychological Counseling on Stress (n=19)

Dimensions	*Mean/ S.D.*	*Before Counseling*	*After Counseling*	*t*
Situational Stress	Mean	93.16	61.79	7.18**
	S.D.	17.79	9.05	
Stress in Body	Mean	35.42	26.53	6.38**
	S.D.	8.68	5.80	
Stress in Mind	Mean	27.63	17.21	5.76**
	S.D.	6.73	5.04	

** $p < .01$.

CONCLUSION

Erectile problems seem to be dependent on the age, education, occupation, income and the smoking habit of the patients. More specifically, younger people with lesser education and working as labor and in the habit of smoking tend to report more ED problems. Situational stress and stress in the body seem to increase with the age and marital status of the subjects. Further, situational stress is highest among the employees followed by the businessmen, labor and farmers. Finally, while the smokers and alcoholics reported higher body stress. However, the educational qualifications of the subjects help to alleviate stress in the mind and the body. Lower stress facilitates erectile functioning. The present study had highlighted the relationship between psychological, social, and physiological factors in sexual difficulties and dysfunctions, particularly male erectile dysfunction. There are numerous psychological issues that impact on an individual's satisfaction and ability to satisfy a partner. The most typical include: low self-esteem, body image issues, past sexual abuse or trauma, relationships difficulties, poor communication and stresses of daily living. A psychologically based treatment of male erectile disorder should include key elements like psycho educational and cognitive intervention, sexual and performance anxiety reduction, behavior modification, conflict resolution and relationship enhancement, and relapse prevention training.

REFERENCES

Avasthi, A.; Basu, D.; Kulhara, P.; Banerjee, S. T. (1994). Psychosexual dysfunction in Indian male patients: Revisited after seven years. *Archives of Sexual Behavior. 1994 Dec Vol 23(6) 685-695.*

Aytac, Isik A.; Araujo, Andre B.; Johannes, Catherine B.; Kleinman, Ken P.; McKinlay, John B. (2000). Socioeconomic factors and incidence of erectile dysfunction: Findings of the longitudinal Massachusetts Male Aging Study. *Social Science & Medicine. 51(5), Sep 2000, 771-778.*

Clerici, Stefano; Orlandini, Alvise; Fossati, Andrea; Montorsi, Francesco; et al (1994). The predictive usefulness of age and kind of onset in discriminating psychogenic from organic impotence. *Sexuality & Disability. 1994 Win Vol 12(4) 279-284.*

Cogen, Raymond; Steinman, William (1990). Sexual function and practice in elderly men of lower socioeconomic status. *Journal of Family Practice. 1990 Aug Vol 31(2) 162-166.*

Derogatis, Leonard R.; Meyer, Jon K.; Kourlesis, Suzanne (1986). Psychiatric diagnosis and psychological symptoms in impotence. *Hillside Journal of Clinical Psychiatry. 1985 Fal-Win Vol 7(2) 120-133.*

Ducharme, Stanley H. (2004) Psychologic factors modulating erectile function. *Sexuality & Disability. 22(2), Sum 2004, 171-175.PsycINFO Database Record (c) 2004 APA, all rights reserved).*

Fahrner, Eva-Maria (1987). Sexual dysfunction in male alcohol addicts: Prevalence and treatment. *Archives of Sexual Behavior. 1987 Jun Vol 16(3) 247-257.*

Goldstein, Irwin (2004). Diagnosis of erectile dysfunction. *Sexuality & Disability. 22(2), Sum 2004, 121-130.*

Granero, Mirta (1990). Assertiveness as a treatment for secondary impotence (erectile dysfunction): A form of therapy: Clinical observations. *Revista Latinoamericana de Sexologla. 1990 Vol 5(1) 55-61.*

Hinchliff, Sharron; Gott, Merryn (2003). Perceptions of well-being in sexual Ill health: What role does age play? *Journal of Health Psychology. 9(5), Sep 2004, 649-660.*

Lendorf, Axel; Juncker, Lise; Rosenkilde, Palle (1995). Frequency of erectile dysfunction in a Danish subpopulation. *Nordisk Sexologi. 1994 Jun Vol. 12(2) 118-124.*

McCarthy, Barry W. (1986). A cognitive behavioral approach to treatment of couples with erectile dysfunction. *Journal of Sex Education & Therapy. 1986 Fal-Win Vol 12(2) 15-19.*

McCarthy, Barry W. (1992). Erectile dysfunction and inhibited sexual desire: Cognitive-behavioral strategies. *Journal of Sex Education & Therapy. 1992 Spr Vol 18(1) 22-34.*

Moore, Todd M.; Strauss, Jennifer L.; Herman, Steve; Donatucci, Craig F. (2003). Erectile Dysfunction in Early, Middle, and Late Adulthood: Symptom Patterns and Psychosocial Correlates. *Journal of Sex & Marital Therapy. 29(5), 2003, 381-399.*

Mulligan, Thomas; Retchin, Sheldon M.; Chinchilli, Vernon M.; Bettinger, Cynthia B. (1988). The role of aging and chronic disease in sexual dysfunction. *Journal of the American Geriatrics Society. 1988 Jun Vol 36(6) 520-524.*

Panser, Laurel A.; Rhodes, Thomas; Girman, Cynthia J.; Guess, Harry A.; et al (1995). Sexual function of men ages 40 to 79 years: The Olmsted County Study of Urinary Symptoms and Health Status Among Men. *Journal of the American Geriatrics Society. 1995 Oct Vol 43(10) 1107-1111.*

Rogers Kirby and Culley Carson, Irwin Gold Stein,(2001.) Erctile Dysfunction. J P Brothers Medical Publishers Ltd. India. 59 ST aldetes oxford OSI 1st UK.

Ronald G. Nathan, Thomas E. Staps. (1987) Instant Stress Relief, USA Ballantine Books, a Division of Random House Inc.New York.

Schiavi, Raul C.; Schreiner-Engle, Patricia; Mandeli, John; Schanzer, Harry; et al (1990). Healthy aging and male sexual function. *American Journal of Psychiatry. 1990 Jun Vol 147(6) 766-771.*

Shrivastava, S.; Kumaraiah, V.; Mishra, H. (1993). Behavioural intervention in the management of male sexual dysfunction. *NIMHANS Journal. 1993 Jul Vol 11(2) 149-153.*

Tengs, Tammy; Osgood, Nathaniel D. (2001). The link between smoking and impotence: Two decades of evidence. Preventive Medicine: *An International Journal Devoted to Practice & Theory. 32(6), Jun 2001, 447-452.*

Urban, Robert; Bela, Marian (2003). Prevalence and psychosocial predictors of erectile dysfunction in representative sample of Hungarian adult males. *Pszichologia: Az MTA Pszichologiai Intezetenek folyoirata. 23(4), 2003, 409-423.*

Wylie, Kevan R.; Steward, David; Seivewright, Nicholas; Smith, Diane; Walters, Stephen (2002). Prevalence of sexual dysfunction in three psychiatric outpatient settings: A drug misuse service, an alcohol misuse service and a general adult psychiatry clinic. *Sexual & Relationship Therapy. 17(2), May 2002, 149-160.*

6

Hatha-Yoga
The Way of Coping with Stress

K. Ramesh Babu*

ABSTRACT

Tensions, conflicts, sorrows and sufferings are common in man's progress. According to yoga stress is imbalance of body mind and spirit. Imbalance is misery. Maharshi Patanjali, the founder of Yoga Philosophy mentioned five afflictions (panchakleshas) viz., ignorance or lack of awareness *(avidya)*, 'I' ness (asmitha), likes (raga), dislikes (dvesha) and fear of death or clinging to life (abhinivesha) which produce imbalance in a man's daily life. These imbalances can lead to conflicts, egocentric behaviors and cause ailments and diseases. Yoga is multi-level discipline and different techniques of Yoga, whether individual or combination with other techniques help to restore balance at various levels of individual, reduce mental stress, and thereby alleviate the symptoms of stress related disorders. Hatha Yoga, the most popular branches of Yoga can help to reduce mental stress, prevent possible break down and enhance the capacity to tolerated crises. The practices of hatha-yoga assume importance because they render this physical body free of toxic elements and influence the psychic centres in man. Every asana exerts mild influence on the hormonal system by

* **Assistant Professor, Institute for Yoga & Consciousness, Andhra University** ***Avidya*** **(lack of awareness or ignorance);** ***Asmitha*** **("I" ness);** ***Raga*** **(likes);** ***Dvesha*** **(dislikes);** ***Abhinivsha*** **(fear of death or clinging or life).**

activating the chakras slightly. Pranayama, which is powerful tool, has a deeper influence on both body and mind.In this paper Hatha yoga techniques like asanas (bodily postures), kriyas (cleansing techniques of internal bodily organs), pranayama (regulation of breathing techniques), yoga nidra (yogic relaxation technique) and nadanusandana (one of the meditation techniques) are described and evaluated for their applicability in relieving stress.

Stress is the gap between expectation and achievement in man's life which leads to tension. Tensions, conflicts and sorrows and sufferings are common in man's progress. Yoga had long back recognized stress as an imbalance between body, mind and spirit. Imbalance is misery. Modern science describes stress as an imbalance of neuro-endocrine system. Yoga philosophy, as well as modern psychology, enumerates three basic tensions or three kinds of stress:

(i) Muscular tensions: are related to the body itself, the nervous system and endocrinal imbalances.

(ii) Mental tensions: are the result of excessive mental activity. The mind is a whirlpool of fantasies, confusions and oscillations. From time to time these explode, affecting our body, mind, behaviour and reactions.

(iii) Emotional tensions: which stem from various dualities such as love and hate, profit and loss, success and failure, happiness and unhappiness are more difficult to erase.

General causes of stress are anxiety, fear, anger, fatigue, depression, ego, attachment, and time pressure. Indian scriptures like *Upanishads, Bhagwad Gita* and *Yoga Sutras* have been described clearly the causes of man's misery and stress.

Concept of Stress (*Pancha kleshas*) in Yoga Sutras

Patanjali Maharshi, the founder of Yoga philosophy, described the concept of stress in his *Yoga Sutras* in a most comprehensive way from the subtlest level (ignorance) to its grossest manifestation. According to him the following five afflictions (named by him as *panchakleshas)*[1] are causes of stress and miseries in men.

These five afflictions (*pancha kleshas*) create imbalance between body, mind and spirit and finally lead to stress and pain. According to Patanjali our original state is stress free and is blissful. He calls it *swaroopa*[2] or Self. When this state is agitated or disturbed then the imbalance occurs. *Avidya* leads to further thinking and we start limiting ourselves, constriction, pressurization or stress is built up. *Avidya* leads to *Asmitha,* the "I" ness, ego, and associated attachments like 'my mind', 'my thoughts', 'my feelings', 'my body' etc., Imbalance at this level leads to disintegration and soon the differentiation takes shape. Attachment and 'I" ness lead to strong likes (raga) and dislikes (*dvesha*). It is then that the emotional expansion starts. Throwing up and down in these emotional imbalance leads to deterioration in the quality of life and loosing all discrimination power and acts from instinctive level. This Patanjali called as *Abhinivisha,* a state of helpless, constriction, slavery or bondage. That is grossest manifestation of stress. He proposes the techniques of Yoga meditation for reducing stress, for thinning of the *kleshas* as under.

> "resorting to yoga for thinning the *kleshas* and achieving higher states of consciousness featured by lesser stresses and emergence of greater capacities"[3]

In describing the process for elimination of stresses, Patanjali has used the term 'thinning' which shows that is not a sudden elimination but a gradual systematic process of moving from higher stress level to lower ones.

Concept of Stress in Bhagwad Gita:

Bhagawad Gita, the scripture of the science of Yoga is regarded as the foundation head of psychology by sages and great thinkers, wherein profound psychological insights are intertwined with philosophical concepts. In *Bhagawad Gita* the whole process of stress origin, development aggravation and consequence was described in the following way.

"A man contemplates sense-objects lead to attachment for them; from attachment to desire for them will be born; from desires (strong likes and dislikes) arises anger (greed, lust, fear, possessiveness, etc.,) from anger comes delusion; from delusion comes loss of memory; from loss of memory comes destruction of discrimination; from destruction of discrimination he perishes."[4]

Concept of Stress in the Upanishads

Psychologists refer to the three dimensions of the mind as the conscious, subconscious and unconscious. In the philosophies of Vedanta and Yoga they are known as the gross, subtle and causal dimensions of the human personality. These three dimensions are again subdivided into the five *koshas* or bodies which constitute a holistic concept of man from the grossest to the most subtle dimensions of existence. The *Taittereya Upanishad*[5] has presented this holistic concept of man systematically as having five major sheaths (*koshas*) of existence. These five *koshas* are related to the psychological dimensions, physiological states and different levels of awareness. According to this Upanishad, stress is interaction among these five *koshas*.

These five *koshas* are:

(i) *Annamaya kosha* (physical sheath): it is physical body of blood, bone, fat and skin, which is perceived through the senses. This is the grossest level of human manifestation. The level of awareness is of the physical plane.

(ii) *Pranamaya kosha* (vital sheath): it is the underlying energy network of the human structure which consists of currents of *prana* or bioplasmic energy. The level of awareness here is of physiological function, e.g. digestion and circulation.

(iii) *Monomaya kosha* (astral sheath): it is layer of conscious operation within the sphere of the mind. Awareness here is of the mental and emotional processes.

(iv) *Vignanamaya kosha* (wisdom sheath): it is the dimension of our personality which is operating on the astral plane. This is the body we experience during dreaming, out-of-body experiences, and the various types of psychic phenomena. Awareness here is of the psychic and causal planes.

(v) *Anandamaya kosha* (bliss sheath): it is the transcendental dimension of human personality existing in total absence of pleasure or pain. This is very important, but difficult to explain. The instrument of experience has been totally transcended.

Emotional imbalances in the form of strong likes and dislikes bring about imbalances in *prana* (the vital energy) in the *Pranamaya kosha* which enter to the *Annamaya kosha* causing stress symptoms and hazards. Origin of desires and action guided by strong likes and dislikes (and not by what is right and wrong) will be the expression of imbalance at *Manomaya kosha*. In *Vignanamaya kosha,* the *Avidya* goes on reducing until in *Anandamaya kosha* it is all bliss. This state is the totally stress-free state which is the aim of Yoga.

Concept of Stress in Relation to Nadies[6]

In Hatha yogic psychology there are two vertically running (forces) nadies, the *Ida nadi* which is corresponds to parasympathetic nerves and responsible for relaxation. *Pingala nadi* which corresponds to sympathetic nerves and responsible for excitation. These two nadies play a vital role in health, disease and in supra-mental achievements. Hatha Yoga aims to bring balance of these nadies i.e balancing the sympathetic and parasympathetic systems which leads balanced condition of body and mind.

Coping the Stress with Hatha Yoga Practices

Hatha Yoga, which is one of the branches of Yoga and most popular in present days thorough out the world is a multi-level discipline and is an antidote to stress. It's practice includes *asanas, kriyas, pranayamas* and meditation and can serve as the best-absorbers against stress. It is the universally accepted system of capable of harmonizing the body, calming the mind and balancing emotions. It helps to bear mental stress and prevent break down by reducing the intensity of mental pressure and enhancing the capacity to tolerate any crises. Different techniques of hatha-yoga, individual or combinations of with other techniques balances at various levels of individual and helps in reducing the mental stress, and thereby remove the symptoms of all other stress disorders. Alternate stress and relaxation is the key to overcome any tension. Tension is never harmful if one is prepared for it and if it is followed by adequate relaxation. The practices of heatha yoga are of primary importance because they render this physical body free of toxic elements and influence the psychic centres in man. Every *asana* and *pranayama* exerts mild influence on the hormonal system and has a deeper influence on both body and mind.

As my profession is teaching and training in Yoga to the students and people of various courses organized by our Yoga

Institute in Andhra University, I have witnessed the people who gained a lot of improvement by hatha-yoga techniques in coping with the stress and related problems. Based on my personal experience in dealing people with stress and its related problems, the following set of *asanas*, combined with *pranayama*, *shatkarmas*, meditation, *Om* chanting and *Yoga nidra*, which are mentioned under the following headings, is most effective in eliminating these knots, tackling them from both the mental and physical levels.

Role of the *asanas* in coping with the stress:

> "*Asanas* are treated of in the first place as they form the first stage of Hatha Yoga. *Asanas* make one get steadiness of body and mind, free from maladies and lightness (flexibility) of the limbs."[7]

As mind and body are not separate entities, the gross form of the mind is the body and the subtle form of the body is the mind. The practice of *asana* integrates and harmonizes both the body and mind. Every mental knot has a corresponding physical, muscular knot and vice versa. The aim of *asana* is to release these knots. *Asanas* release mental tensions by dealing with them on the physical level i.e through the body to the mind. For example, emotional tensions and suppression can tighten up and block the smooth functioning of the lungs, diaphragm and breathing process. Muscular knots can occur anywhere in the body: tightness of the neck as cervical spondylitis, the face as neuralgia, etc. Practice of *asanas* would be ideal thing to deal the psychosomatic problems. The results of *asanas* are achieved by directly influencing the body organs like muscles, joints, ligaments, visceral organs, etc, and by influencing the autonomic nervous system.

Asanas will remove these tensions and give the practitioner real muscular relaxation. If the *asanas* viz., *Tadasan, ardha katchakrasana, hastchalanasana, katichakrasana, sirshasana, sarvangasana, halasana, matsyasana, paschimottanasan, bhujangasana, shalabhasana, ardha matsyendrasana, shashankasana, yogumudra*, and *jataraparivrittanasana* are done with concentration, relaxation and with internal awareness, they will quickly eliminate mental tension and induce tranquility of mind.

Role of *shat karmas* (six acts) in Coping with the Stress:

> "these six acts (*shat karms*) are named *Dhauti, Vast, Neti, Trataka, Nauli* and *Kapalabhati*. These six acts that purify the body should be kept secret, as they produce various wonderful results, and (as such) are held in high esteem by great yogin.."[8]

Hatha Yoga is also known as the science of purification. In Hatha-Yoga there are six cleansing techniques which are called *shat- karmas* or *kriyas*. They clean internal organs of various corners of the body such as eyes, nasal passage esophagus, stomach, large intestines and frontal brain. These shat karmas are used to balance these three *doshas* (humours) in the body. In order to purify the mind, it is necessary for the body as a whole to undergo a process of absolute purification. Then the energies move like wave frequencies throughout the channels within the physical structure, moving right up to the brain.

The following are the *shat karmas*:

Dhauti: cleans stomach and digestive system

Vasti: cleans the large intestines

Neti : Helps to relieve allergies, colds and sinusitis disorders of eyes, ears and throat.

Alleviates, migraine, anxiety, anger and depression; Removes drowsiness and makes the head feel light and fresh. Improves the activities of the brain. Gives good relief from nervous tension, head ache and migraine.

Trataka: clean the eyes, improves vision and concentration

Nauli: churning the abdominal organs

Kapalabhati: cleans frontal brain and lungs purification. Stimulates the brain cells and improves memory; Energies the mind for mental work. Irrelevant thoughts will be reduced.

Balances and strengthens the nervous system.

In above techniques *dhauti kriya, neti kriya, kapalabhati* are very useful in coping with the stress.

Role of *Pranayama* in Coping with the Stress

> "when breath (*prana*) wanders (i.e is irregular), the mind (*chitta*) is unsteady, but when breath is still, so is the (mind) still and the yogin obtains the power of stillness. Therefore the breath should be restrained."[9]

> "through the proper practice of *pranayama* there is freedom all diseases"[10]

Hatha Yoga states that all the diseases are ultimately caused by improper distribution of *prana* in the physical body. Even those diseases which are regarded as psychological in nature are acatually caused by an imbalance in *pranic* distribution. All these illness are treated by supplying *prana* through the practice of pranyama. Swami Satyananda Saraswathi, regarded as an authority on Hatha-Yoga, averred that *prana*yama influences the cerebral fluid in the brain. When energy is generated, it changes the chemical structure of the cerebral fluid. When this fluid is chemically influenced, it acts on behaviour of the brain. *Prana*yama helps in striking a balance between the two components of the Autonomic Nervous System- the sympathetic and para-sympathetic and thus established emotional stability.

Disease can originate either in the body or in the mind. Diseases originate in the mind and travel into into the body are known as psychosomatic diseases. Diseases which originate in the body and then travel into the mind are called somato-psychic. Hatha Yoga have prescribed techniques for dealing with both somato-psychic and psychosomatic illness. The science of hatha yoga recognises that the body is the base and *prana* is its force; that both body and mind are dependent on *prana*, the life force.

In this regard, Yogic breathing, *Anuloma* and *Viloma, Bhastrika, Bhramari* and *Sheetali pranayamas* are very useful in coping with stress.

Role of Yoga Nidra in Coping with Stress

Yoga nidra is a systematic method of inducing complete physical, mental and emotional relaxation. Yoga means union or one pointed awareness, and *nidra* means sleep. Yoga *nidra* is sleep with a trace of awareness, a state of mind between wakefulness and dream. Langley Porter[11] Neuropsychiotric Institute in California, found the reduction in blood pressure and anxiety levels in hypertensive patients continued for twelve months after yoga *nidra* training. It is usually performed in *Shavasana,* but in a therapeutic role it may be performed in sitting position also. Instructions are normally given throughout by a Yoga teacher or tape recording or with experience one can give the instructions to himself.

The practice of *Yoga Nidra*[12] consists of following parts:

(i) Preparation for the practice: here one may lie in *shavasana* position and prepares the consciousness for practicing *yoga nidra*.

(ii) Resolve: here one makes a resolve of precise, positive and clear statement according to his need and inclination.

(iii) Rotation of Consciousness: here rotation of the consciousness is to be done in definite sequence, beginning with the right thumb and ending with the little toe of right foot and then the circuit from the left thumb to the little toe of the left foot.

(iv) Awareness of breath: in this part one may watch his breath at the nostrils, at the chest, at the throat, and at the navel which promotes relaxation and concentration.

(v) Feelings and sensations: usually this is practiced with pairs of opposite feelings such as heat and cold; heaviness and lightness; pain and pleasure; joy and sorrow; love and hate which helps to harmonizes the opposite hemispheres of the brain.

(vi) Visualization: in this part one could be asked to visualize the images named or described by the instructor.

(vii) Ending the practice: the practice of *yoga nidra* is concluded by gradually bringing the mind from the condition of psychic sleep to the waking state.

Influence of "OM" CHANTING in Coping the Stress

The sound 'Om' is regarded as powerful sound in Hindu scriptures and there is vast literature on it. The letter 'A', 'U' and 'M' constitute the 'OM' sound. Medical researches experimenting on hundreds of people have shown that 'Om' can be used a therapy.

When 'O' sound is uttered and the vibrations of the sound reach the brain, alpha waves are increasingly registered in the brain, leading to rest and relaxation. When the vibrations of the 'M' sound reach the brain, beta waves are increasingly registered in the brain, leading to dynamism and inspiration. When 'O' and 'M' sounds vibrations enter the brain for equal periods, dynamic tranquility is produced through alpha and beta waves being registered in similar quantities.

Role of Meditation in Coping with Stress

Herbert Benson,[13] Prof. of Medicine at Harward University (1969) declared that meditation increases energy and efficiency in performing any kind of work. It also helps to reduced physical and mental tension and increases calmness. He also reported creativity, productivity, inventiveness, discrimination, intuitiveness and concentration.

Meditation will help create balance in the nervous system and mind. This will enable the glands to return to a correct state of hormonal balance and thereby overcome the feeling of depression. The effects of meditation in clinical condition are encouraging. It helps to change internal response to external demands. The basic principle involved in meditation is to developing of internal awareness.

Even though there are so many meditative techniques, among them *svasaanusandana* (breath awareness or watching the breath) is suitable for all walks of people and especially recommended those with stress and its related problems. Technique is simply sitting in any comfortable position, one may watch his own breath at the nostrils with feeling of sensation. One may repeat mentally "Sooo... and "Hamm" ... with his inhalation and exhalation respectively.

Conclusion

Hatha Yoga has succeeded as an alternative form of physical and mental therapy, because of the balance created in the nervous and endocrine system which directly influences all the other systems and organs of the body and helps very much in coping with the stress in men's daily life. To know more about physiological responses to Hatha Yoga and Meditation one may refer the book 'Science Studies Yoga'[14] and *Yoga Mimamsa*[15].

REFERENCES

1. *Bhagawad Gita* ch. II. 62, 63.
2. Cited by Swamy Satyananda Saraswathi, *Yoga Nidra*, Bihar School of Yoga, Munger, 1998, p. 214.
3. Cited by Yogi Ram, *Stress the Killer—Counter and Conquer*, Yoga Academy, Hyderabad, 1997, p. 152.
4. Funderburk James, *Science Studies of Yoga* (A Review of Physiological Data), Himalayan International Institute of Yoga Science & Philosophy, U S A, 1977.
5. I.K. Taimni, (Eng. Commentary), *The Science of Yoga*, Ch. II. 3, The Theosophical Publishing House, Adyar, 199, p. 130.
6. Ibid., Ch. I.3, p.
7. Ibid., ch. II. 16, p. 25.
8. Ibid., Ch. II. 2 &11, pp. 129,155.
9. Ibid., ch. II. 2, p. 13.
10. Ibid., Ch. II. 22, 23, p. 26.
11. Iyanger Srinivasa (Tr) *The Hatha Yoga Pradipika of Svatmarama*, Tr. Revised by Ramanatham, A.A. and Burner Radha, Madras, Adyar Library Resarch Centre, 1994, ch. I. 17, p. 11.
12. Swamy Satyanada Saraswathi, *Asana Pranayama Mudra Bandha*, Yoga Publications, Munger, 1996, p. 523.
13. Swamy Satyananda Saraswathi, *Yoga Nidra*, Bihar School of Yoga, Munger, 1998 pp. 69-73.
14. *Taittereya Upanishad, Briguvalli*, ch.III. 2-6.
15. *Yoga-Mimamsa*, A Quarterly Journal Devoted Scientific and Philosophic—Literary Research in Yoga, Kaivalyadhama, Lonavala.

7

Marital Adjustment of Working Women

Shivaraj.B.K*, Prakash Huggi**

ABSTRACT

The major intention of this study is to find out the marital adjustment of working women in Gulbarga city. Nowadays women are facing more problems in their families because of the dual burden of work. Women working within and outside the home experience more stress and this influences marital adjustment. For the present study a total of 300 respondents consisting of three categories of working women including doctors, teachers and clerks were selected (100 respondents from each category). The following were the major objectives - to assess the adjustment of working women belonging to different sub-group samples, to study the effect of educational level of working women on adjustment, to study the effect of occupational status on the marital adjustment of the sample, to examine the effect of length of marital life (number of years of marriage) on the adjustment and to know the effect of other relevant factors like age, religion, experience, family type and income on marital adjustment and analysis made by using relevant statistical tools and presented data in the form of tables.

* Guest Lecturer, Department of Women's Studies Gulbarga University, Gulbarga – 585 106 (KARNATAKA)

** Research Scholar, Department of Women's Studies Gulbarga University, Gulbarga – 585 106 (KARNATAKA).

The definition of marital adjustment will depend upon the conception of marriage and the standards of adjustment prevalent in a particular society at a particular time. Since a very few studies in India have been carried out on marital adjustment, it has not been specifically defined in the Indian context.

Landis in his study of marital adjustment has used the term adjustment to refer to the state of accommodation, which is achieved in different areas where conflict may exist in marriage (Landis, 1946). Locke and Williamson have defined marital adjustment as the presence of such characteristics in a marriage as a tendency to avoid or resolve conflicts, a feeling of satisfaction with the marriage and with each other, the sharing of common interests and activities, and the fulfilling of the marital expectations of the husband and wife (Locke and Williamson, 1958).

OBJECTIVES OF THE STUDY

The following are the main objectives of the study:

1. To assess the adjustment of working women belonging to different sample sub-groups.
2. To study the effect of educational level of working women on adjustment.
3. To study the effect of occupational status on the marital adjustment of the sample.
4. To examine the effect of length of marital life (No. of years of marriage) on the adjustment.
5. To know the effect of other relevant factors like age, religion, experience, family type and income on marital adjustment.

METHODOLOGY

The fieldwork for the present study is carried out in Gulbarga city, selecting randomly the required sample. The reason for selecting Gulbarga is that Gulbarga is the District Cum-Divisional Headquarter and is the center place for Hyderabad Karnataka Region. Hyderabad-Karnataka Region Consists of Five Districts – Gulbarga, Bidar, Raichur, Koppal and Bellary.

Being the head quarter, Gulbarga covers several Govt. as well as private offices and a large number of workers are seen in the city center. In recent years, due to educational expansion, Gulbarga has witnessed a number of changes in the mentality and life style of its people. Because of higher education attained, women are joining several workforces and serving for the cause of welfare. Consequent upon joining service, women are likely to face several difficulties including problem of adjustment. Hence an attempt is made to study the marital adjustment of married working women. For the purpose the respondents were selected randomly based on the occupations i.e., Doctors, Teachers and Clerks (clerical staff). They were administered Personality Questionnaire and the Marital Adjustment Inventory was administered on categorized sample of independent variables. Thus the total sample includes both working wives and husbands. The sample distribution is given in the following Table -1.

Table 1

Sample Design

Category	*Wives*	*Husbands*	*Total*
Doctors	50	50	100
Teachers	50	50	100
Clerks	50	50	100
Total	150	150	300

MARITAL ADJUSTMENT INVENTORY

This scale is developed by H.M. Singh (1987). It consists of two forms A & B, for wives and husbands separately, with 10 questions in each form.

The questions/items are to be answered either 'yes or no', and then again for each item (of Yes or No) on one point out of ten points on rating scale, ranging from +10 to -10 (Most favorable to least favorable). The items are scored according to scoring key given in the manual. The total score indicates marital adjustment score of the sample.

The reliability (r = 0.85) and validity of the scale are quite satisfactory.

Statistical Analysis

The following statistical tests are used in the present study:

1. t-tests to compare the sample sub-groups.
2. r – test to find out correlation between dimensions of the scale items.

MARITAL ADJUSTMENT IN DIFFERENT SAMPLE SUBGROUPS

The major objective of the present study is to assess the amount marital adjustment of workingwomen of different occupational status.

Accordingly, the data are prepared and presented. Marital adjustment is assessed by computing the mean scores of sample subgroups on categorized independent variables. This kind of comparison enables to understand relative status of women/sample on dependent variable i.e., marital adjustment.

Studies on marital adjustment of workingwomen have highlighted that employment to a wife strengthens her relations with husband. It is believed that married woman's employment helps to improve good marital conditions (Iephcott, Seer & Smith, 1962). Similarly, Ross (1964) opines that marriage is strengthened and enriched by a wife's return to work/employment. However, it is observed that there is no difference in marital adjustment between wives who are working and those who are not employed (Locke & Mackeprang, 1949). Therefore, the studies in relation to marital adjustment are inconclusive and need an extended inquiry.

As mentioned earlier, marital adjustment can be assessed by computing mean scores. Accordingly, the mean scores, SDs and t-values are computed and presented in Table- 2.

Table 2

Means, SDs and t-values of Marital Adjustment of Working Women in Three Occupations (N = 150)

Sl. No.	*Occupations*	*Mean*	*SD*	*t-value*
1.	Doctors	69.06	10.27	4.42** (1 & 2)
2.	Teachers	61.06	13.39	0.76 (2 & 3)
3.	Clerks	59.10	12.21	3.35** (1 & 3)

** Significant at 0.01 level.

Table 2 gives mean scores, SDs and t-values of marital adjustment of working women belonging to three different occupations. It can be noticed that the mean score of Doctors is higher (69.06) than those of Teachers (61.06) and Clerical staff (59.10). And clerical staff has scored lower (59.10) than teachers (61.06). This reveals that women who are in the highest occupational status (i.e., Doctors) are found to have highest marital adjustment followed by teacher women. The t-values of 4.412 and 3.35 which are significant at 0.01 level clearly reveal that there is significant difference in marital adjustment between doctors and clerks, doctors and teachers. However the difference between teachers and clerks is not significant. Thus women who enjoyed highest occupational status are found to have greater marital satisfaction. It appears that higher job produces harmony and cordial and warm relations in marital life.

Women teachers and clerks appear to enjoy more or less similar amount of adjustment in their family life. They have more comfort, harmony and quiet and enjoy their profession as a result of which they could achieve greater marital satisfaction that leads to better adjustment.

Hence it can be argued that marital adjustment is mediated by occupational status, which the wife embraces. Similar results are noticed by certain researchers (Ross, 1964, Locke, et.al., 1949.

Further attempt is made to categorize the sample of working women (wives) depending upon the education, experience, married years, age, religion, income, family type and personality dimensions. Accordingly women belonging to different sub-groups are classified and means, SDs and t-values are calculated and presented in Tables to follow.

Table-3 gives the mean score, SDs and t-values of marital adjustment of working women belonging to different levels of education. The mean score of professional course is higher (70.06) than those of post graduates (66.10), under graduates (61.45) and pre-university (60.88) course. Workingwomen's who had pre-university level of education have scored lower (60.88) than those of UG level of education. This clearly indicates that women who completed their professional course and post-graduate course are found to have higher marital adjustment than the women of pre-university and under graduate education.

Table 3

Mean, SD and t-values of Martial Adjustment of Working Women in different Educational Levels

Sl. No.	*Education*	*Mean*	*SD*	*t-value*
1.	PC (N= 50)	70.06	8.62	1.11 (1 & 2)
2.	PG (10)	66.10	16.62	1.10 (2 & 3)
3.	UG (48)	61.45	11.79	1.03 (2 & 3)
				4.03** (1 & 3)
4.	PU (42)	61.45	11.79	4.15** (1 & 4)
				0.22 (3 & 4)

** Significant at 0.01 level.

The t-values 4.03 and 4.15 which are significant at 0.01 level clearly reveals that there is a significant difference in marital adjustment between women with professional course and under graduate, professional course and pre-university level of education. There is no significant difference in marital adjustment between women who had professional course and post graduate; post graduate and under graduate; pre-university and under graduate course.

The women who have higher level of education and who completed the professional course have greater martial adjustment than the women who completed the under graduate and pre-university level of education. Higher level of education produces better adjustment in marital relationship because higher knowledge promotes mutual understanding.

Table 4

Mean, SD and t-values of Marital Adjustment of Working Women in Three Groups of Work Experience

Sl. No.	*Experience (in years)*	*Mean*	*SD*	*t-value*
1.	0 – 4 (47)	68.17	12.35	0.81 (1 & 2)
2.	5 – 9 (56)	66.30	10.81	3.50** (2 & 3)
3.	10 and above (47)	58.51	11.73	3.88** (1 & 3)

** Significant at 0.01 level.

Table 4 shows mean SDs and t-value of marital adjustment of working women having different years of work experience. Women who have 0-4 years of work experience have more marital adjustment than those who have 5-9 and 10 and above years of work experience. The mean score of 0-4 years of work experience group is higher (68.17) than that of 5-9 (66.30) and 10 and above (58.51) years of work experience. This reveals that women whose work experience is less have higher marital adjustment than the women with more work experience. It appears that women who have less work experience have minimum responsibilities in the workplace. They can complete their work early without much strain. This helps them to pay more attention to the family and this will make them more contended and happy in their marital life. Whereas women who have more work experience have more responsibilities in workplace, and therefore spend much of their time in their office work. It appears that their priority is office work. Further, they don't get enough time and patience to pay required attention to their family. The t-value of 3.50 is significant at 0.01 level which indicates that there is a significant difference in marital adjustment between working women with 5-9 and 10 and above years of work experience as much as the t-value of 3.88 which is significant at 0.01 level reveals a significant difference in marital adjustment between 0.-4 years and 10 and above years of work experience.

Table-5 gives mean score, SDs and t-values of marital adjustment of working women having different years of married life. The mean score of working women with 1-5 years of married life is more (69.0) than 6-10 (66.0) 11-15 (59.08) 16-20 and 20 and above (52.23) years of married life. The mean score of 20 and above years of married life group is less in comparison with other groups. The mean score clearly indicates that women who have less years of married life have more marital happiness than the women whose length of married is more. The t-value (4.34) is significant at 0.01 level which clearly reveals that there is a significant difference in marital adjustment between the women who have 1-5 and 20 and above years of married life. The t-values of 3.74 and 2.72 which are significant at 0.01 level indicate that there is a significant difference in marital adjustment between 6-10 and 20 above years of married life groups and between 11-15 years group and 20 and above years group. Further the t-value of 2.83 which is significant at 0.01 level reveals significant difference between 1-5 years and 16-20 years group of married life. The t-values of 2.53, and 2.01 that are significant at 0.05 level indicate that there is a significant difference in marital adjustment between working women of 1-5 & 11-15 and between women of 6-10 and 16-20 years of married life.

Table 5

Mean, SD and t-values of Marital Adjustment of Working Women with Different Years of Married Life

Sl. No.	*Married years*	*Mean*	*SD*	*t-value*
1.	1-5 (48)	69.0	11.91	1.26 (1 & 2) 1.44 (2 & 3)
2.	6-10 (46)	66.0	11.03	0-98 (3 & 4) 1.39 (4 & 5)
3.	11-15 (30)	62.4		4.34** (1 & 5) 9.91 2.53* (1 & 3)
4.	16-20 (13)	59.08	10.83	2.72** (3 & 5) 3.74** (2 & 5)
5.	20 and above (13)	52.23	13.92	2.83** (1 & 4) 2.01* (2 & 4)

* Significant at 0.05 level.

** Significant at 0.01 level.

In the beginning of marital life husband and wife talk to each other openly and give respect to the feelings of each other. They have more positive feelings about each other. In the beginning women maintain a balance in both the place. They cannot perceive any problem in managing the two roles simultaneously. This may because of the dreams they had seen about their marital life. Husband and wife, in the starting years of marital life, give importance to each other and value each other's professions and overlook minor problem and tackle it efficiently. As their married years increase their duties and responsibilities towards family become more complex as much as in workplace there is increased responsibilities with the strains on both sides and subsequently, they experience mental tension. They fail to communicate, share feelings, expectations and personal needs.

Table 6

Mean, SD and t-values of Marital Adjustment of Working Women in Different Age Groups

Sl. No.	*Age*	*Mean*	*SD*	*t-value*
1.	25-29 (37)	67.97	12.52	0.09 (1 & 2)
2.	30-35 (45)	68.22	10.83	2.51* (2 & 3)
3.	36-40 (30)	62.20	9.12	1.44 (3 & 4) 0.04 (4 & 5)
4.	41-45 (16)	57.63	12.06	2.98** (1 & 5) 2.11* (1 & 3) 2.79** (1 & 4)
5.	46 and above (20)	57.45	13.02	1.51 (3 & 5) 3.47** (2 & 5) 3.26** (2 & 4)

* Significant at 0.05 level.

** Significant at 0.01 level.

Table-6 presents the mean score, SDs and t-value of marital adjustment of working women belonging to different age groups. It can be noticed that the mean score of women in age group of 30-35 years is higher (68.22) than those who are in age group of 25-29 years (67.97). The women in age group 36-40 years scored more (62.20) than those belonging to age group of 41-45 years (57.63) and 46 and above years of age (57.45). This reveals that women who are in the age of 25-29 and 30-35 years of age are better adjusted in their married life than the older women. The t-value (2.51) is significant at 0.05 level which shows that there is a significant difference in marital adjustment between women in age group 30-35 and 36-40 years of age. The t-values of 2.98, 2.47, 3.47 and 3.26 which are significant at 0.01 level clearly indicate that there is a significant difference in marital adjustment between 25-29 & 46 and above; 25-29 & 41-45 years; 30-35 & 46 and above; 30-35 and 41-45 years of age. Couples in their early years of marriage are better adjusted to each other. They have more intimacy and closeness in their relationship. They communicate each other's feelings, thoughts etc and this gives them to know and solve each other's problems. Happiness or unhappiness in marriage depends primarily upon the relationships of the spouses that strengthens each other for emotional security.

As the years (age) increase, there will be more commitments in the family. The couples do not get enough time for communication that creates a psychological gap in their relationship. This leads to lack of intimacy and mutual understanding. They have to spend more time in their children's upbringing, paying less attention to each other. This may cause marital unhappiness in the couples, of increasing age.

Table 7

Mean, SD and t-values of Marital Adjustment of Working Women in Two Religions

Sl. No.	*Religion*	*Mean*	*SD*	*t-value*
1.	Hindu (118)	64.71	12.16	0.51
2.	Muslim(32)	63.47	12.61	

Table-7 shows the means, SDs and t-value of marital adjustment of working women belonging to two religions. It can be noticed that the mean score of women belonging to Hindu religion (64.71) is more than the women belonging to Muslim (63.47) religion. The higher mean scores indicate that Hindu women have more marital adjustment than the Muslim women. But the t-value is not significant. It appears, therefore that religion has no 'say' in making couple better adjusted. According to Hindu tradition marriage was considered to be a sacrament, joining together two human beings in eternal and indissolvable union, was in itself responsible for making people accept their marriage. Marriage was not meant mainly for individual gratification interests and aspirations, but was rather a social duty towards the family and community everyone was expected to do one's duty. With these goals there was hardly any room for marital frictions. Through the socialization process, individuals has learnt to respect the marriage and have a good relationship with the partner, respect each others feelings, and to share the duties and responsibilities etc. This made them to have a better adjustment in their marital life. Therefore women, whether Hindu or Muslim, are found to acquire similar amount knowledge for making better adjustment. Hence being Hindu or Muslim does not product differences in marital harmony.

Table 8

Mean, SD and t-values of Marital Adjustment of Working Women in Three Income Groups

Sl. No.	*Income(in lakhs)*	*Mean*	*SD*	*t-value*
1.	> 0.50 (97)	62.35	12.86	2.08* (1 & 2)
2.	1.0 – 1.5 (2.0)	68.21	11.92	0.21 (2 & 3)
3.	1.5 > (25)	67.60	8.07	1.86 (1 & 3)

* Significant at 0.05 level.

Table 8 indicates the mean, SDs and t-value of marital adjustment of working women's belonging to different income levels. The mean scores indicates that the marital adjustment of women whose income is between 1.0 - 1.5 lakhs is better than the women's whose income is 0.50 and above 1.5 lakhs. The mean score is higher in 1.0 – 1.5 lakhs income group. It is low in 0.50 lakh income group. Thus it indicates that women whose income is high are better adjusted in their marital life. The t-value (2.08) is significant at 0.05 level which indicates a significant difference in marital adjustment between 0.5 and 1.0 – 1.5 lakhs of income group. However, in other income groups, the marital adjustment is found to be insignificant

Money has become an increasingly important factor in marriage. The more disappointed couples are with their index of overall income, the less satisfied they are with their relationship. Women who have high income are financially secured and had a prestigious position in the society. This increases their self-esteem and makes them to handle their roles and responsibilities in society. This helps them to have good relationship in their married life. Whereas women with low income group has to work hard to maintain their family. However there is a marginal difference between the two groups of higher income as regards adjustment.

Table 9

Mean, SD and t-values of Marital Adjustment of Working Women in Two Types of Family Structure

Sl. No.	*Family type*	*Mean*	*SD*	*t-value*
1.	Nucleus (109)	64.28	11.67	0.25
2.	Joint (41)	64.88	13.743	

Table 9 demonstrates the mean, SD and t-values of marital adjustment of working wives belonging to two types of family structure. It can be noticed that the mean score of women in nucleus family type is lower (64.28) than those of joint family (64.88). The t-value of 0.25 is not significant at any level. Thus, the results clearly speak the fact that there is no significant difference in marital adjustment between the two sample groups. It appears that the type of family in which the working wives live in, has no profound influence on the amount of marital adjustment and happiness. In any type of family structure, the women seem to lead a contented married life and hence are more adjusted.

FINDINGS

1. There is a significant difference in the marital adjustment of working women in different occupational status.
2. The marital adjustment of doctors is significantly higher than teachers and clerks.
3. Working wives with higher educational level are better adjusted than those with lower level of education.
4. Work experience has a positive influence on marital adjustment of working women.
5. There is a better adjustment in the couple in the initial or beginning years of marriage.

6. The marital adjustment is significantly higher in the sample of 25 to 35 age than those with above 36 years of age.
7. Higher income is found to produce significant differences in marital adjustment. Higher the income greater is the adjustment.
8. Educated couples have equal marital adjustment.
9. Occupational status has not produced any significant sex differences in marital adjustment.
10. In the sample of different work experience, the differences in marital adjustment are found to be insignificant.
11. Husbands in the age group of 25 – 29 years have significantly higher marital adjustment.
12. Religion has nothing to do with the marital adjustment of the couple.
13. The type of family produces no significant sex differences in marital adjustment; but females found to outscore males in both the types of family, insignificantly.
14. The family income has not produced any significant sex differences in the marital adjustment.

LIMITATIONS AND SUGGESTIONS

1. The study was conducted in the area like Gulbarga in which there is a paucity of larger sample of working women. Had the study comprised of large sample of working wives, the diversity and dimensionality of the magnitude of marital adjustment would have been more clear, specific and adequate. Therefore an extended enquiry in this regard is necessary to fill in gaps and pitfalls, if any.

2. The results would have been still more promising if statistical techniques like ANOVA, multiple regression analysis, multiple classification analysis and path analysis were employed in the study to assess the impact of each independent variable on dependent variables. Lack of such resources in the study area needs to be won over in further research endeavours.

3. Marital adjustment is not unidimensional, rather, it is multiphasic in nature. Hence exploration of several other factors contributing to marital adjustment is necessary. It is obvious that further research may unfold all such factors related to marital adjustment and harmony of the couple of this backward region.

REFERENCES

1. Locke, Harvey J., and Williamson, Robert (1958) Marital adjustments, a factor analysis study, American sociology review, Vol. 23, No. 1, pp. 562-9.
2. Landi, Jvdson T. (1946) Length of time rednired to achieve adjustment in marriage, American sociological review, Vol. II, No. 6, pp. 666-77.
3. Ross, Aileen D., (1961) The Hindu family in its urban setting, Bombay, Oxford University Press.
4. Rossi, Alice S. (1964) A good woman is hard to find, transaction, community leadership project of Washington university.
5. Jephcott, Pearl, Seear, Nancy, and Smith. John H. (1962) Married women working London, George Allen and Unwin Ltd.
6. Kapadia, K.M. (1959) "The family in transition, sociological, Bulletin, Vol. 8, No. 2.
7. Kapoor P. (1972) Marriage and Working Women in India Vikas publications, Delhi.

8

Senior Citizens – Adjustments

T.J.Mouni Suvarna Raju*, T. Indira Rani, D. Ramesh*****

ABSTRACT

The present study was conducted to assess various dimensions of adjustments among senior citizens. The study was conducted on senior citizens above 60 years of age residing at old age homes in Guntur district. The study was conducted on a sample of 100 senior citizens among them 50 were males and 50 were females. They were administered a Senior Citizens Adjustment Questionnaire with various adjustment dimensions like home, health, social, emotional and financial adjustments. The results indicated that there were considerable significant differences among senior citizens in regard to gender, age and pension able demographic variables.

Ageing is a natural phenomenon common to all human beings. The last period of ageing is old age and ultimately it is a closing period. Generally we can consider age sixty, as the starting period of old age.

Chronologically after retirement, we can consider old age or retirement age, that is, the age of sixty. According to the norms of the state or central governments, the old age people who cross age

* **Principal, K.P.N. College of Education, Gantyada-535 215, Vizianagaram District, A.P., South, India.**

** **6/12 Brodiepet, Guntur - 522 002 (A.P.)**

*** **Asst. Professor, Department of Anthropology, Andhra University, Visakhapatnam - 530 003 (A.P.)**

sixty are treated as senior citizens. The senior citizens are honored by giving railway concessions, seats in buses, old age pensions, higher interest rates for fixed deposits etc. There is a quotation saying that" ***Grey hair is respected***".

According to Hindu mythology, ***"Vridhatyam-Jarasa Vina"*** which means, let the old age be without senility or disability. (Poet Kalidasa, II century B.C.).

According to new American Standard Bible version, Moses states, ***"As for the days of our life, they contain seventy years, or if due to strength, eighty years, yet their pride is, but labor and sorrow for soon it is gone and we fly away."*** (Psalms 90: 10).

If a man has a total life span of seventy years, during this period, a decade will be old age. If a man possesses high energy he will be having another decade more.

The high energy means, if a man obeys the rules and regulations of the government as well as God, then he can gain ten years more for his life span. The variations of age are according to the will of God.

After crossing sixty years of age, senile dementia will occur. It is the loss of cognitions. When the age increases slowly, the human potentialities like remembering, reasoning, problem solving, memory, thinking, etc., will gradually decreases. So even if a professor having high potentialities of knowledge, losses every thing in his old age.

During old age, the person has to become dependent on somebody. At the same time, he has to spend his life in lonely atmosphere. Sometimes, the older people are alone in their homes. So, there is a lot of variation between his worked conditions, in relationship with retirement age or old age. Hence, the old person has to adjust himself, to the environmental dimensions. A proper adjustment will make him a better and comfortable life. An improper adjustment will lead him a problematic life.

AIM

1. To study the difference between the adjustments of the aged people based on gender.

2. To study the adjustment among 60-69 years and 70 & above years.
3. To study the difference between the pensioners and non-pensioners.

TOOLS

The Senior Citizens Adjustment Questionnaire was developed by R.A.Sharma (1998).The SCAQ assesses five dimensions of adjustment covering home, health, social, emotional and financial adjustments. There are 50 questions; each dimension consists of 10 questions. The low score indicates poor adjustment and high score indicates better adjustment.

SAMPLE

The study was conducted on a sample of 100 senior citizens at five old age homes of Guntur urban limits. The sample consisted of 50 and 50 females. The investigators approached the managements of old age homes and got permission to conduct study. Then the researchers approached the senior citizens and requested them to participate in this study. The subjects were made to feel at ease and an initial rapport was established. The questionnaire was given to the senior citizens and they were asked to fill them as per the instructions laid down in the questionnaire.

DATA ANALYSIS

The data obtained from the sample of 100 senior citizens was scored and analyzed with the help of a computer. The analysis involved Mean, Standard Deviation and application of t-tests.

RESULTS AND DISCUSSION

The critical value is 0.48. There is no significant difference between male and female senior citizens in home adjustment.

The critical value is 14.66. There is a significant difference in home adjustment between the age groups of 60-69 yrs and 70 and above yrs.

The results indicate that there is a considerable difference in home adjustment between pensioners and non-pensioner senior citizens.

Table 1
Home Adjustment and Variables

Variable		*Sample*	*Mean*	*S.D*	*M.D*	*C.R*
Gender	Male	50	24.82	2.60	0.24	0.48
	Female	50	24.58	2.51		
Age	60-69	60	23.05	1.81	4.12	14.66
	70 above	40	27.17	1.00		
Financial support	Pensioners	30	24.00	2.05	1.00	2.67
	Non-Pensioners	70	25.00	2.69		

Table 2
Health Adjustment and Variables

Variable		*Sample*	*Mean*	*S.D*	*M.D*	*C.R*
Gender	Male	50	25.62	3.49	0.86	1.34
	Female	50	24.76	2.97		
Age	60-69	60	27.18	2.31	4.98	11.82
	70 above	40	22.20	1.89		
Financial support	Pensioners	30	26.33	3.16	1.63	2.39
	Non-Pensioners	70	24.70	3.19		

The critical ratio is 1.34.There is no significant difference between male and female regarding the health adjustment.

The critical value is 11.82 There is significant difference between the age groups of 60-69 and 70 and above, in health adjustment.

There is significant difference between pensioners and non-pensioners in health adjustment.

Table 3

Social Adjustment and Variables

Variable		*Sample*	*Mean*	*S.D*	*M.D*	*C.R*
Gender	Male	50	25.38	2.94	1.18	2.31
	Female	50	26.56	2.26		
Age	60-69	60	24.31	1.71	4.13	11.50
	70 above	40	28.45	1.81		
Financialsupport	Pensioners	30	24.66	2.61	1.62	2.94
	Non-Pensioners	70	26.51	2.57		

There is considerable difference between male and female of senior citizens in the aspects of social adjustment.

There is significant difference between the age groups of 60-69 and 70 & above in social adjustment.

There is considerable difference between pensioners and non-pensioners in social adjustment.

Table 4

Emotional Adjustment and Variables

Variable		*Sample*	*Mean*	*S.D*	*M.D*	*C.R*
Gender	Male	50	24.90	2.65	0.32	0.69
	Female	50	25.22	2.20		
Age	60-69	60	23.48	1.56	3.94	14.07
	70 above	40	27.42	1.33		
Financial support	Pensioners	30	24.66	2.44	0.56	1.09
	Non-Pensioners	70	25.22	2.43		

There is no significant difference between male and female regarding emotional adjustment.

There is considerable difference in senior citizens between 60-69 and 70 & above age groups in emotional adjustment.

The results show that there is no significant difference between the pensioners and non-pensioners in emotional adjustment.

Table 5

Financial Adjustment and Variables

Variable		*Sample*	*Mean*	*S.D*	*M.D*	*C.R*
Gender	Male	50	23.80	3.66	0.24	0.40
	Female	50	24.04	2.33		
Age	60-69	60	25.43	1.81	3.78	6.88
	70 above	40	21.65	3.15		
Financial support	Pensioners	30	25.53	2.40	2.30	4.10
	Non-Pensioners	70	23.22	3.06		

There is no considerable difference between male and female in financial adjustment.

There is significant difference between the age groups of 60-69 and 70 & above in financial adjustment.

The above table shows that there is considerable difference between pensioners and non-pensioners in the aspects of financial adjustment.

CONCLUSION

There is significant difference in age groups and financial support in home adjustment. In health adjustment there is significant difference in age groups and financial support. In social adjustment gender, age groups and financial support variables are significantly varying. In respect of emotional adjustment age is more influenced. There is statistical significant difference in age groups and financial support in financial adjustment.

REFERENCES

Bhatia, H.R. (1965), Elements of Social Psychology. Bombay, India: Manaktalas.

Lazarus, R.S. (1976), patterns of adjustment. Tokyo, Japan: Mc Graw – Hill, Kogakusha Pvt. Ltd.

Lindgren, H.C. (1959). Psychology of Personal and Social Adjustment, (2nd). New York: American Book Company.

New American Standard Bible, (1976), (Psalms 90:10), Study Edition, A.J. Holman Company, Philadelphia.

Ruch, F.L. (1970), Psychology and Life. Bombay, India: D.B. Taraporewala sons and co.

Shaffer, L.F and Shoben, E.J. (1956). The Psychology of Adjustment. Boston: Houghton Mifflin Co.

Sharma,R.A.(1998).The Senior Citizens Adjustment Questionnaire. Agra psychological research cell, Agra.

Smith, H.C. (1961). Personality Adjustment. New York: Mc Graw – Hill Book Co.

9

Music Therapy

The Present Scenario

V.Gowri Rammohan*

ABSTRACT

Human beings in the modern world are on the constant strive to rise higher and higher on the material plane with the result that they have no time to realize their pathetic condition at a time when they become helpless and need the help of an expert in the area of medicine and if that doesn't seem to yield positive results they tend to seek the help of a psychiatrist or a psychologist. Although music has been used from the time civilization started it is only in the recent years that people seem to realize the importance of music to relieve them from the tress that they unknowingly under go in their struggle to overcome the obstacles and the problems they experience everyday. Today many people talk about music therapy as a means of receiving ones stress and as a tool that creates a way of relaxing the body and mind. People who talk and realize music as a stress reliever seem to outnumber those who actually show empirically that music is a useful tool to relieve one's stress. Empirical studies with music as a therapeutic tool entails a number of practical problems as well as theoretical issues. The present paper examines music therapy in the Indian and the western contexts and discusses the issues and problems involved in using music as a therapeutic device.

* **Professor, Department of Psychology, Andhra University, Visakhapatnam.**

Music as a therapeutic tool has its roots in ancient history irrespective of the culture. The effect of music on the behavior was mentioned in the Vedas, Bible, and in the early Buddhist texts. Music therapy was used in almost all the parts of the world and it may be of interest to note that music was used not for treating the mental disorders but for the physical disorders. The Egyptians and other Greek physicians used music to restore the health of the patients. The Arabs used music therapy in the thirteenth century and the French in the nineteenth century in their hospitals (Sharma, 2000).

A primitive practice known as *Shamanism* that refers to the treatment of various diseases using music therapy believed that diseases develop due to imbalance in the rhythm of the body and mind. Music was used to regain and restore the balance. Music was organized during the World War I to relieve the physical and mental disturbances among the soldiers. The term 'Melotherapy' was coined by Launagein (1924) to refer to the use of music for the treatment of diseases. The terms musicotherapy and later psycho rhythmo therapy were used to refer to the power of the sound patterns in music. The powerful effect of the repetition of a single musical phrase in helping one to relax and avoid unwanted sub-alpha brain waves, and influence of rhythm in synchronizing the functions of the body was noticed in the early nineties (Pinto,1994).

Music as a therapeutic device has been understood from two modalities, one, as a passive form where importance is given to listening, and two, active form where there is active participation in the musical activity, such as training in music, participating in group singing, and so on. In either form the sound and the vibrations of the music were said to have impact on the participant and music was thought to be used effectively in two ways: one, as a therapeutic means to cure a disease and two, as a Prophylactic or preventive measure (Sharma, 1996 & Sharma, 2000). Several studies come to light where music was used as a therapeutic tool.

Thomas (1968) discussed the use of music therapy in the treatment of mentally ill and also in the emotionally disturbed children. Clark (1968) reported musical rhythm motivation as a technique for creating a sense of self-efficacy among the institutionalized retarded boys. Feign and Povilenco (1969) reported studies where music was used as a therapeutic measure in dental surgery, obstetrics, and psycho-neurological practices.

Shapiro (1969) described therapeutic use of music with the aged individuals and enhanced socialization among various nationality culture groups was established and also by assigning rhythm instruments to the patients on the basis of their physical needs helped them to relieve some of the stiffness of arthritis, increased muscular movements and improved personal satisfaction. Michel and Martin (1970) reported that among the elementary school boys development of musical skill could aid in increasing the self esteem of the disadvantaged problem students which could generalize into increased self confidence in other tasks.

Other studies among several others where music therapy was implemented in the West include Kaser's (1991) study in which pedophelia was treated with drum set, Sydensticker (1991) who used music therapy in the treatment of patients with psycosis and Stanton (1975) and Fogelson (1972) who found that highly anxious subjects increased their performance with music as opposed to without music.

Various other aspects that have been studied include such aspects as emotion in children's songs (Adachi Trehub,2000), musical and religious experiences related to happiness (Hills and Argyle,1998), personality, creativity and aesthetic preference (Rawlings, Twomey, Burns and Morris,1998) and the beneficial quality of music to the individual in terms of cognitive aspects, (Graziano, Peterson and Shaw,1999; Shaw, Rauscher, Levine, Wright, Dennis and Newcomb,1977; Sergent, et al,1992).

From the Indian point of view the whole universe is considered to be made of sound, called *nadabrahma* alias *Shabda Brahma* which means that the whole universe and the creator of the universe are just the sound (Sharma, 1996). Indian music system consists of *nada* as the pivot whether it is Hindustani music (the music of the northern part of the country) or Karnatik music (the music of the southern part).

Nada refers to the cosmic sound, which is perceived inwardly. Two kinds of *nada* have been delineated in the Indian system namely, *ahata* and *anahata*. The former refers to the sound perceived externally, audible to the ears as in the case of the musical notes and the latter *anahata* that refers to the sound that is heard inwardly as in the yogic and meditative practices. If universe is made of sound why do the people fail to hear is answered by the fact that we cannot hear it because our hearing range is just a small band of frequencies; anything below called 'subsonic' and anything above called 'ultrasonic' is inaudible and what we hear is 'sonic' which is audible to the human ear (Vasudev, 2007).

Indian music is rendered on the basic seven notes, namely, S R G M P D N in the ascending order and N D P M G R S in the descending order. S is described as *adhara shadja* or the basic note from which the other notes have emerged. At the end of the seven notes the S is repeated at the *tara sthayi* or the higher pitch to make a complete octave. Within this octave the scale consisting of seven notes or *saptaswaras* is delineated into 12 notes called *Dwadassa swara sthanas,* 16 notes called *shodasa swara sthanas* and finally an octave can be divided into 22 *dwavimsathi swaras* or the microtones. Division of the octave into 22 minute tones or microtones was done in the 1st century AD by a unique experiment by Bharata the author of the first treatise on Dance, Drama and Music, *Natya sastra.* It is believed that the seven musical notes encompass everything and the seven charkas which are the meeting points in the human system correspond to the seven musical notes. Concentration on the seven notes can vitalize the energy in the human body.

Indian music has evolved with two broad systems namely, *raga* and *tala* each having a highly evolved complex pattern. Thus based on the 22 *srutis* thousands of *ragas* could be delineated. The *tala* system also has emerged with complex patterns taking the lead from seven basic *tala*s. Each can be varied into five kinds resulting in 35 *talas* which in turn can evolve into 105 types by varying each of the 35 *talas* into three types each. (Parthasaradhi and Parthasaradhi, 1965/2003.

Indian music can be traced back to the *Vedas* and Bharata in his treatise attributes the origin of the arts to the three gods Brahma, Vishnu and Maheswara as the creators of *raga, tala* and *bhava,* respectively. As Vasudeva (2007) remarks for a Hindu right from the time one is born the only goal is *mukti* or liberation. Everything else is secondary. The path to liberation is spiritual realization and music which is nothing but nada has been extolled as the easier way to attain *jivan mukti* or liberation from the body to attain the supreme consciousness. *Nadabindupanishad* speaks about the power of *Nada* for disciplining the mind. The mind that which looses itself in nada does not get disturbed by other things and remains stable. The worship of *Nada* is a very powerful means of disciplining the mind just like the reins to a horse. (Musalagaonkar, 1975).

In India, references to the use of music as a therapeutic tool could be traced to the 12th to 14th centuries by Jayadeva, Narayana Tirtha, Annamacharya and others who used music through their songs to bring the deceased persons to life. During the period 1750 to 1850 the time of the musical trinity, Tyagaraja, Muthuswami Dikshitar and Syama Sastry, Tyagaraja brought to life a person declared dead by singing a composition *Naa Jeevadhara* in the raga *Bilahari*. Muthuswami Dikshitar who saw his student suffering from a stomach ailment composed a song *Brihaspate* in the raga *Attana* on the planet and suggested his disciple to sing the same to alleviate him from his stomach ailment. Several other anomalous instances and references to music therapy were reported in the lives of the musical trinity (Rammohan, 2006).

Till about 2000 A.D.not many studies have been reported to see the effect of music as a therapeutic tool in India as much as it is found in the west. This view seems to be shared by a few who have attempted to conduct systematic studies in this area of research. Sharma (2000), for example wrote, "no substantial work has been done in the field of investigating the relaxation value an therapeutic efficacy of music on psychological and psychophysiological disorders"(pg.40). She referred to the few studies conducted in India during 90s that include those of Khumar and Kaur (1992) and Sharma (1992). Khumar and Kaur (1992) who did a single case study to see the efficacy of instrumental music in the treatment of insomnia failed to find positive outcomes. In yet another study, Sharma (1992) found that groups of subjects from music discipline as well as non music disciplines showed positive influence on psycho physiological changes with the preferred music. Sharma, (1996) who used music as special education program for the mentally handicapped children obtained promising results to the point that whether classical or folk-popular songs had exhibited identical effects on the school achievement and school adjustment of the students. Sharma (2000) who used music and biofeedback techniques for relaxation in her study found that biofeedback training and music treatment had adequate relaxation value. She found that the musicality group showed more relaxation under music treatment and low musicality group under biofeedback treatment.

In recent years there seems to be an upsurge and concern to use music therapy as a therapeutic tool with various disorders in their respective clinics as evinced by the work reported by Mythily (2007a; 2007b and 2007c.) In one study, Mythily (2007a) with hyperactive children, music therapy was introduced by making the children learn classical music songs. The results suggested that music therapy was an effective and viable alternative for children who receive medication for hyperactivity. The quality of improvement in the behavior of children after music training sessions was quite satisfactory and parents were overwhelmed with the effectiveness of music therapy. The treatment was effective in changing social behavior, and improvement in attention skills other aspects such as handwriting and completing school assignments, etc.

Mythili (2007b) used specific musical notes of classical music to treat patients with depression. A ten week therapeutic program yielded positive results and the patients with depressive moods were able to come out of their depressive state of mind slowly and steadily. After the period of ten weeks almost all the patients enrolled in the therapeutic session have felt the brighter side of their mind. Subjects who were not given the music therapy program remained in their darkness and in the words of the experimenter, she felt that the subjects in the control could not have the pleasure of coming out of the depressive mood for the purpose of the experimental design. However, after the research period, later on she has given them a free music therapy CD for overcoming the depression.

In a third study, Mythily (2007c) used classical music ragas as therapeutic means to students and some business men to relieve them of the examination stress and the routine business activities, respectively. In both the groups the effect of listening to classical music regularly for some sessions showed marked improvement. Both boys and girls could shed off their anxiety for examination; the professionals who were exposed to two or three classical music sessions were rejuvenated. Based on her results the experimenter concluded that classical music proved as a stress reliever for the participants; music therapy enhanced the students' approach to examinations considerably in a positive direction; professionals were able to overcome their stress easily; music therapy created mental freshness to all the participants and there was no sex difference with regard to relieving from stress.

In a study by the author of this paper (Rammohan 2002) children in the age group of eight to thirteen were tested in two sessions with a gap of nine month period. Music students (those who were attending music classes) were compared with non music students (those who were not attending any music classes) on variables such as intelligence, attention span, dependence proneness, personality, Om chanting time duration and parents' and teachers' rating on hyperactivity check list. No significant outcomes were noticed in the study. However, the music students showed increased dependency proneness at the end of the nine month period; the ability to hold the breath was more among the music students compared to the non music students; music and the non music students showed an increased span of attention after the training period; the ratings on hyperactivity given by the parents of music students were lower than the non music students and the personality pattern of music students was found to be similar to that of the non music students.

Working with mentally handicapped children Saraswathidevi of Lebenshelfe (Visakhapatnam), a school for the mentally handicapped, found that music could act as a stimulant to bring activity among the profound mentally retarded and those who were otherwise unable to involve any regular activity could participate in rendering classical music songs in good tune and rhythm with positive feelings of self worth. In a study by Rekha (2006) classical music (Pancharatna kritis) was presented to the HIV?AIDs patients and normal subjects for a duration of fifteen minutes. They were tested for anxiety and well being before and after the music session. Results showed that the anxiety was reduced and the well being scores were enhanced after listening to classical music for about fifteen minutes.

Although the number of empirical studies using music as a therapeutic tool in the West outnumbers those in the East, there is a growing awareness today among the academicians, musicians as well as the lay public about the efficacy of music as a therapeutic means. Recognizing music as a beneficial tool in the treatment of actual diseases in different ways Sharma (1996) enlists several uses of music in various ways. Music can be used as a sedative. It can replace the use of tranquilizers or sleeping pills. A dentist can use it as a diversionary tactics. In case of physiological trauma, as in war time, the right type of music diverts the mind of the patient from brooding on the horrors of past experience. Music helps by directing the behavior of neurotics and other mental patients towards positive side. Music is used to invigorate and stimulate the action of physiotherapy. Participating in group singing develops a sense of belonging and develops good personal relations with others. As an avenue of self expression music is even better than language. The great desire to be admired by teenagers is achieved by giving music performance on stage or among friends. Music creates a sense of security among the patients who are afraid of either loneliness or from big gathering.

The major catchphrase and concern in the present day modern times is stress which is on rise in everyone' life. Stress as a harmful factor for the physical and mental well-being of the individuals is highlighted in all the cultures today and people are becoming open-minded to alleviate stress by paramedical practices such as yoga and meditative practices. If untreated, stress can result in severe consequences and leave the body vulnerable to a number of disorders that could end up in incurable diseases. Music therapy was found to replace medication with long-term positive effects but was found to be more expensive than drug treatment in the sense that it requires more involvement and commitment on the part of both the parents and children and the therapists (Mythili, 2007a).

The overall benefits that music can have on people in different walks of life was studied by The National Association for Music Education. The benefits conveyed by music education was grouped into four categories, success in society, success in school, success in developing intelligence and success in life. Music education was found to be superior to computer education in enhancing abstract reasoning skills (Shaw et al., 1977).

In the studies cited so far music was found to help people of different age groups to alleviate them of their problems or help them improve their cognitive skills or help them in a general way to improve their interpersonal relations and social life and so on. One aspect was that the classical music was recognized for its beneficial effect in some of the empirical studies referred to in the present paper conducted in India. There seem to be some problems associated with the use of music as a therapeutic tool. The first question that arises is what kind of music should be used. The concept of music gives rise to a variety of music in the minds of people. Is it classical music, light or film music. The concept of music encompasses a broad spectrum with so many different types of music. People tend to have their own preferences for particular music. The tendency to react to music generally varies with the personality of the person concerned.

In Indian classical music where ragas forms the pivot in Karnatic as well as Hindustani music. A well rendered raga in Indian classical music can create total engrossment in the mood of the listener. The effect of music on the listener takes a cyclic form As Holroyde (1972) said, Indian music moves in spirals "from the musician inwards to the climax of the music and outwards to the audience who listen, so taking hold of each listener and working again to the musician. The development is not linear as in a symphony but swirling and whirling as galaxies of sounds in progression (pg 46).

Indian ragas can create different moods in the listener has been well accepted by a number of researchers working in that direction. Sharma,(1996) listed out six primary ragas of Hindustani music that tend to have been associated with particular qualities, sentiments and moods. These ragas include Hindola, Shri, Meghmalhar, Deepak, Bhairav, and kaushik. Among south Indian ragas, ragas like Kalyani can produce energy, Thodi can bring melancholy, Hamsadhvani can create positive feelings and sri can bring feelings of auspicious moods. The ancient music sholars have attached some powers to some ragas. For example, singing raga Madhyamavathi at the end of a music concert can alleviate the doshas (mistakes) committed by the musician unknowingly. One should not forget the fact that individual differences exist in the preferences to the music and to the ragas in particular. Forcing one to listen to some kind of music for relaxation might itself create stress in the individual.

While music seem to have positive effect on the listener, giving due credit to one's preference for the kind of music that will have positive impact, musicians themselves seem to undergo anxiety and hardships for giving music performances. Here it may be relevant to consider people who tend to consume music and those who tend to produce music. It appears that consumers of music are certainly at their beneficial end while the producer of music especially one who has to perform under go what may be termed as 'performance anxiety' Taylor (2007). In spite of the demand for hardships one has to undergo to become a musician people who have a genuine interest for music prefer to suffer rather than give up music as their serious interest, be it in the west or east.

Researchers in the area of music therapy may be suggested to see the specific power of the ragas and their effect on the various ailments. Empirical studies should focus on specific ragas and their impact on the specific disorders. Raga Shankarabharanam, for example, has been considered to create sober, calm, tranquil and composed feelings. So, to create the feeling of self-poise, self-confidence, etc., a listener may be presented with this raga for the desired effect. Therefore, the researchers should probably aim to find out the exact raga for a particular ailment.

A look into the chemistry of the raga reveals that it is not a single note nor a single beat of rhythm but a compound of several notes with various frequencies. Each note seem to be associated with a particular feeling. For example, *Prathi Madhyama* gives the feeling of pain and disaster while *sudha rishabha* gives the feeling of sorrow or sleepiness. The minimum notes in a raga generally range between a combination of five to seven. With different individual notes giving rise to different moods and feelings what mood can be expected from a raga with a combination of different notes. In a Karnatic music concert, generally, the performer renders at least a dozen songs which when delved deeply, individually, could produce different moods. Here it may be pertinent to consider the global effect of the ragas and their overall impact on the listener.

Considering the above then the day will not be far to prescribe a music concert for overall benefits to a person having any kind of problem or a suitable raga to alleviate a particular disorder. At that point of time a music therapist, in future, can very quickly assess the requirement of the individual and give a prescription of the raga that can work wonders.

REFERENCES

Adachi, M., and Trehub, S.E. (1998). Children's expression of emotion in song. *Psychology of Music.* 26, 133-153.

Clark, L. (1968). Musical rhythm motivation. Journal of Psychiatric Nursing and Mental Health Services. 6(5),287, 290-293.

De Obaladia, M and Best,G.A. (1971). Music therapy in the treatment of brain damaged children. *Academic Therapy.*

Fogelson, S. (1972). Music as a distracter on reciting test performance of grade students. *Perceptual and motor Skills*, 34, 981-990.

Feign, V. and Povilenco, R. (1969). Music as a means of medical treatment. *Journal of Medical Profession,* Psychological abstracts, 65.

Graziano, A.B., Peterson, M., and Shaw, G.L. (1999). Enhanced learning of proportional math through music training and spatial-temporal training. *Neurological Research*, 21, 139-152.

Hills,P., and Argyle, M.,(1998). Musical and religious experiences and their relationship to happiness. *Personality and Individual Differences.* 25, 91-102.

Holroyde, P. (1972). *The Music of India.* Praegar Pubishers inc.

Kaser, V.A. (1991). Music therapy treatment pedophilia using the drum set. *Journal of Psychotherapy,* 18, 7-15.

Khumar, S.S. and Kaur, Manjit (1992). Efficacy of instrumental music for treatment of insomnia: A single case study.Unpublished practicum report, Punjabi University, Patiala.

Launagein. (1924). Music therapy for mentally ill. *The Journal of General Psychology,* 62, 311-318.

Michel, D.E. and Martin, D. (1970). Music and self esteem research with disadvantaged, problem boys in an elementary school. *Journal of Music Therapy.* 7, 124-127.

Musalagaonkar, V. (1975). Music and sound in yoga. In R.C. Mehta (ed.), *Psychology of music.* Indian Musicological Society, Baroda, pp. 44-65.

Mythily,T. (2007a). Effects of music therapy and withdrawal of stimulant medication with hyper active children. http:www.emusictherapy.com/rhyper.html (a)

Mythily, T. (2007b). Effects of music therapy in overcoming depression. http:/ www.emusictherapy.com/rdepression.html

Mythily, T. (2007c). Effects of music therapy in overcoming stress.http:/ www.emusictheray.cm/rstress.html

Parthasaradhi, N. C. and Parthasaradhi, D. (1965/2003). *Ganakalabhodhini*. Tagore Publishing House, Hyderabad.

Pinto, J. (1994). High frequency medicine. The Sunday review. *The Times of India*, August 14.

Rammohan, V.G. (2002). *Effect of south Indian music training on physical and mental abilities.of students*. Report of major search work, Andhra University. (Unpublished manuscript)

Rammohan,V.G. (2006). *An insight into the lives and works of the musical trinity Tyagaraja Muthuswami Dikshitar and Syama Sastry*. Andhra University Press, Visakhapatnam.

Rawlings, D., Twomey, F., Burns,E., and Morris, S.(1998). Personality, creativity and aesthetic preference; comparing psychotism, sensation seeking, schizotypy and openness to experience. *Experimental studies of the Arts*, 16, 153-178.

Rekha, Suvarna I. (2006).Comparative study of the effect of music on HIV/ AIDS patients and normal subjects. M.Phil. Dissertation in Counseling Psychology, Andhra University. (Unpublished dissertation)

Sergent, J. Zuck, E., Tenial, S., and Mac Donall, B. (1992). Distributed neural network underlying musical sight reading and key board performance. *Science*, 257, 106-109.

Shapiro, A (1969).A pilot program in music therapy with residents of a home for the aged. *Gerontologist*. 9,128-133.

Sharma, Mamta. (1992). A study of preferred music on psychophysiological changes among normal university students. Unpublished M. Phil. dissertation, Punjab University, Patiala.

Sharma, Manorma. (1996). *Special Education Music Therapy*. APH Publishing Co. Darya Ganj, New Delhi.

Sharma, Mamta. (2000). *Mental Relaxation - Music Therapy, Extraversion and Neuroticism*. Arun Publishing House, Chandigarh.

Shaw, G.L., Rauscher, F.W., Levine, L.J., Wright, E. L., Dennis. W. R. and Newcomb, R. (1977). Music training causes long term enhancement of preschool children's spatial temporal reasoning. *Neurological Research*, 19, 1, 1-18.

Stanton, H.E. (1975). The effect of music on test anxiety. *Australian Psychologist*, 10, 220-228.

Sydensticker,T (1991).Music therapy: An alternative for psychosis treatment. Brasileiro-de-Psiguiatria, 40, 509-513.

Taylor, L. Performance anxiety and our motivation for performing. (http:// eeshop.unl.edu/anxiety.html)

Thomas, M. (1968). The challenge of music therapy. Provo papers, 4, 12-21.

Vasudev, S.J. (2007) Tune your world. *Eternal Solutions- manual of life*. 4, 12, 54-56.

10

Myriad Moods and Music

Srujana Satish*

ABSTRACT

This paper examines the meaning and importance of music in the lives of people and gives an insight into the various moods created by different kinds of music. It also pays particular attention to the ways in which music contributes to quality of life and wellbeing. Music is a way of expression. It is a language of emotions. The healing power of music is not unknown to man-primitive or modern. It is a medicine for the body, mind and soul. People have understood the significance of the mind and its influence on the individual from time immemorial. Even a perfectly normal human being can never stay in a balanced state of mind throughout his life. Every person, due to various factors has different moods- he may be very excited and happy at times and may also be stressed out and be depressed. Studies reveal that music provides people with ways of relieving stress, understanding their mind and developing a mental state of balance and acts as a companion and lessens feelings of isolation and loneliness. In today's world, deciding which music to listen to is a serious concern too. Listening to the right form of music in a given situation can help a person experience and maintain his wellbeing. The paper argues that music can be used to maintain and promote a better quality of life for people in general.

* Research Scholar, Department of Music, Andhra University, Visakhapatnam.

MEANING AND IMPORTANCE OF MUSIC

'Music', is a very short word to encompass all that one would want to say about the art. Music has been there from the birth of the universe. From the evolution of mankind, music has always been a part of our lives. We hear music everywhere. It is believed that even the planets eminate sound which is musical while revolving around the sun. What does music really mean?

Music has been defined and understood in numerous ways. An oft cited definition of music, made by Wynton Marsalis among others, is that it is "sound organized in time." The fifteenth edition of the *Encyclopaedia Britannica* describes that "while there are no sounds that can be described as inherently unmusical, musicians in each culture have tended to restrict the range of sounds they will admit."

The word *music* comes from the Greek *mousikê (tekhnê)* by way of the Latin *musica*. It is ultimately derived from *mousa*, the Greek word for muse. In ancient Greece, the word *mousike* was used to mean any of the arts or sciences governed by the Muses.

Aristotle (384-322 BC), a disciple of Plato, asserted that the function of art is not merely an imitation of nature but a rather consummation of what nature has left unfinished. He firmly regarded music as significant of life values and as capable of stimulating one's affective responses. Homer, Euripides and other ancient Greeks attributed qualities such as amusement and relaxation to music. The importance of music is its power to transcend time, emotion, culture, and language as we connect with others. Like food and water, music has nourished man for generations.

Every culture, nation, and for that matter every individual has music around him knowingly or unknowingly. From the chimes at the door step to the ring tone on our mobile we hear music right from the time we wake up in the morning. So how important is it in our lives? One would have got the answer by now.

Music is basically used as a form of entertainment. But now a days people are slowly beginning to discover the many uses that music bestows upon us. Music therapy is a field of research which has gained importance in recent time. However, it mostly deals with the cure of mental and physical ailments which I would like to keep aside for the moment. We are here to talk about how music can help people in general, to maintain and promote a better quality of life and well-being.

MUSIC AS A WAY OF EXPRESSION

Rousseau and other music critics such as Riemann, great musicians like Beethoven, Schumann and Liszt, all believed the essence of music to be 'self-expression'. Guy Madison, in his 'Emotion and meaning in music', says, "Music is an extremely versatile means of communication. It is capable of exploiting all the acoustic features that are used in verbal communication. Moreover, it does so in an explicit and structured way, which makes it an interesting and useful window into human communication in general."

Music is a way of expression. It is a language of emotions. Be it love, sorrow, joy, valour, devotion, or any feeling, there is no better way to express it than through music. It leaves ample space for thought and scope for imagination in the listener. It may be worth mentioning one of Johann Sebastian Bach's most striking organ representations, '*Durch Adams Fall ist ganz verderbt*' (Through Adam's fall, all is spoiled; NAWM 82). A jagged series of dissonant leaps in the pedals depicts the idea of "fall", departing from a consonant chord and falling into a dissonant one as if from innocence into sin, while the twisting chromatic lines in the inner voices suggests at once temptation, sorrow, and the sinuous writhing of the serpent. (Donald Jay Grout & Claude V. Palisca, 1996).

HEALING POWER OF MUSIC

Music has not only been a means to express one's feeling but has also been serving as a great healer. The healing power of music is not unknown to man-primitive or modern. It is a medicine for the body, mind and soul. It is believed that St. Tyagaraja sang his composition 'Naa jeevadhara' in the raga Bilahari and brought back a person to life. Another composer of the 18th century of South Indian classical music, Muttuswami Dikshitar had asked his disciple to sing his (Dikshitar's) composition 'Brihaspate', an invocation to the planet Mercury who is believed to be the God of health, in the Raga Attana, to cure the disciple of a stomach ailment. [Gowri Rammohan, 2006].

Healing with music continues to date in this so called scientific era. Sonali S. Sokhal, in her article "Music: Nourishment for the soul" says that psychologist Dr. Sanjay Chugh, consultant at Delhi's Apollo Hospital uses music as part of his therapy.

"Music therapy," he says, "has helped me in treating many people with problems like dementia, dyslexia and trauma." He further points out that many children with learning disability and poor coordination have been able to learn to respond to set pieces of music. Dr Chugh recommended a mini-synthesizer to play on for a five-year-old child who was withdrawn and unsociable with his peers because of a slight retardation. Soon, he noted a marked improvement in the child's social and interpersonal skills.

Sonali also mentions in her article about Dance critic Ashish Khokar, who cites an experiment as proof: "Music is produced from sound, and sound affects our sense perception in many ways. Even fish in an aquarium were once made to listen to different kinds of music and it was found that their movements corresponded with the beat of the music. Mind you, fish do not hear, they only felt the vibrations of the sound through water. So you can imagine what a profound effect sound and music might have on the human mind."

Music was also found to reduce the pain during dental procedures.

MUSIC AS STRESS RELIEVER

Music is widely used as a stress reliever too. Some are of the opinion that everyone has different tastes in music therefore, one has to listen to the music that one feels comfortable with. Sitting down and forcing oneself to listen to relaxation music that one doesn't like may create stress, not alleviate it. Which music can relieve stress?

Many experts suggest that it is the rhythm of the music or the beat that has the calming effect on us although we may not be very conscious about it. They point out that when we were a baby in our mother's womb, we probably were influenced by the heart beat of our mother. We respond to the soothing music at later stages in life, perhaps associating it with the safe, relaxing, protective environment provided by our mother.

Playing music in the background while we are working, seemingly unaware of the music itself, has been found to reduce the stress.

Music was found to reduce heart rates and to promote higher body temperature - an indication of the onset of relaxation. Combining music with relaxation therapy was more effective than doing relaxation therapy alone.

However complex, music is readily appreciated by the mind without the need for formalized knowledge.

CONCEPT OF "QUALITY OF LIFE"

Before we see the relationship with music, let us briefly see what the term 'Quality of life' means.

"Quality of Life" has been defined as *subjective well-being*. it has also been said that *physical* health contributes relatively little to 'Quality of life'. For instance, *emotional well-being* and *life satisfaction* (two constructs that determine quality of life) have been found to be the same for people with serious physical disability as for those in the general population. (Balfour M. Mount MD, McGill University, 2004).

Here we might say that just like a=b & b=c .: a=c; similarly, quality of life depends more on mind and mind can be influenced by music therefore quality of life can be influenced by music.

One of the most influential writers on the concept of "quality of life" in Scandinavia has been the Norwegian psychologist Siri Næss. According to Næss, quality of life has four main components: 1) *Activity*, which contains the dimensions of engagement, energy, self-realisation and freedom. 2) *Good interpersonal relations* which are realised through friendship and intimate relations. 3) *Self-confidence*, which has to do with self-esteem and self-acceptance, and 4) *A basic sense of happiness* which is maintained through emotional experiences, safety and joy. (Even Rudd, 1997). I shall deal with the same and their relationship with music later on in this paper.

Another Norwegian writer, Tone Rustøen, discusses — from the perspective of nursing science — how an enduring state of happiness, deeper feelings, love and social life have importance in making our life feel better. In her conceptual clarification, Rustøen comes up with four dimensions, which from her professional background seems relevant to the concept of quality of life: *hope, meaning, feelings of communality and identity.*

Without going too much into the details regarding the concepts of quality of life and well being which have been extensively dealt with by a number of psychologists and others, I will now quickly proceed into our main topic which deals with the relationship of music with quality of life.

MUSIC – QUALITY OF LIFE AND WELL-BEING

In the modern times, music has a wider scope and a broader meaning. The study of music does not only involve its power to heal and act as a stress reliever but is being studied in the light of 'Quality of life' and the well-being of a person.

In his article 'Music and the Quality of Life', first published in *1997 in* ***Nordic Journal of Music Therapy****, 6(2), pp 86-97., Even rudd* suggests how music may contribute to the quality of life in the following four areas: (1) Music may increase our feelings of vitality and awareness of feelings, (2) music provides opportunity for increased sense of agency, (3) music-making provides a sense of belonging and communality, and (4) experiences of music creates a sense of meaning and coherence in life.□ He further gives the last definition offered by the World Federation of Music Therapy:

> *"Music Therapy is the use of music and/or its musical elements (sound, rhythm, melody and harmony) by a music therapist, and client or group, in a process designed to facilitate and promote communication, relationship, learning, mobilisation, expression and organisation (physical, emotional, mental, social and cognitive) in order to develop potentials and develop or restore functions of the individual so that he or she can achieve better intra and/or interpersonal integration and, consequently, a better quality of life"* (Barcello 1996).

Rudd opines " it is understandable that music therapy, when it first established itself among other academic disciplines in the US in the fifties, had to depart from all kinds of meta-physical or idealistic types of theory in order to gain respect in the prevailing scientific community. However, in creating the science of music therapy, along with the *profession* of the music therapist, the question of the general role and value of music in everyday life seemed to be somewhat left out of focus. The concept of music as therapy won much scientific credibility but lost its historically important role as a field of knowledge seeking to utilize music as an important source of information about how to live and relate to the world."

MYRIAD MOODS & MUSIC

As I mentioned earlier, I wouldn't want to go too much into music therapy per say. In order to understand and know how music can help people in general we need to know the numerous moods that music can create and the relation between the mind, its moods and music. People have understood the significance of the mind and its influence on the individual from time immemorial. Even a perfectly normal human being can never stay in a balanced state of mind throughout his life. Every person, due to various factors has different moods-he may be very excited and happy at times and may also be stressed out and be depressed. The human mind is usually unstable. It has the tendency to keep swinging. It is always in search of the balance- a state of stability but often fails. Music loves to swing too. It loves to play with the mind. If the mind goes down, it could enlighten it, if its too excited, music could bring it down. Music gives scope for a person to express his emotions and feelings, at the same time can help him overcome the same and transcend his mood.

Talking of the various moods of the mind, the aesthetic emotions or Rasas and the responsive emotions or bhavas were well enumerated by Bharata in his Natyashastra (300BC-200AD), in the sixth chapter.

The following table shows the rasa-bhava, meanings of these terms and even colours assigned to these emotions as given in the treatise.

NavaRasa

RASA	STHAYI BHAVA	MEANING	COLOUR
Shringar (amorous)	Rati	Love	Pale Light Green
Hasya (Humorous)	Hasa	Mirth	White
Karuna (Pathetic)	Shoka	Sorrow	Grey
Raudra (Furious)	Krodh	Anger	Red
Veera (Valorous)	Utsaha	Enthusiasm	Pale Orange
Bhayanaka (Horrific)	Bhaya	Fear	Black
Bibhatsa (Repugnant)	Jugupsa	Disgust	Blue
Adbhuta (Wonderous)	Vismaya	Surprise	Yellow

The ninth Rasa, Shanta-Calm was added later on to the above eight by Abhinavagupta.

Let me give a brief introduction to the term 'Raga' which is extensively used in Indian music and which I would be using hereafter in this paper.

Brihaddeshi of Matanga (AD 500-800), provides a special chapter on Ragas. This treatise is considered to be an important landmark in the history of ragas, since it is here that the expression raga was used and defined for the first time in the sense it is understood to date. Although Bharata does not use the expression raga as defined by Matanga and his followers, Bharata's jatis provide the genus out of which ragas have evolved. Matanga defines raga as :

"Svara-varna-visesana dhvani-bhedena va punah.

Rajyate yena yah kaschit sa ragah sammatah satam."

(Brihaddeshi, v. 263)

It means, "that which colours the mind of the good through a specific svara (interval) and varna (melodic movement) or through a type of dhvani (sound) is known by the wise as raga."

Suvarnalata Rao, in her book 'Acoustical Perspective on Raga-Rasa Theory' states that G.S.Tembe in his article 'Raga and Rasa' supports the idea of notes (tones) bearing the latent power of producing an aesthetic effect. He insists that notes alone contribute to the rasa creation. He even attaches emotional attributes to different notes. For example, shadja = like a yogi beyond any attachment; antara gandhara = fresh and pleasant; suddha daivata = grief, pathos; kaisiski nishada = gentle, happy, affectionate and kakali nishada = piercing appeal. Using his hypothesizes he says that when suddha madyama is made to dominate a melody, it leads to a serene and sublime atmosphere. Example, Malkauns, Lalitha, Bageshri and Kedara.

She further gives a table which suggests that the assigning of emotional attributes is not only an Indian concept but was also suggested by Westerners.

Emotional attributes for musical notes

Notes (Indian)	Rasas attributed by Bharata	Notes (Western)	Emotional attributes suggested by Western musicians
Shadja	Vira, Roudra, Adbhuta	Do	Strong, firm
Rishabha	Vira, Roudra, Adbhuta	Re	Rousing, hopeful
Gandhara	Karuna	Mi	Steady, calm
Madhyama	Sringara, Hasya	Fa	Desolate, awe-inspiring
Panchama	Sringara, Hasya	So	Grand, bright
Daivata	Bibhatsa, Bhayanaka	La	Sad, weeping
Nishada	Karuna	Ti	Piercing, sensitive

Coming back to Navarasas and Ragas, according to Somanatha's *Raga Vibhoda, Kalyana* is presented in the portrait of a king. The textual and oral sources regarding rasa of this raga suggest that it has been predominating associated with the Sringara Rasa or amorous mood. However, expressions such as joyful, contended, bright, active, Bhakti etc. have also been linked with this raga. The findings of psycho-acoustical experiments conducted by B.C.Deva report rasas such as sringara, vira, raudra to be associated with raga *Yaman*.

One more interesting feature of North Indian music is the association of ragas to time of the day and seasons of the year. It is said that one can experience the same feeling of the day or night as specified by the musical manuscripts. For example, a tune in the raga *Ahir bhairav/Chakravakam*(in the South Indian music, hereafter Carnatic Music-CM), or *bhowli* (CM) gives the feeling of the pleasantness of the morning. Similarly, a tune in *Purvi* and *Yaman* give the effect of dusk and evening respectively. A very popular raga *Desh, Jaijaiwanthi,* and *Durga* are related to late evening; *Behag* and *Bageshree* to night and *Malkauns, Darabari kanada* and *Sahana* to mid night.

Many other ragas have been associated to different things and interestingly they do give the same feel; like raga *Pahadi* to mountains and *Malayamarutham* (CM) to the cool breeze of the mountains.

MUSIC AND QUALITY OF LIFE: A RELATIONSHIP

Let us now see how music can help a person maintain this quality of life, keeping in view the components given by Siri Næss.

1. ***Activity,*** [which contains the dimensions of engagement, energy, self-realisation and freedom]:

According to Leonard Meyer, a well known composer,critic and aesthetician of music, 'musical mood gestures' may be similar to 'behavioural mood gestures' since both, the emotional behaviour and music involve motions differentiated by the same qualities such as energy, directions, tension, continuity and so forth. Further, he adds, "because moods and sentiments attain their most precise articulation through vocal inflection, it is possible for music to imitate the sounds of emotional behaviour with same precision." However, he points out that since musically affective stimuli are obviously diferent from the referential stimuli of real life, there will always be a generic difference between musical affective experience and the experience of everyday life, and hence musical experience is unique.[Suvarnalata Rao, 2000]

Music is engaging, it has energy and can energize. Music has been a favourite pass-time of several people irrespective of their age, creed, race or region. Primitive man was also said to have used music by way of Drums and other instruments to celebrate, as well as to drive away all the strain after a hard day's work. It has been a source of solace, a means of rejuvenating and a celebration of victory and freedom.

For example, Raga *Mohana*, a five notes (Oudava) Raga which is also found in Chinese and Japanese music and other parts of the world, has been used in South Indian music(CM) to convey emotions of victory, happiness and is full of energy.

Example: 'Nannupalimpa ndachivachchitivo Naa Prananaadha' of Tyagaraja.

Other ragas like *Nata* and *Aarabhi* in which Tyagaraja had composed his famous Pancharatna Kritis are full of energy and are engaging.

It is true that 'an idle mind is a devil's workshop'. Even if you have nothing to do, you may not be relaxed or at ease. In such cases music helps as an activity in the sense that it keeps the mind occupied. Ghazals are thought provoking, but of course one needs to understand the language. Plain music, say a tune in a raga like *Malayamarutham* may give a feeling of wandering in the mountains. Symphonies of Bach, Sonatas of Mozart or even drum music can energize or soothe the mind depending on the state of mind of the listener. Self-realisation and freedom may be experienced when one listens to the devotional bhajans etc.

2. ***Good interpersonal relations*** [which are realised through friendship and intimate relations.]

Music can create a great bonding. I have come across people requesting me to sing some particular kritis in my concerts. Musicians are often asked to perform some numbers, which become favourites among some audiences. Why? It could perhaps be because they find a sense of belonging to those songs or they associate them to a thing, event or person.

Examples

An oft-requested kriti is 'Samajavara gamana' in Raga *Hindola* (CM). "Within Attraction", a number by Yanni is a piece which one would like to hear again and again. "Once Upon a Time" is another piece by the same composer that truly takes you into the past and reminds you of something very special and close to your heart.

The experience that one has while listening to some musical works is not describable. They take you to a distant place and time from where one would not like to return. They feed the listeners with a certain kind of intimacy which makes the listener feel wanted and loved.

As stated by Even Rudd, music provides a sense of belonging. One may associate his favourite songs with a person, place or thing. Listening to a particular tune may make him feel secured or he may relate it to an event in the past. Music has been proved to expel feelings of lonliness and isolation.

3. *Self-confidence* [which has to do with self-esteem and self-acceptance].

Music is one such tool which acts as a companion, friend and helps a person be alone yet not lonely. It helps a person introspect and find for himself his strengths thereby boosting sef-confidence. The process involved herein could either be by giving him a feeling of belonging, reminding him of the past or simply soothing and relaxing his stressed out and tense mind or it could also energize him if he is too timid and feels inferior to others.

The Overtures and Symphonies of Mozart, Bach, Vivaldi, Haydn et al offer a variety of moods. Ragas like *Begada, Aarabhi* etc show a certain amount of strength and confidence.

Example: In 'Gattiganu nannu' of Tyagaraja in *Begada,*the term 'Gattiga' – 'strong' or 'with strength' itself depicts the raga bhava of *Begada*.

Almost all of Dikshitar's kritis have a self-confidence of their own. They (all ragas) are treated so maturely by Dikshitar that even a kind of dull raga or ragas with low notes used by other composers to convey a feeling of sympathy, have been used by Dikshitar with dignity and are mostly used to describe or praise a Deity in a mature and dignified manner.

Example: *Subhapantuvarali* (*Todi* in Hindustani music-HM) is often heard on Television and Radio on the demise of some famous personality. However, interestingly, the same Raga has been used by Dikshitar, very beautifully to express his reverence to Lord Satyanarayana in his kriti 'Sri Satyanarayana Upasmahe nityam'.

Inferiority complex is developed in individuals with a low self-esteem and self-confidence. Music helps such individuals by taking them into a different plane of thought. All vital energies are recharged in the body by listening to a vibrant raga/ piece, which boosts up the self-confidence in the person.

4. ***A basic sense of happiness*** [which is maintained through emotional experiences, safety and joy]:

Almost all compositions of Indian Classical music are regarding 'God'- Addressing God, praising God, pleading with God or requesting Him etc. all of which have some relation to emotional experiences or joy. The bliss experienced by the saints in Classical music is at a much higher level of understanding.

Ragas like *Pantuvarali* (*Purva Dhanashree* in HM), *Purikalyani,* have much more to explain than words can. One has to experience it to understand what it means. A very soothing and peace loving raga which has been used several times to express devotion as well , is *Jaijaiwanthi*(HM). A very famous and a favourite song of the Father of our Nation, Mahatma Gandhi in this raga is 'Raghupati Raghava Rajaram Patita Pavana Sitaram' and a film song 'Mana Mohana bade jhute' is also based on this raga.

There surely is a large amount of unexplainable joy in music. On the normal plane, anyone listening to the FM Radio will agree that music gives joy. We might have all experienced a chill down the spine or goose pimples at some point of time while listening to music. If you have, you would have understood what I meant. The joy that music can create can be experienced better than described. Musicians would be full of such narrations to offer when we speak of the bliss that music can bestow.

CONCLUSION

Each one of us could be listening to music but, in today's world, deciding which music to listen to is of paramount importance too. Listening to the right form of music in a given situation can help a person experience and maintain his well-being. Choosing what will work for any individual is difficult, most will choose something they 'like' instead of what might be beneficial. In doing extensive research on what any given piece of music produces in the physiological response system many unexpected things were found. Many of the so-called Meditation and Relaxation recordings actually produced adverse EEG patterns, like Hard Rock and Heavy Metal does in some individuals. The surprising thing was many selections of Celtic, Native American as well as various music containing loud drums or flutes were extremely soothing. The most profound finding was, any music Performed Live and even at moderately loud volumes even if it was somewhat discordant had very a beneficial response. Whenever the proper sounds were experienced an amazing right/left brain hemisphere synchronization occurred. The normal voltage spiking pattern changed to a smooth sinusoidal waveform and the usual voltage differential equalized.

We often find people saying 'this music is good' or 'that music is boring', which I feel is not justifyable because music, like beauty, depends on the beholder, in this case the mood of the listener and what is good for one may not necessarily be to another's liking. Raghava Menon a noted musicologist, makes an interesting observation: "I believe that the nature of music therapy would depend not so much on the music, but on the person playing or producing the music". He avers that it is the nature of the *sadhana* (dedication) of the musician that would differentiate the quality of his music.

Many people also believe that any music you respond to *positively* will work for you, regardless of its content. Thus, even pop music might work for you. Dr. Chugh often asks his patients to select the tape they wish to listen to during a counseling session.

One important aspect to keep in mind is that the mood of the performer and the mood of the listener play a crucial role in producing results. A same raga performed by different people produce entirely different results among listeners. Thus, a piece of music could end up producing desirable, undesirable or even no mood at all! Interestingly, the same raga performed by the same person at different times could give different moods according to the mood of the performer.

Pieces of instrumental music be it Yanni, Kenny G, Vivaldi, Bach, Mozart, Bismillah Khan, Hari Prasad Chaurasia, Shiv Kumar

Sharma, Pt Ravi Shankaror vocalists like Pt Jasraj, Bhimsen Joshi, Parveen Sultana, Balamurali krishna or Yesudas can effect the mind of the listener to a large extent and soothe the body, mind and soul regardless of the audience. This innate power of music is what makes it a balm to soothe the human emotions.

I completely agree with Dr. Chugh and say "Music is manna for the soul". Music can help you better the quality of your life by integrating itself with your thoughts, moods and feelings. It is for you to extract what you want out of music because music can create, sustain or transcend the mood of the listener.

REFERENCES

Cook, Nicholas, (1998), *Music A Very Short Introduction*, Oxford University Press Inc., New York. p. 5.

Grout, Donald Jay & Palisca, Claude V., (1996), *A History of Western Music*, W.W.Norton & Company, New York. p. 369.

Madison, Guy, (2004), *Emotion and meaning in music*, http://www.psyk.uu.se/hemsidor/guy.madison/emomus.htm

Mount, Balfour M., (2004), *The Healing Power of Music*, http://www.scena.org/lsm/sm10-1/guerisseur-musique-en.htm

Music-therapy, (1998), http://www.holisticonline.com/stress/stress_music-therapy.htm

Rammohan, Gowri V.,(2006), *An Insight into the Lives and Works of the Musical Trinity Tyagaraja, Dikshitar and Syama Sastry*, Andhra University Press, Visakhapatnam.

Rao, H.P.Krishna, (1984), *The Psychology of Music*, Asian Educational Services, New Delhi. p. 18, 30.

Rao, Suvarnalata, (2000), *Acoustical Perspective on Raga-Rasa Theory*, Munshiram Manoharlal Publishers Pvt. Ltd., New Delhi. p. 3, 4, 7, 39-40, 46,62.

Ruud, Even (1998), *Music and the Quality of Life*, in Nordic Journal of Music Therapy, 6(2), pp. 86-97.

Sokhal, Sonali S., (1998), *Music: nourishment for the soul*, Life positive, http://www.lifepositive.com/body/new-age-therapies/music-therapy/music-therapeutic.asp

The Importance of Music, (2004), http://www.greenhill.org/facultyfolders/finearts/performance_hall/band/news%20stories/0405/walsh%20essay.htm

11

Prenatal Stress Among Pregnant Woman

C. Mohana Sundari*, T. Mohan**, B. Prasad Babu***

ABSTRACT

The present study was conducted to assess the prenatal stress among pregnant women. The study was conducted on a sample of 50 pregnant women at Southern Railway Hospital, Chennai. They were administered Allen Cameron's Stress assessment questionnaire. The study indicates that there is no significant difference in the level of stress among pregnant women irrespective of their age and also the results shows that there is a significant difference in the level of stress among the pregnant women irrespective of their number of pregnancies.

INTRODUCTION

Science and Technology bring improvement in the quality of human life in many ways, it also resulted in many new crises. Crowding, noise pollution, competition, social insecurity, unemployment, violence, loneliness etc., are all accompaniments of modern living. Stress is an integral part of our lives. While stress is

* Counsellor, Integrated Counselling and Testing Centre, Southern Railway Hospital, Chennai – 600 001.

** Psychologist, Government of India, Ministry of Labour, Vocational Rehabilitation Centre for Handicapped, Puducherry – 605 007.

*** Rehabilitation Counsellor, Government of India, Ministry of Labour, Rural Rehabilitation Extension Centre for Handicapped, Thiruvallur – 602 001.

considered a major cause of mental and physical health problems, its effect is not always undesirable. In fact, stress is a basic ingredient of life.

Today, people are living longer and healthier lives than ever before. In contrast to the diseases that were prevalent in the early 1900's, the most common causes of death and illness today are strongly related to the behaviors in which a person chooses to engage. Unhealthy behaviors, from smoking and poor diet, to sedentary lifestyle and poor coping skills, are all major contributors to illness. Fortunately, we can learn ways to control negative thoughts and the behaviors in which we choose to engage. By learning specific skills, we can make positive, healthy changes in our lives.

Stress is a common problem in modern life, but extreme levels of stress can cause fatigue, irritability, burnout and even illness. Health psychology attempts to define, measure and treat stress.

Stress in Psychology is used in at least two different ways. First it is defined as the state of Psychological upset or disequilibrium in the human beings caused by frustrations, conflicts and other internal as well as external strains and pressures. In a more serious condition of the stress, the individual reaches a point where the Physical processes are seriously affected and mental processes are confused, and the emotional state is chaotic.

Stress can be described as the pattern or response an organism makes to stimulus event that disturbs the equilibrium and exceeds a person's ability to cope. The stimulus events include a large variety of external and internal conditions called stressors if they are perceived to threaten one's well-bring and demand some kind of adaptive response.

During stress, women tend to care for their children and find support from their female friends. Women's bodies make chemicals that are believed to promote these responses. One of these chemicals is oxytocin, which has a calming effect during stress. This is the same chemical released during childbirth and found at higher levels in breastfeeding mothers, who are believed to be calmer and more social than women who don't breastfeed. Women also have the hormone estrogen, which boosts the effects of oxytocin. Men, however, have high levels of testosterone during stress, which blocks the calming effects of oxytocin and causes hostility, withdrawal, and anger.

According to Selye (1956), "any external event or internal drive which threatens to upset the orgasmic equilibrium" is stress. He has defined stress as the non-specific response of the body to any demand made upon it.

METHODOLOGY

The present study was conducted to examine the prenatal stress among pregnant women. The study was intentionally done on pregnant women since the follow up of clients to the hospital is encouraging. Earlier studies have indicated that the pregnant women had stress and anxiety about their pregnancy and prenatal development of child.

Aim

The aims of the present study are following:

1. To study the stress level of pregnant women belonging to different age groups.
2. To study the stress level of the first, second and third pregnancy in a pregnant women.

Hypothesis

1. There will not be significant difference among the stress levels of pregnant women belonging to different age groups.
2. There would be significant difference among the stress levels of pregnant women on the basis of number of pregnancies.

Sample

The study was conducted on a sample of 50 pregnant women at the Southern Railway Hospital, Perambur, Chennai. The sample included those who had undergone pregnancy testing and were confirmed and those who referred to counseling and HIV testing. The investigator approached Chief Medical Officer and explained about the study and got permission. Then the investigator approached these pregnant women and requested them to participate in this study. The patients were made to feel at ease and an initial rapport was established. The questionnaire was given to pregnant women and they were asked to fill them as per the instructions.

Scale

Stress Assessment Questionnaire (SAQ)

The Stress Assessment Questionnaire (SAQ) was developed by Allen Cameron's aims to help people recognize and manage stress in their daily lives. The SAQ assesses seventeen dimensions of stress covering possible Sources, common symptoms, coping style, personality factors and the impact on mental health. The SAQ is designed for the counselee to understand the things that may be coping stress in their life and how they respond to pressure and stress. There are 128 questions and it should take her about 30 -35 minutes to complete.

Data Analysis

The data obtained from the sample of 50 pregnant women was scored and analyzed. The analysis involved Mean, Standard Deviation and the application of t-tests, analysis of variance.

RESULTS AND DISSCISSION

Table 1

The table shows the stress level among the pregnant women at different age groups

Sl. No.	*Group*	*Mean*	*SD*	*F-value*
1.	Up to 25 years	400.18	39.42	
2.	Between 25 and 30 years	387.31	37.21	1.85
3.	Above 30 years	415.83	50.97	

AGE GROUPS

The Table 1 indicates that there is no significant difference in the level of stress among pregnant women irrespective of their age. In the age group of below 25 years, the reason may be their lack of mental maturity and fear of labour pain. In the second age group of 25 to 30 years of age, though they are physically and mentally mature the fears and in some cases lack of social support can increase their stress in pregnancy. In the above 30 years of age group, the chances of complicated pregnancy are more compare to younger age group.

Table 2

The table shows that the stress level among first, second and third time pregnant women

Sl. No	*Group*	*Mean*	*SD*	*F-value/ t-value*
1.	1st pregnancy 2nd pregnancy 3rd pregnancy	389.40 393.68 443.00	40.70 39.70 25.86	5.45*
2.	1st pregnancy 2nd pregnancy	389.40 393.68	40.70 39.70	0.33
3.	2nd pregnancy 3rd pregnancy	393.68 443.00	39.70 25.86	3.53*
4.	1st pregnancy 3rd pregnancy	389.40 443.00	40.70 25.86	4.27*

Note: *p= 0.01.

NUMBER OF PREGNANCY

The table 2 indicates that there is a significant difference in the level of stress among the pregnant women irrespective of number of pregnancies. There is no significant difference in the level of stress between the pregnant women having 1st and 2nd pregnancies. The reason for the stress in the 1st pregnancy may be due to the anxiety for the condition 'pregnancy' and lack of knowledge and experience about it. Same way, in 2nd pregnancy, though they know the process yet the syndrome occurring during the pregnancy period and the outcome of labour make them develop stress.

The above table indicates that there is significant difference in the level of stress between the women having 2nd and 3rd pregnancies. In this table the 'mean' shows that the women having 2nd pregnancy are also having much stress, but 3rd time pregnant women are more stressed. The reason could be that now-a- days the third baby increases the pressure on the women's health as well as on the family's finances.

The result shows that there is significant difference in the level of stress between the women having 1st and 3rd pregnancies. The reason could be that in first pregnancy, despite all the stressful factors, enthusiasm is there for the first baby. But in the third pregnancy it somehow feels like a burden. Which she has to carry, in most of the cases, either unwanted pregnancy or for a 'boy' baby.

CONCLUSIONS

In the age group of below 25 years, the reason may be their lack of mental maturity and fear of labour pain. In the second age group of 25 to 30 years of age, though they are physically and mentally mature, the fears and in some cases lack of social support can increase their stress in pregnancy. In the above 30 years of age group, the chances of complicated pregnancy are more compare to younger age group.

The reason for the stress in the 1st pregnancy may be due to the anxiety for the condition 'pregnancy' and lack of knowledge and experience about it. Same way ,in 2nd pregnancy, though they know the process yet the syndrome occurring during the pregnancy period and the outcome of labour make them develop stress. 3rd time pregnant women are more stressed. The reason could be that now-a- days the third baby increases the pressure on the women's health as well as on the family's finances.

REFERENCES

Allan Cameraon (2002) Professional manual of stress assessment questionnaire. *The test Agency*, UK.

Dunkel Schetter, C. (1998) Maternal stress and preterm delivery . *Prenatal and Neonatal Medicine,* 3 , 39-42.

Forde. R. (1992) Pregnant women's ailments and psychosocial conditions. *Family Practitioner*. 9(3) 270-3.

Geogas.J., Giakoumaki.E., (1984). Psychological stress and its relation to obstetrical complications. *Psychotherapy psychosomatic* 41(4) 200-206.

Joffee, H. (1989) Emotional factors in pregnancy. *Australian family physician* 18(5)493: 496-7.

Vimala, T.D., Prasad Babu, B. & Bhaskara Rao, D. (2007). Stress, Coping and Management. *Sonali Publications,* New Delhi.

12

Self-Esteem and Self-Efficacy in Dual Earner Couples with an Information Technology Professional Spouse

Sangeetha M*, Sheela. J**

ABSTRACT

The study aims at assessing the Self-esteem and Self-efficacy and to investigate whether there is a relationship between Self-esteem and Self-efficacy in dual earner couples with an Information Technology Professional spouse. An ex post facto survey research was adopted for the present study. The sample size for the study was 40 (N=40), of whom 25 were professionals in the field of Information Technology with a Non Information Technology professional for a spouse and 15 were Non Information Technology professionals with an Information Technology professional for a spouse. The method of purposive sampling was used for the selection of sample. The Rosenberg Self-Esteem Scale (1962) and The General Self-Efficacy Scale (GSE)-English version (Matthias Jerusalem & Ralf Schwarzer 1981) were the tools used for the study. The t-test and Pearson's product moment correlation were the statistical techniques used for data analysis. The results revealed that there is a significant difference in self-esteem between dual

* **Sangeetha Makesh Research Student. Department of Psychology Women's Christian College, Chennai.**

** **Sheela Julius Reader & Head, Department of Psychology Women's Christian College, Chennai.**

earner Information Technology and Non Information Technology professionals. However there was no difference with regard to Self Efficacy. There is no significant relationship between self-esteem and self efficacy in dual earner Information Technology professionals and Non Information Technology professionals.

In today's world there seems to be an increase in dual earner couples. In dual career couples, both husbands and wives struggle to balance the demands of work and family and both report that work commitments often interfere with family responsibilities (Hochschild 1997, Milkie and Peltola 1999). When pressures increase at work, husbands and wives report more role conflicts and often feel overwhelmed by their multiple commitments (Crouter et al 1999). Spouses' stress at work can have a substantial negative effect on their marital interactions (Perry Jenkins, Repetti and Crouter 2001). This is more so for the Information Technology Professionals who have reported exhaustion predominantly due to work overload (Moore 2000).

Research has shown that self-esteem can be regarded as a variable that holds an important status in stress management. The National Association of Self-Esteem (NASE) defines self esteem as "the experience of being capable of meeting life's challenges and being worthy of happiness". According to Joubert (1990) self esteem can be defined as a "person's judgement of general self-worth that is a product of an implicit evaluation of self approval or self disapproval made by the individual". High self-esteem contributes to an overall sense of psychological well-being, mainly because high self-esteem seems to be linked to feelings of optimism and of being able to exert some control over events. It is also linked to being able to face difficulties and set backs in life, whereas low self-esteem seems to be linked to pessimism and lowered expectations. Self-efficacy is an important psychological variable in stress tolerance and adjustment. The construct of Perceived Self-efficacy reflects an optimistic self-belief. Perceived Self-efficacy facilitates goal setting, effort investment, persistence in the face of barriers and recovery from setbacks (Bandura 1990), receptiveness to technological training (Christoph, Schonfeld and Tansky 1998) and is related to positive responses to stress (Bandura 1997). It can be regarded as a positive resistance resource factor.

Operational Definitions

Self-esteem is "the evaluation which the individual makes and customarily maintains with regard to himself expressed as an attitude of approval or disapproval". Rosenberg (1979). Self efficacy is "the belief that one can perform a novel or difficult task or cope with adversity in various domains of human functioning". Schwarzer (1992)

OBJECTIVES

1. To explore self-esteem and self-efficacy in dual earner couples with an information technology professional spouse.
2. To find the relationship between self-esteem and self-efficacy in dual earner couples with an information technology professional spouse.

HYPOTHESES

1. There will be no significant difference in self-esteem between dual earner Information Technology and Non Information Technology professionals.
2. There will be no significant difference in self-efficacy among between dual earner Information Technology and Non Information Technology professionals.
3. There will be a significant relationship between self-esteem and self-efficacy in dual earner Information Technology professionals.
4. There will be a significant relationship between self-esteem and self-efficacy in dual earner Non Information Technology professionals.

METHODOLOGY

An ex post facto survey research was adopted for the present study.

Sample

The method of purposive sampling was used for the selection of sample. The sample consisted of dual earner couples, one of whom (either the husband or the wife) was a professional in the field of Information Technology. The couples who took part in the study were essentially living together. The sample size for the study was 40 (N=40), of whom 25 were professionals in the field of Information Technology with a Non Information Technology professional for a spouse and 15 were Non Information Technology professionals with an Information Technology professional for a spouse.

Tools

1. The Rosenberg Self-Esteem Scale (1962)

This scale was developed by Morris Rosenberg. The scale has 10 items, each with 4 response categories namely, Strongly Agree, Agree, Strongly Disagree and Disagree.

There is no time limit for completing the scale. Items 1, 3, 4, 7, 8 and 10 get a negative scoring of 4, 3, 2 and 1. Items 2, 5, 6 and 9 get a direct scoring of 1, 2, 3 and 4. The score ranges from a minimum of 10 to a maximum of 40. Higher the score, higher the self-esteem.

Reliability

The test-retest reliability of the scale is .88.

2. The General Self-Efficacy Scale (GSE)-English version (Matthias Jerusalem & Ralf Schwarzer 1981)

The scale was first developed in 1979 by Matthias Jerusalem and Ralf Schwarzer in German. Later in 1981, owing to its need in various psychological studies, the scale was revised by the same authors with the help of the regional co-authors and adapted in 26 languages including English. The scale was created to assess general sense of perceived self-efficacy with the aim in mind to predict coping with daily hassles as well as adaptation after experiencing all kinds of stressful life events. It is designed for the general adult population. The scale has 10 items, each with 4 response categories namely, Not at all True, Hardly True, Moderately True and Exactly True. It takes 4 minutes on average to answer this questionnaire. The response Not at all True gets a score of 1, Hardly True gets a score of 2, Moderately True gets a score of 3 and Exactly True gets a score of 4. The score ranges from a minimum of 10 to a maximum of 40. Higher the score, greater the self-efficacy.

Reliability and Validity

Cronbach alpha coefficient ranges from .76 to .90. . Criterion related validity is established for the scale.

Procedure

The Rosenberg Self-Esteem Scale (1962) and The General Self-Efficacy Scale (GSE) which had the standardized instructions printed on them were administered to the sample in their work places. The data collected was statistically analyzed using t-test and Pearson's product-moment correlation.

RESULTS

Table 1 shows the mean, standard deviation, t-value and the level of significance for Self-esteem between dual earner Information Technology and Non-Information Technology professionals

SELF-ESTEEM

Sample	*N*	*Mean*	*S.D*	*t*	*Level of significance*
IT Professionals	25	35	1.8	3.52	P<0.01
Non IT Professionals	15	29.93	3.24		

P<0.01 Significant at 0.01 level.

Table 1 shows that there is a significant difference in self-esteem between dual earner Information Technology and Non-Information Technology professionals. Hence, *Hypothesis no 1* which states that *"There will be no significant difference in self-esteem between dual earner Information Technology and Non Information Technology professionals"* is *rejected*. The mean shows that the Information Technology professionals have a higher self-esteem than the Non Information Technology professionals. The field of Information Technology is one of the fastest growing areas within the Indian economy and perpetually creates new challenges and new opportunities. A high degree of technical knowledge is required to be a part of the Information Technology profession. They will have to work as part of a team and carry on managerial functions.and so, it is logical that they score high on their self-esteem. High self-esteem contributes to an overall sense of psychological well-being, mainly because high self-esteem seems to be linked to feelings of optimism and of being able to exert some control over events. It is also linked to being able to face difficulties and set backs in life. According to Tesser (2000), "self esteem is a global evaluation reflecting our view of our accomplishments and capabilities, our values, our bodies, other's responses to us, and events, or occasions, our possessions". A high self esteem goes to show that Information Technology professionals have a positive evaluation of their accomplishments and capabilities, values, bodies, other's responses, events or occasions, and possessions.

Table 2 shows the mean, standard deviation, t-value and the level of significance for Self-efficacy between dual earner Information Technology and Non-Information Technology professionals

SELF-EFFICACY

Sample	*N*	*Mean*	*S.D*	*t*	*Level of significance*
IT Professionals	25	34.32	4.36	0.017	NS
Non IT Professionals	15	31	3.38		

NS- Not Significant.

Table 2 shows that there is no significant difference in self efficacy between dual earner Information Technology and Non-Information Technology professionals. Hence, *Hypothesis no* 2 which states that *"There will be no significant difference in self efficacy between dual earner Information Technology and Non Information Technology professionals"* is *accepted*. Perceived Self-efficacy affects how well individuals manage requirements and challenges of occupational pursuits (Bandura 2005). It also facilitates goal setting, effort investment, persistence in the face of barriers and recovery from setbacks (Bandura 1990). In the present competitive world, both Information Technology and Non Information Technology professionals are likely to show the same commitment and involvement at work. They need to show a lot of dedication at work if they desire for career advancement. From a family front, irrespective of the profession, dual earner families face a lot of stress and self-efficacy becomes a requirement that helps to handle stressful situations by enhancing better coping skills. Self efficacy enhances confidence in their potential to meet challenges and to have a higher degree of sense of control which leads to better well-being (Wenzel 1993). Both the Information Technology and Non Information Technology professionals do not show a difference in their self-esteem because although their professions are different the demands placed on them from their profession and family remains the same.

Table 3 shows the significance of correlation between Self-esteem and Self-efficacy between dual earner Information Technology professionals and Non Information Technology professionals

RELATIONSHIP BETWEEN SELF ESTEEM AND SELF EFFICACY

Sample	*N*	*r*	*Level of Significance*
IT Professionals	25	0.02	1.20 (NS)
Non IT Professionals	15	0.41	

NS- Not Significant.

Table 3 shows that there is no significant relationship between self esteem and self- efficacy both in dual earner Information Technology and Non-Information Technology professionals. Hence, *Hypothesis nos 3 and 4* which state that *"There will be a significant relationship between self esteem and self efficacy between dual earner Information Technology and Non Information Technology professionals"* is *rejected.*

Self esteem is the sense of value or worthiness individuals attach to themselves. From this sense of worthiness will be born the conviction that they can perform even a difficult task. In fact, self - esteem forms the basis of self efficacy. However, the present study does not show a significant relationship. The reason for an insignificant relationship between self esteem and self efficacy in dual earner Information Technology professionals in spite of them showing high self esteem could be because even when the self-esteem is high, their belief about their competency might still stand questionable for them.. For both dual earner Information Technology professionals and Non Information Technology professionals though there can be self efficacy, a person's sense of worthiness is not associated only with the belief in competency and hence it need not be related to self esteem. The study further shows that in both dual earner Information Technology professionals and Non Information Technology professionals there is no significant difference in relationship between self esteem and self efficacy.

SUMMARY

A study was done to assess the Self-esteem and Self-efficacy and to investigate whether there is a relationship between Self-esteem and Self-efficacy in dual earner couples with an Information Technology Professional spouse among 25 professionals in the field of Information Technology with a Non Information Technology professional for a spouse and 15 were Non Information Technology professionals with an Information Technology professional for a spouse using The Rosenberg Self-Esteem Scale (1962) and The General Self-Efficacy Scale (GSE)-English version (Matthias Jerusalem & Ralf Schwarzer 1981). The t-test and Pearson's product moment correlation were the statistical techniques used for data analysis. The results revealed that there is a significant difference in self-esteem between dual earner Information Technology and Non Information Technology professionals. However there was no difference with regard to Self Efficacy. There is no significant relationship between self-esteem and self efficacy in dual earner Information Technology professionals and Non Information Technology professionals.

CONCLUSION

The findings of the present study show that there is a significant difference in self-esteem between dual earner Information Technology and Non Information Technology professionals with the Information Technology professionals showing greater self-esteem. This is a positive note both in terms of their career advancement and personal life especially when they are dual earner couples. Self esteem enhancement training programmes can be suggested for the Non Information Technology professionals. A noteworthy finding is that there is no significant difference in self-efficacy between dual earner Information Technology and Non Information Technology professionals. This only goes to show that irrespective of the profession, the demands placed on individuals both from the professional and family front remains the same and hence for both the groups self efficacy becomes a requirement for progress. There is no significant relationship between self-esteem and self efficacy in dual earner Information Technology professionals and Non Information Technology professionals. This finding is contrary to the research (Azar and Vasudeva 2006) which shows a strong relationship between these two variables.

REFERENCES

Azar, I.A.S, and Vasudeva, P. (2006). Self esteem and Self-efficacy: A comparative study of employed and unemployed married women in Iran. Iran journal of psychiatry, 1, 104-111.

Bandura, A.(1997). Self efficacy: The exercise of control. New York, Freeman.

Bandura, A. (2005). Self efficacy: The exercise of control: an outline composed by Geo Valiant. Emory University, Communications of the International Information Management Association, 3:1.

Christoph, Richard T, Schoenfeld, Gerald A., Jr., Tansky, Judith W. (1998). Overcoming Barriers to Training Utilizing Technology: The Influence of Self-Efficacy Factors on Multimedia-Based Training Receptiveness. Human Resource Development Quarterly, v9 n1, p. 25-38, Springer.

Crouter, A.C., Bumpus, M.F., Maguire M.C., and McHale, S.M. (1999). Linking parents' work pressure and adolescents' well-being: Insights into dynamics in dual earner families. Developmental Psychology, 35 (6), 1453-1461.

Hochschild, A.R.(1997). The Time-bind: When work becomes home and home becomes work. New York, Holt.

Joubert, C.E. (1990). Relationship among self esteem, psychological reactance and other personality variables. Psychological reports, 66, 1147-1151.

Matthias Jerusalem & Ralf Schwarzer. (1981). The General Self-Efficacy Scale (GSE)-English version. web.fu-berlin.de/.../Turkish/General_Perceived_Self-Efficac/hauptteil_general_perceived_self-efficac.htm

Milkie, M.A., and Peltola, P. (1999). Playing all the roles: Gender and the work-family balancing act. Journal of marriage and the family, 61, 476-490.

Moore, J. (2000). One Road to Turnover: An Examination of Work Exhaustion in Technology Professionals. Management Information Systems Quarterly, Vol. 24, No. 1 pp. 141-168.

Perry-Jenkins, M., Repetti,R.L., and Crouter, A.C. (2001). Work and family in the 1990s: In R.M. Milardo (9Ed), Understanding families into the new millineum: A decade in review (pp.200-217). Minneapolis, MN, National Council on Family Relations.

Rosenberg. (1962). Manual of the Rosenberg Self-Esteem Scale: www.bsos.umd.edu/socy/Research/rosenberg.htm

Tesser, A. (2000). The Encyclopedia of Psychology Behaviour of Science. 3,213-216, Iran journal of psychiatry, 1, 104-111.

Wenzel, SL. (1993). The relationship of psychological resources and social support to job procurement self efficacy in the disadvantaged: Journal of Applied Psychology, 23(18), 1471-1497.

13

Stress and Coping Among Parents of Children with Hearing Impairment

A Socio-economic Approach

Nalluri Krishna Murthy*

ABSTRACT

The objective of the present study was to examine the influence of socioeconomic factors on stress, coping and depression among parents of children with hearing impairment. Data was collected on 150 parents (age range 18-42 yrs, mean age was 27.28 yrs.) of children with hearing impairment. Results show that mothers with lower education and family income having children with hearing impairment reported significantly high stress on domains such as acceptability about the disabled child, more demanding work, more difficulties with their sense of competence, more efforts put into relationship with their spouse, isolation, more depression, than mothers with high education and family income having children with hearing impairment. Depression was significantly high in lower maternal education and family income group than high maternal education and family income group. The results of this study suggest early intervention programs, preschool education, family therapy and counseling for parents of children with hearing impairment to reduce maternal stress and depression.

* **Psychologist, Ali Yavar Jung National Institute for the Hearing Handicapped, Southern Regional Centre, (Ministry of Social, Justice and Empowerment, Govt. of India), Manovikas Nagar, Secunderabad.**

Deafness in childhood has devastating effects. It is a hidden disability, which often remains unnoticed for an unreasonably long time. Children with congenital deafness are handicapped in many ways. The most obvious handicap is seen in the development of speech and language.

THE MAGNITUDE OF THE PROBLEM

The NSSO (National Sample Survey Organisation) reports indicate that there are over 3 lakhs children in India suffering from deafness, in the age range of 0-4 years. A Multi Centric Study by ICMR (Indian Council of Medical Research)-1983 reported that 1out of 1000 children born in India was deaf.

As a part of rearing a child with a hearing impairment, the added tasks that a caretaker may have to perform can lead to an increase in stress, irritability, depression, anxiety, aggression and all types of abuse, all of which are signs of mismanaged stress. These emotions and behaviors can have a dramatic impact on the family.

According to Hintermair and Horsch (1998), a hearing impairment is a stress factor for the entire family. The results of hearing loss with disturbed or delayed speech and communication development influence the other family members and the entire family system. Constant confrontation with the disability may arouse in family members and other involved persons such feelings as grief, disappointment, helplessness, and aggression (Wunsch & Bengel, 1998).

Obtaining a better understanding of factors that influence this form of stress in hearing mothers of children with hearing loss is critical because parental stress has been linked to negative parent and child outcomes. Early childhood deafness is a significant medical problem that alters the educational and psychological development of the child and has major implications for family adjustment (Greenberg, 1980; Meadow, 1980; Moores, 1987). Research has consistently shown that deaf children are at greater risk for behavioral and emotional disturbances, language delays, and more frequent hospitalizations than children with normal hearing (Freeman, 1979).

Raising a deaf child, parents are faced with a number of chronic stresses. These include frequent visits to speech therapists, controversies about oral versus manual communication, and decisions about educational placement. Mothers, in particular, are frequently asked to assume the dual role of parent and language teacher, spending an average of two hours per day on language training from age two through twelve (Schlesinger & Meadow, 1972). These chronic stresses may substantially drain parents' energy, time, and financial resources, potentially leading to emotional reactions of frustration, depression, and social isolation (Meadow, 1980).

If marriage and family bonds are strong, they do help the parents of children with disabilities to cope. If this kind of support system-for whatever reason-does not exist, or does not properly function, it is, for obvious reasons, considered to be negative. In this case, support systems outside the family become effective and are felt to be more helpful (Brand & Coetzer, 1994; Segal, 1985). In essence, most of the studies stress the importance to successful coping of both a well-functioning family system and good relationships with non-family members (Bradley, Rock, Whiteside, Caldwell & Brisby 1991; Morgan-Redshaw, Wilgosh, & Bibby, 1990; Wyngaarden Krauss, 1993).

Finally, separate from the characteristics of the child and his or her hearing loss, some characteristics and perceptions of the mother may influence parental stress. For example, previous research with hearing children has found that increased stress is related to lower levels of maternal education (Deater-Deckard & Scarr, 1996; Singer, Song, Hill, & Jaffe, 1990) and decreased income (Deater-Deckard & Scarr, 1996; Pianta & Egeland, 1990). Generally, it has been found that resources, in terms of income and education, may act as mediating factors in stress reactions of individuals (Palfrey, Walker, Butler, & Singer, 1989).

Limited work has been done in examining how socioeconomic status (education and family income) may have a negative impact on parents having children with hearing impairment, particularly with reference to stress and depression. Brand and Coetzer (1994) found that parents with more education reported less stress than those with less education. Chen and Rubin(1994) reported that parents with less education and less monthly family income are more likely find parenting stressful.

Gowen et al. (1989), examined maternal depression and feelings of parenting competence longitudinally among mothers of handicapped and non-handicapped infants, and who were assessed multiple times during infancy. Despite notable differences in the care giving needs of the two groups of infants, there were no significant differences in feelings of depression or parenting competence between their mothers. Further, between both groups of mothers, about half evidenced clinically significant depressive symptoms at least once in the series of assessment points. These findings suggest a waxing and waning pattern of maternal depression in response to the challenge of having an infant (with or without disabilities). In contrast, feelings of parenting competence and quality of family relationships were stable over time in both groups.

A few important points need to be considered with regard to studies done in this area. First, early childhood deafness is a significant medical problem that has major implications for parenting and family adjustment across the life span (Meadow, 1980). Parents are faced with a number of stressors, including frequent visits to speech therapists, controversies about oral versus manual communication, and decisions about educational placement (Moores, 1987).

Second, Prelingual deafness among children of normally hearing parents is a condition that is randomly distributed across the population (Brown, 1986). There is little reason to believe that the incidence of childhood deafness will be higher among parents with particular demographic characteristics (e.g., lower income), who may also be vulnerable to stressful life events or psychopathology (Thoits, 1982b). Thus, a confounding of parental stress with predisposing factors such as low income has been precluded in the present study. Finally, the chronic, inescapable nature of deafness may result in less biased estimates of stress effects because parents can neither select themselves *into* or *out of* the stressful situation. These sampling factors pose distinct advantages for untangling causal associations between the stressor and outcome variable (Kessler, 1987).

OBJECTIVES

The main objective of the present study was to examine the influence of socioeconomic factors (education and family income) on levels of stress, coping and depression in parents having children with hearing impairment.

The hypotheses for this study are as follows:

1. Mothers of children with hearing impairment and higher levels of education will have lower levels of stress and depression than mothers with hearing impaired children but with lower levels of education.
2. Mothers of children with hearing impairment and of higher levels of income will have lower levels of stress and depression than mothers of children with hearing impairment but with lower incomes.

METHODOLOGY

Sample

The sample consisted of 150 mothers (age range is 18-42 years) of hearing impaired children aged 1 to 5 years. Criteria for inclusion in the hearing impaired children were severe or profound hearing loss (defined as a loss of 70 db or greater across the speaking range) and no other physical disabilities. The hearing impaired children were in the age range of 14 to 60 months (M= 43.79 months, SD= 13.60 months). On an average the children were identified with hearing loss at 19.57 months (SD=10.10). Mean age at intervention for hearing loss was 29.08 months (SD=13.34 months). There was almost equal sex representation with 64 (53.3%) children was male and 56 (46.7%) children were female.

Mothers were identified in Audiology section and preschool at Southern Regional Centre, Ali Yavar Jung National Institute for the Hearing Handicapped, Secunderabad, different preschools and hospitals from Secunderabad and Hyderabad in Andhra Pradesh, India. Mothers mean age was 27.28 years (SD=4.07) and family income between Rs.800/-pm to Rs. 60000/-pm. Their average income is Rs.7417/-pm (SD= Rs. 7417/-). A majority of mothers were up to tenth class education.

INSTRUMENTS

The following test materials were used to assess stress, coping and depression. All the scales were translated from English to the regional language, namely Telugu in order to facilitate the subjects to comprehend the items easily. A description of the scales employed is as follows:

Parental Stress Index (PSI) (Abidin, 1995)

The Parental stress index is a 120-item clinical and research questionnaire designed to identify sources of stress in parent child subsystems. The PSI yields stress score in three domains: child domain, parent domain, and life stress. In the child characteristics domain, sub scales measured are child-related stressors such as child's adaptability (adaptability), acceptability of child to the mother (acceptability), demandedness, moodiness, and distractibility (demanding, child mood, and Distractibility-Hyperactivity) and degree to which the mother found the child reinforcing (Reinforces parent). In the parent characteristics domain, sub scales measured are parent attachment to the child (attachment), restrictions imposed by the parental role (Restriction of role), depression, social isolation, relationship with spouse/parenting partner, parental health and parent's evaluation of their competence (sense of competence). Finally, the life stress scale assessed the occurrence of 19 stressful life events over the previous 12 months, weighted for their potential impact. Eleven of the 19 life events are negative (e.g., death of the family member). The PSI demonstrated acceptable internal consistency, with alpha values ranging from.60 to .95, and adequate test-retest reliability ranging from .70 to .90 for a 3 to 4 week interval.

The Norbeck Social Support Questionnaire (NSSQ; Norbeck, Lindsey & Carrieri, 1995): The NSSQ is a self-administered measure rating extent of perceived emotional support (e.g., Affect, Affirmation, and Aid (tangible support)) and network structure (i.e., size and frequency of contact). In an interview format, the respondent is asked to generate a list of significant others in his or her life (network size) and then to answer a series of structured questions that allow for measurement for the parent's satisfaction with each person nominated. The NSSQ may be scored to obtain information on the sources of support and the relative contributions of friends, family members, and health care professionals to perceptions of support. Internal consistency estimates have ranged from .69 to .98. The test-retest reliabilities of .85 to .92 have been reported.

Family Support Scale (Dunst, Jenkins, & Trivette, 1984) consists of 18 sources of family support, including parents, friends, spouse, co-workers, church/temple, professional agencies, and so on. Parents are also invited to rate others if source of support is not included in the questionnaire. Parents rated whether each source of support was available, and, if available, whether the source was not at all helpful to extremely helpful on a scale of 0 to 4. The final score was obtained by adding together the ratings on each of the items.

Centre for Epidemiological Studies Depression Scale (CES-D; Radloff, 1977). The CES-D is a 20- item scale designed to measure current levels of depressive symptoms and mood in the general population. Several field studies have reported internal consistency coefficients of .84 to .90, and there is evidence of the CES-D's convergence with other measures of depression.

Procedure: Following an initial screening, prospective subjects were notified for the project by a letter mailed to the local schools and hospital. They were requested to participate in the research program by furnishing required information as given in the questionnaire. After taking their oral consent, a structured interview was conducted in which demographic information as well as ratings of child-rearing and disability specific stress was collected from mothers. Several standardized questionnaires were also filled in by the mothers to assess the following variables: parenting stress, coping and depression. Questionnaires that were not completed by the subjects were discarede.

RESULTS

Data was analyzed with the help of 't ' test to find the differences between the high and low level socioeconomic levels among parents of children with hearing impairment in terms of stress, coping, and depression.

The mothers were divided into 2 groups based on their education levels.

1. *Low education level:* This sample belong to the group of mothers who had education level up to tenth class; and
2. *Higher education group:* This sample consisted of mothers who had college/graduate level education.

Table 1

Comparison of stress between education levels for mothers of children with hearing impairment

Variable	*Lower level education(n=89)*		*Higher level education(n=61)*		*T*
	Mean	*SD*	*Mean*	*SD*	
Child Domain	135.95	18.56	125.13	18.65***	
Adaptability(AD)	32.42	6.35	30.37	6.35	1.94
Acceptability(AC)	19.84	4.84	17.24	4.67	3.29***
Demandingness(DE)	26.20	5.10	23.55	5.29	3.05***
Mood(MO)	13.69	3.56	11.59	3.67	3.49***
Distractability/ Hyperactivity(DI)	28.79	4.46	28.95	4.37	-.21
Reinforces Parent(RE)	14.98	3.85	13.40	3.04	2.80**
Parent Domain	154.26	25.91	140.16	24.72	3.37***
Depression(DP)	27.38	6.17	24.32	5.46	3.19**
Attachment(AT)	16.96	4.36	16.01	3.83	1.37
Role Restriction(RO)	21.28	5.59	20.62	5.52	.71
Competence(CO)	39.48	5.54	35.16	6.39	4.28***
Isolation(IS)	15.93	4.95	14.06	4.04	2.53*
Spouse(SP)	19.22	5.94	16.59	5.18	2.88**
Health(HE)	14.00	4.09	13.37	3.46	1.00
Total Stress	290.22	40.37	265.29	39.59	3.76***
Life Stress(LS)	17.28	9.39	14.77	8.16	1.74

* p <.05.

** p <.01.

*** p <.001.

Table 1 shows differences in terms of stress between lower and higher education levels. Parents of low education level among children with hearing impairment reported significantly higher stress levels on the child domain scales (t=3.50, p<.001) pertaining to acceptability(t=3.29, p<.001), demanding ness(t=3.05 p<.01), mood(t=3.49 p<.001), reinforces parent(t=2.80, p<.01) and on the parent domain scales (t= 3.37 p<.001) pertaining to depression(3.19 p<01), sense of competence(t=4.28 p<.001), isolation(t=2.53 p<.05), relationship with spouse(t=2.88 p<.01) and total stress (t=3.76 p<.001) than parents of higher education level/college education group among children with hearing impairment.

Table 2

Comparison of emotional coping and family support between education levels for mothers of children with hearing impairment

Variable	*Lower level education(n=89)*		*Higher level education(n=61)*		*T*
	Mean	*SD*	*Mean*	*SD*	
Affect	43.74	11.63	44.27	10.46	.29
Affirmation	43.02	11.99	43.80	11.46	.40
Emotional Support	86.79	22.83	88.08	20.92	.35
Aid	32.89	10.35	33.65	11.01	.40
Total Functioning	119.68	30.78	120.19	32.85	.10
Duration	30.21	7.94	31.13	7.94	.70
Frequency	29.65	7.50	29.47	6.86	.15
List	8.37	1.86	8.34	1.98	.08
Total Network	68.23	15.13	68.95	14.66	.29
Family Support	30.33	13.43	29.55	9.41	.42

Table 2 reveals comparison in terms of emotional coping and family support between lower level education and higher level of education for mothers of children with hearing impairment. The results, however, show no significant differences between the two groups on measures of emotional coping, instrumental aid and family support.

Table 3

Comparison of depression between education levels for mothers of children with hearing impairment

Variable	*Lower level education(n=89)*		*Higher level education(n=61)*		
	Mean	*SD*	*Mean*	*SD*	*T*
Depression	22.04	8.76	16.45	9.10	3.75***

*** p <.001.

Table 3 indicates a comparison of depression between lower level of education and higher level of education for mothers of children with hearing impairment. Mothers of low level education group had significantly more depression ($t=3.75$ $p<.001$) than mothers of higher education group. Thus, hearing impairment is found to be associated with depression/psychological distress in the mother's lower level of education but not for the higher education group.

Further the mothers of children with hearing impairment were divided into two groups as per their monthly family income level.

1. *Lower income group:* This sample comprised of those mothers who had a monthly family income up to Rs. 5000/-, and
2. *Higher income group:* This sample consisted of those mothers who had a monthly family income is Rs. 5001/- and above.

When a comparison was made between lower income and higher income for mothers of children with hearing impairment (as represented in table 4, table 5, and table 6 respectively), it was found that there was significant differences in terms of stress and depression for the both groups of mothers among children with hearing impairment.

Table 4

Comparison of stress between lower income and higher income mothers of children with hearing impairment

Variable	*Low Income Group(n=109)*		*High Income Group(n=41)*		*T*
	Mean	*SD*	*Mean*	*SD*	
Child Domain	133.49	18.19	126.39	21.31	2.03*
Adaptability(AD)	31.74	6.21	31.19	6.99	.47
Acceptability(AC)	19.22	4.81	17.60	5.10	1.81
Demandingness(DE)	25.69	5.15	23.60	5.53	2.17*
Mood(MO)	13.33	3.64	11.53	3.73	2.67**
Distractability/ Hyperactivity(DI)	28.88	4.47	28.80	4.30	.09
Reinforces Parent(RE)	14.16	3.56	13.63	3.70	1.48
Parent Domain	151.76	24.71	139.95	28.67	2.49**
Depression(DP)	27.11	5.70	23.53	6.30	3.33**
Attachment(AT)	16.68	4.20	16.29	4.11	.52
Role Restriction(RO)	21.22	5.14	20.43	6.55	.78
Competence(CO)	38.66	5.55	35.21	7.33	3.09**
Isolation(IS)	15.44	4.68	14.46	4.65	1.14
Spouse(SP)	18.67	5.58	16.75	6.10	1.83
Health(HE)	13.93	3.87	13.24	3.80	.98
Total Stress	285.25	38.80	266.34	46.34	2.26**
Life Stress(LS)	16.69	9.78	15.09	6.27	.97

* p <.05.

** p <.01.

*** p <.001.

Table 4 shows that the mean score differences between the lower income group and the higher income group for these samples in terms of the parental stress. Significant differences were noticed in terms of child domain (t=2.03 p<.05), parent domain (t=2.49 p<.01) and total domain (t=2.26 p<.01), pertaining to demanding ness(t=2.17 p<.05), mood(t=2.67 p<.01), depression(t=3.33 p<.01), and sense of competence(t=3.09 p<.01) for lower income group mothers.

Table 5

Comparison of emotional coping and family support between lower income and higher income mothers of children with hearing impairment

Variable	*Low Income Group(n=109)*		*High Income Group(n=41)*		*t*
	Mean	*SD*	*Mean*	*SD*	
Affect	43.69	11.44	44.65	10.39	.49
Affirmation	42.99	11.60	44.26	11.58	.60
Emotional Support	86.68	22.24	89.00	21.55	.57
Aid	32.96	10.24	33.85	11.60	.46
Total Functioning	111.64	30.16	120.56	33.91	.16
Duration	30.02	7.45	32.07	8.99	1.41
Frequency	29.31	7.34	30.29	6.54	.74
List	8.31	1.88	8.48	1.96	.50
Total Network	67.65	14.58	70.85	15.65	1.17
Family Support	29.59	12.75	31.26	9.45	.76

Table 6 which indicates differences in terms of emotional coping, instrumental aid and family support between the two groups reveals that none of these mean score differences is significant, thus showing that two groups do not differ with respect to coping.

Table 6

Comparison of depression between lower income and higher income mothers of children with hearing impairment

Variable	*Low Income Group(n=109)*		*High Income Group(n=41)*		*T*
	Mean	*SD*	*Mean*	*SD*	
Depression	21.66	9.20	14.75	7.57	4.29***

*** p <.001.

A comparison in terms of depression between the two groups as shown in table 6 reveals that the low income group was found to be significantly higher on depression (t=4.29 p<.001), when compared to their higher income group counterparts.

DISCUSSION

The findings of the study clearly shows that, overall, mothers of lower education level and monthly family income having children with hearing impairment reported higher levels of stress and are more depressed than mothers of higher education and higher income group having children with hearing impairment. These results are in agreement with results of earlier studies found that lower levels of maternal education and family income are related to increased stress in mothers of children with hearing impairment (Chen & Rubin, 1994; Brand and Coetzer, 1994; Deater-Deckard & Scarr, 1996; Singer et. al., 1990; Pianta & Egeland, 1990). Mothers of low education level and lower family income among children with hearing impairment reported feeling more depressed and had more difficulties with their sense of competence, more strain in their relationship with their spouse and social isolation. They also rated their children as more moody, unhappy, less acceptability of the child to the mother, reinforcement from their child and demanding ness when compared to higher education and higher family income mothers of children with hearing impairment. This is understandable when the life situations of these mothers are considered. These parents often have to take care of their children under economic hardship. They also demonstrate less parental acceptance of their children.

As regards the dimension of maternal depression, mother's lower level education and family income among hearing impaired child were found to be significantly more on depression as compared to their counterparts. The overall results indicate that mothers of lower education and family income among children with hearing impairment felt distress, feeling of inadequacy and inferiority feeling, self-depreciation and self-doubt , depressed, nervousness, negative and anger about their deaf child compared to mothers of higher income and education. A number of studies have reported that mothers of children with hearing impairment experience high psychological distress than parents of children with normal hearing (Watson, Henggeler & Whelan, 1990; Gowen et.al., 1982).

IMPLICATION

The findings of this study suggest that there is a need to pay more attention to the situation of mothers with children who are hearing impaired and to seek ways to help them in a positive way. The present situation in India is still focussed on finding the "right way" for educating both, the child who is hearing impaired, and the parents.

The finding shows very clearly that parents with a lower level of education and family income having children with hearing impairment experienced higher levels of stress and depression. This calls for quality intervention methods to deal with the new challenge faced by the parents of the disabled child. The findings therefore speak very strongly for a thorough analysis of the situation of the mothers concerned and for an evaluation of their needs.

It is important to suggest to professionals that they provide early intervention programs, parent education classes and parent discussion groups, compliance training, group therapy and individual counseling approaches, parental therapy, assertive training and family therapy for parents of children with hearing impairment to reduce their higher stress and depression, to develop maternal attachment to the hearing impaired child, to develop positive relationship between mother and child, parent-child bonding, increase in practical child development knowledge and child management skills, to develop emotional support, child care responsibilities, to develop emotional bonding with deaf child, and to develop maternal self-esteem in mothers of children with hearing impairment.

RECOMMENDATIONS FOR ADDITIONAL RESEARCH

The results of the present study suggest several important areas for additional research. Although some of the literature indicates that stress is a major factor in the lives of parents and families with children who have disabilities, others show that the phenomenon is more complex. The results of the present study indicate that the mothers of children with severe and profound hearing loss indicated high stress and emotional support at the time of the study. A review of other studies supports this conclusion. Future research should survey parents of deaf or hard of hearing children within the first few weeks after they have been informed of their child's disability.

The study focused on a particular population and age group. Hearing-impaired children as a sample were chosen for several reasons, one being the specific and extremely taxing nature of the disability (Meadow, 1980) and its implications for disruptions in parenting. Further, the preschool age was selected because of the salience and importance of the parenting role during this period, and because the parenting tasks for this age are specific and easily defined. A large body of developmental research indicates that parenting issues vary across the lifespan suggesting that the parenting stresses reported by mothers of older or younger children that is 6 to 10 years period would likely be different from those found in the present study in Indian context.

Finally, the current study focused exclusively on mothers' reports of stress, emotional support and depression in Indian condition. The perspectives of fathers and siblings were not included. A father's adaptation to a hearing-impaired child may differ greatly from that of his spouse (Cummings, 1976). Comparisons of mothers and fathers in terms of stressors, emotional support and depression may aid in differentiating patterns of maternal and paternal adjustment in Indian context.

REFERENCES

Abidin, R.R. (1995). *Parenting stress index* (3rd ed.). Odessa, FL: Psychological Assessment Resources.

Brand, H.J., & Coetzer, M.A. (1994). Parental response to their child's hearing impairment. *Psychological Reports*, 75(3), 1363-1368.

Bradley, R. H., Rock, S. L., Whiteside, L., Caldwell, B.M., & Brisby, J. (1991). Dimensions of parenting in families having children with disabilities. *Exceptionality*, 2, 41-61.

Brown, S.C. (1986). Etiological trends, characteristics, and distributions. In A.N.

Schildroth & M.A. Karchmer (Eds.), *Deaf Children in America* (pp.33-54). San Diego, CA: College-Hill Press.

Chen, X., & Rubin, K.H. (1994). Family conditions, parental acceptance, and social competence and aggression in Chinese children. *Social Development*, 3, 269-290.

Cummings, S., Bayley, N., & Rie, H. (1966). Effects of the child's deficiency on the mother: A study of mothers of mentally retarded, chronically ill, and neurotic children. *American Journal of Orthopsychiatry, 36*, 595-608.

Deater-Deckard, K., & Scarr, S. (1996). Parenting stress among dual-earner mothers and fathers: Are there gender differences? Journal of Family Psychology, 10, 45-59.

Dunst, C.J., Jenkins, V & Trivette, C.M. (1984). The Family Support Scale: Reliability and Validity. *Journal of Individual, Family and Community Wellness, 1,* 45-52.

Freeman, R.D. (1979). Psycho social problems associated with childhood hearing impairment. In L.J. Bradford & W.G.Hardy (Eds.), *Hearing and hearing impairment* (pp. 405-415). New York: Grune and Stratton.

Gowen, J.W., Johnson-Martin, N., Goldman, B., & Appelbaum, M. (1989). Feelings of depression and parenting competence of mothers of handicapped and non-handicapped infants: A longitudinal study. *American Journal on Mental Retardation, 94,*259-271.

Greenberg, M.T. (1980). Hearing families with deaf children: Stress and functioning as related to communication method. *American Annals of the Deaf, 125,* 1063-1071.

Hintermair, M., & Horsch, U. (1998). Hearing impairment as a critical life event. Aspects of stress and coping with parents of children with a hearing impairment. Heidelberg. Groos.

ICMR (1983), *Collaborative study on prevalance and Actiology of hearing impairement,* New Delhi: ICMR and DST

Kessler, R. (1987). The interplay of research design strategies and data analysi procedures in evaluating the effects of stress on health. In S.V.Kasl & C.L.Cooper (Eds.), *Stress and health: Issues in research methodology* (pp.113-140). San Diego, CA: Wiley.

Meadow, K.P. (1980). *Deafness and child development.* Berkeley: University of California Press.

Moores, D.F. (1987). *Educating the deaf: Psychology, principles, and practices.* Boston: Houghton Mifflin.

Morgan-Redshaw, M., Wilgosh, L., & Bibby, M.A. (1990). The parental experiences of mothers of adolescents with hearing impairments. *American Annals of the Deaf,135,* 293-298.

Norbeck, J.S., Lindsey, A.M., & Carrieri, V.L. (1983). Further development of the Norbeck Social Support Questionnaire: Normative data and validity testing. *Nursing Research, 32,* 4-9.

NSSO (1981 & 1991) as quoted by R.S. Pandey and Lal Advani (1995) *Perspectives in Disability and Rehabilitation,* New Delhi: Vikas Publishing House Pvt., Ltd.

Palfrey, S. Walker, K.D., Butler, AJ., & Singer, DJ. (1989). Patterns of response in families of chronically disabled children: An assessment in five metropolitan school districts. American Journal of Orthopsychiatry, 59(1), 94-104.

Pinata, R.C., & Egeland, B. (1990). Life stress and parenting outcome in a disadvantaged sample: Results of the Mother and Child Interaction Project. *Journal of Clinical Child Psychology, 19,* 329-336.

Radolff, L.S. (1977). The CES-D Scale: A self-report depression scale for research in the general population. *Applied Psychological Measurement, 1,* 385-401.

Schlesinger, H.S., & Meadow, K.P. (1972). *Sound and sign: Childhood deafness and mental health.* Berkeley: University of California Press.

Segal, M.M. (1985, December). An interview study with mothers of handicapped children to identify both positive and negative experiences that influence their ability to cope. Paper presented at the meeting of the National Center for Infants' Programs, Washington, DC.

Singer, L.T., Song, L.Y., Hill, B.P., & Jaffe, A.C. (1990). Stress and depression in mothers of failure-to-thrive children. *Journal of Pediatric Psychology, 15,* 711-720.

Thoits, P.A. (1982b). Life stress, social support, and psychological vulnerability: Epidemiological considerations. *Journal of Community Psychology, 10,* 341-362.

Watson, S.M. Henggeler, W.H., & Whelan, J.P. (1990). Family functioning and the social adaptation of hearing impaired youths. *Journal of Abnormal Child Psychology,* 18(2), 143-63.

Wunsch, A., & Bengel, J.(1998). Psychologische Aspekte von Korper und Sinnebehinderung (Psychological aspects of physical and sensory disabilities).

In L. von Rosenstel, C. M. Hockel, & W. Molt (Eds.), *Handbuch der angewandten Psychologie: Grundlagen-Methoden-Praxis* (Handbook of applied psychology: Foundations, methods, practice) (pp. 1-14) Landsberg/ Lech,Germany: Ecomed.

Wyngaarden Krauss, M. (1993). Child-related and parenting stress: Similarities and differences between mothers and fathers of children with disabilities. *Journal on Retardation, 97,* 393-404.

14

Identifying Stressors Among University Students

N.Vijaya Lakshmi*

ABSTRACT

Students are generally prone to stress during the transition phase from graduate colleges to university stage. They face enormous pressure as they try to perform at post graduate level while constantly thinking about settling in good career immediately after completion of post graduate program. In order to assess this stress, a study was conducted on first year university students in the very first month of their admission. The objective of the study is to identify the stressors among the university students and also to examine which category of stressors were more prevalent in the representative sample. The sample consisted of 120 male students who were pursuing Masters of Business Administration program in a private university. A survey was conducted on first 120 students who showed high anxiety on the global factor as per the Cattells 16 personality factor questionnaire which is administered as part of the curriculum. These students were further asked to list out the various stressors they were experiencing in the last one month. The stressors listed by the students were appropriately grouped into four broad categories such as intrapersonal, interpersonal, academic and environmental stressors. Based on this information descriptive statistics that is frequency distribution and percentages were calculated for the responses given by the students, which showed

* **Faculty Member, IBS, Hyderabad.**

that there were more intrapersonal stressors listed as compared to the other three categories. The most common stressors reported in the total sample was found to be overload of assignments (66.7%), followed by inability to manage time effectively (50%), pre placement fear (43.3%) and home sickness (40%). The results were discussed accordingly.

INTRODUCTION

Stress is a common condition in our day to day lives. It stems from our daily efforts to achieve goals, adapt to the new environment and also to adjust to the demands of living in an ever changing world. We often view stress as a negative impact in our lives and tend to reduce or eliminate it. However, there can be a great deal of learning which takes place when exposed to the stressful situations. Dr. Hans Selye (1978), an expert in this area has said, "Our aim shouldn't be to completely avoid stress, which at any rate would be impossible, but to learn how to recognize our typical responses to stress and then try to modulate our lives in accordance with it".

Stress is any situation that evokes negative thoughts and feelings in a person. The same situation may or may not be stressful to different people and also in the same person on different occasions. Numerous studies were conducted in this area. In the field of education, several studies have shown that college students especially freshmen are prone to stress (D'Zurilla & Sheedy, 1991) due to the transitional nature of college life (Towbes & Cohen, 1996). The dynamic relationship between the person and environment in stress perception and reaction is especially magnified among college students. Particularly, during the transition phase from college to the university level, they are exposed to new challenges such as seeking a job of their choice, settling early in career, trying out opportunities in employment and so forth. Students react to the university education in a variety of ways. For some students, it is stressful because it is a sudden change from college level to the higher university level, with different challenges. For others, separation from home is a source of stress. They must adjust to being away from home for the first time, maintain a high level of academic achievement and adapt to a new social environment. .Although, an optimum level of stress is necessary to achieve desired goals, but often quite a few students face more stress than what is desirable and this may overwhelm them and affects their ability to cope with difficult circumstances.

Stress among students has an effect on learning. The Yerkes-Dodson law (1908) states that individuals under low and high stress learn the least and those under moderate stress learn the most. Several Studies have been conducted which proved that excessive stress is harmful to student's performance. There are various studies which showed that if stress is not dealt with effectively, feelings of loneliness and nervousness, as well as sleeplessness and excessive worrying may result (Wright, 1967). Romano in 1992 has stated that stress results from the interaction between stressors and the individual's perception and reaction to those stressors. Studies have shown that the environment at college is quite different as compared to a non-student population where they are exposed to continuous evaluations through tests, presentations and so forth. (Wright , 1964) . The pressure to earn good grades and to earn a degree is normally very high among the students (Hirsch & Ellis, 1996). Earning high grades is not the only source of stress for students. Other potential sources of stress include excessive homework, unclear assignments and uncomfortable classrooms (Kohn & Frazer, 1986). In addition to academic requirement, relations with faculty members, and peer as well as time pressure may also be other key sources of stress to the students (Sgan-Cohen & Lowental, 1988). Relationship with family and friends, eating and sleeping habits, loneliness may affect some students adversely (Wright, 1967).

Assessing the stress levels among students is a topic often studied by the researchers in the field of psychology. Towbes and Cohen (1996) conducted a study to find out the sources of stress and which category of students was more prone to stress. They found out that first year students showed more stress levels as compared to their seniors. The present study is conducted on the first year MBA students during the first month of their admission. The stressors were grouped under four categories, the first one being Intrapersonal stressors which result from internal sources, such as, changes in eating habits, lack of self-esteem etc. The second category is Interpersonal stressors which result from interactions with other people such as conflicts with friends, pressures from parents, peers etc. The third category pertains to Academic stressors, which arise from college related activities and academics. Finally, the forth category relates to Environmental stressors. They result from problems in the environment and outside academics. The objective of the study is to

- To identify the stressors faced by the students.
- To examine which category of stressors are more prevalent.

METHOD

Sample: Participants were 120 male graduate students pursuing Post Graduate program in a well reputed Business School in India.

Description of sample: Students are from various regions of India. They come from different cultural backgrounds, educational background and from different socio-economic status. The students reside in the hostel provided by the university and most of the students are staying away from home for the first time.

Materials and Procedure: The students were administered the **16 PF** questionnaire as part of the regular counseling procedures to help the students identify their strengths and weaknesses. This questionnaire was administered a few days after the students joined the course. In this regard, the researcher identified first 120 students showing high anxiety which was obtained from one of the global factors in the 16pf questionnaire. The students were called by the researcher individually and were asked to list down all the stressors. Before this the participants signed the consent forms that indicated that all data furnished by them would be kept strictly confidential.

After the data was collected from 120 participants, the stressors mentioned by the students were grouped under the above mentioned four categories i.e., Intrapersonal, Interpersonal, academic and environmental stressors

RESULTS AND DISCUSSION

Table – 1 (See Appendix-1) shows the frequency distribution and percentage of stressors identified and categorized under these four broad categories. The total number of stressors reported by the total sample was found to be 47. Out of which 16 stressors are intrapersonal, 11 are interpersonal stressors, 12 academic stressors and the remaining 8 reported were environmental stressors. This shows that the most prevalent category of stressors were intrapersonal stressors which accounted for 34% of the stressors reported. A similar study done by Shannon E Ross et al (1999) found that there were more intrapersonal stressors (38%) as compared to the other category of stressors.

Appendix-1

Table 1

Frequency Distribution and Percentage of Stressors Identified

Type of Stressors	*Frequency Distribution*	*Percentage*
INTERPERSONAL		
Fear of rejection	4	3.3
Unable to socialize	6	5
Taking care of aged parents	4	3.3
Lack of negotiation skills while working in teams	12	10
ACADEMIC		
Frequent class tests	8	6.7
Low marks in test	7	5.8
Unhappy with internal assessments	2	1.7
Coping with new subjects	20	16.7
Vast syllabus	4	3.3
Not clear in choosing specialization	8	6.7
Exam anxiety	16	13.3
Having low attendance	12	10
Overloaded with class assignments	80	66.7
Pre-placement fear	52	43.3
Unable to complete team assignments	4	3.3
Hectic schedule	32	26.7

(Contd...)

Type of Stressors	*Frequency Distribution*	*Percentage*
ENVIRONMENTAL		
Lack of time for recreational activities	10	8.3
Problems with internet connections	20	16.7
Post lunch classes	5	4.2
Long queue in canteen	5	4.2
Acclimatization	6	5
Campus away from the city	15	12.5
Shuffling from one building to another in the campus	4	3.3
Large strength of students in the class	20	16.7

Among University Students

Type of Stressors	*Frequency*	*Percentage Distribution*
INTRAPERSONAL		
Home sickness	**48**	**40**
Decline in personal health	12	10
Unable to concentrate	16	13.3
Financial difficulties	16	13.3
Feelings of dissatisfaction for self-performance	12	10
Feeling guilty for not supporting family	4	3.3
Unable to overcome shyness	16	13.3
Change in sleeping habits	20	16.7
Change in food habits	20	16.7
New responsibilities	12	10
Not able to meet deadlines	**60**	**50**
Fear of failure	16	13.3
Poor communication skills	20	16.7
Unable to make decisions	4	3.3
Low self-esteem	8	6.7

(Contd...)

Low motivation levels	5	4.2
INTERPERSONAL		
Being taken granted by friends	12	10
High expectations from parents	16	13.3
Conflict with friends/room mates/ girl friend	21	17.5
Family problems	12	10
Unequal participation in teams	12	10
Pressure to compete with friends	28	23.3
Infrequent phone calls from home	4	3.3

The frequency distribution of the stressors reported by the total sample in all the categories shows that the four most prevalent stressors reported by the students was found to be that they were pressurized with assignments which accounts for 66.7% of the stressors reported followed by their inability to meet deadlines (50%), Pre-placement fear (43.3%) and homesickness (40%). As the data was collected in the first month of their admission the students felt that they were overloaded with assignments as they were not exposed to this kind of pressure during their graduation (college) days. Another reason probably, could be that they are new to the subjects and may have felt difficult to cope up with the assignments. Further, in professional courses like MBA, the curriculum is rigorous and the competition very stiff unlike that of any graduation programs at college level. This clearly puts pressure on the students to perform under strict deadlines. This is exactly corroborated by the present study which clearly showed that the students were not able to manage time properly due to which they were not able to meet deadlines which is reported to be the second major stressor.

The MBA program being a two year residential course with on campus placements during the second year puts a great amount of pressure on the students to perform and excel in order to achieve a better placement. Most of the time they find it difficult to complete assignments due to their poor time management and in turn they fear that this may affect their semester exams and finally the placements. This primarily may have lead to pre-placement fear. Since the principal objective of the students taking up the two years MBA program is to get a good placement and the fact that the strength of the batch is too large, there is enormous peer pressure faced by the students and they mostly feel that they may not be able to cope with the competition. Homesickness is another major stressor reported by 40% of the sample as the students joining the MBA program have to stay in the hostel provided by the university. A majority of the students were staying away from home for the first time. Staying away from home requires lot of things to be done by them on their own and most often they may or may not have support from peers. Another factor could be that the student may not have been exposed to taking responsibility. Since the students take time to settle down and also take time to know each other, they may be hesitant to ask for help in the initial stages. Hence, getting through classes in a new place while living away from all the comforts of home is found to be stressful to some students.

To conclude the major stressors reported by the students which have had impact on their performance in the present sample were high overload of assignments, followed by the inability to meet deadlines, pre placement fear and homesickness. Further research in this area can be carried out using other variables like birth order, type of family, academic performance and so on to find out the impact of stress on the students.

REFERENCES

D'Zurilla, T.J., Sheedy, C.F. (1991). Relation between social problem-solving ability and subsequent level of psychological stress in college students. *Journal of Personality and Social Psychology, 61* (5), 841-846.

Hans, S. (1978). On the real benefits of eustress. Interview by Laurence Cherry. *Psychology Today*, March, p. 60.

Hirsch, J.K., & Ellis, J.B. (1996). Differences in life stress and reasons for living among college suicide ideators and non-ideators. *College Student Journal*, 30, 377-384.

Kohn, J.P., & Frazer, G.H. (1986). An academic stress scale: Identification and rated importance of academic stressors. *Psychological Reports*, 59, 415 – 426.

Romano, J.L. (1992). Psycho educational interventions for stress management and well-being. *Journal of Counseling and Development*, 71, 199-202.

Sgan-Cohen, H.D., & Lowental, U. (1998). Sources of stress among Israeli dental students. *The Journal of the American College Health Association*, 36, 317-321.

Shannon, E.R., Bradley, C.N., & Teresa, M.H. (1999). Sources of stress among college students. *College Student Journal.* Truman State University.

Towbes, L.C., & Cohen, L.H. (1996). Chronic stress in the lives of college students: Scale development and prospective prediction of distress. *Journal of Youth and Adolescence,* 25, 199-217.

Wright, J.J. (1964). Environmental stress evaluation in a student community. The *Journal of the American College Health Association,* 12 (5), 325 -336.

Wright, J.J. (1967). Reported personal stress sources and adjustment of entering freshmen. *Journal of Counseling Psychology,* 14 (4), 371-373.

Yerkes, R.M., & Dodson, J.D. (1908). The Relation of strength of stimulus to rapidity of habit-formation. *Journal of Comparative and Neurological Psychology,* 18 Nov, 459-482.

15

Quality of Family Environment, Stress and Coping Skills Among Offspring of Chronically ILL Parents

A.J. Wadkar*, Sunitha Thampi**

ABSTRACT

Parenting and family relationships are important factors shaping a child's development. Parents who are unable to carry out parental roles because of chronic illnesses can have a significant influence on children's social and emotional well-being. Present study examines how parental chronic illness is related to quality of family environment, stress and coping skills among offspring. This study was conducted on adult (18-25 yrs.), unmarried offspring of mentally ill parents, physically ill parents and that of normal parents. It was hypothesized that offspring of normal parents have better quality of family environment, experience less stress, and have better coping skills compared to offspring of chronically ill parents. Analysis of data revealed that offspring of normal parents have better quality of family environment and experience significantly less psychological symptoms of stress compared to offspring of chronically ill parents. Data also revealed that there is no significant difference between offspring of chronically ill parents and that of normal parents in their coping skills. Further analysis

* Reader, Department of Psychology, Pune University, ajw@unipune.ernet.in

** Doctoral Student, Department of Psychology, Pune University, svthampi@yahoo.com

of data revealed that offspring of mentally ill parents have significantly poor quality of family environment and significantly higher psychological symptoms of stress, than the other two groups. Future research should investigate the mediating factors that help to cope with stress effectively in the context of parental mental illness.

Home is the most important place where a child first experiences feelings of sharing, nurturance and acceptance. During developmental stages, the family remains as a crucial guiding influence in personality development of children. Healthy family relationships and interactions foster new competencies, as well as positive attitude in children, which serve as the basis for social relationships formed by children later.

Parenting is a complex activity that include many specific behaviors that work individually and together to influence child outcomes. Primary role of all parents is to influence, teach, control and ultimately provide maximum physical as well as mental protection to children. Parents who are unable to carry out parental roles because of mental as well as physical illnesses can have a significant influence on children's social and emotional well-being. A child who faces such adverse situations can precipitate trauma, insecurity and future psychological and behavioral problems (Davies & Windle, 1997; Garber & Little, 1999; Mowbray, Oyserman, MacFarlane, Bybee, & Rueda-Riedle, 2001). Alternatively, such challenges can produce enhanced family communication, compassion, and better coping skills that can last a lifetime (McCue & Bonn, 2003).

The models proposed by Rolland (1987), Lewis et al. (1989), and Armistead et al. (1995) hypothesized that some combination of illness, individual, and family variables influence child and or family functioning with illness (Korneluk & Lee,1998). Rolland's model explained family functioning with illness in a family member. Lewis et al.'s (1989) family-focused model placed emphasis upon family coping with parent illness. Similarly, the model proposed by Armistead et al., (1995) was designed primarily to explain child functioning with parent illness.

Numerous research studies found that children of parents with chronic illnesses have more negative outcomes than those with normal parents. Offspring of parents with chronic illness may lack adequate models for appropriate development of offspring (Mowbray and Oyserman, 2003). Numerous studies have been conducted on children of mentally ill parents show that the children are at risk of having diagnosable psychiatric conditions (Fendrich, Warner, & Weissman, 1990; Jacobsen, Miller, & Kirkwood, 1997; Neff, 1994), academic difficulties (Davies&Windle, 1997; Garber & Little, 1999) and child behavior problems (Maria & Beverly 2003; Mowbray, Oyserman, MacFarlane, Bybee, & Rueda-Riedle, 2001; Rutter & Quinton, 1984; Zahn-Waxler, Cummings, McKnew & Radke-Yarrow, 1984) . David (2000) studied experiences of family members of mentally ill and found striking similarities in the experiences of caregivers like feeling of shame, fear, guilt and powerlessness.

Most of the literature addressing impact of parental physical illness on children comes out of the field of oncology (e.g. Birenbaum, Yancey, Philip, Chand & Husten, 1999; Morgan, Stanford & Johnson 1992). During last two decades, healthcare research has increasingly paid attention to children whose parents suffer from physical illness, resulting in the publication of 3 reviews (Armistead, Klein & Forehand, 1995; Kelley, Sikka & Venkatesan, 1997; Korneluk, & Lee, 1998). Armistead, Klein & Forehand(1995) noted that the way parents' physical illnesses affect children's functioning can vary with a number of different dimensions of illness like onset (acute or gradual), course (progressive, constant, episodic), impairments (physical or cognitive) and outcome (morbidity or mortality).

Parental illness has to be considered within the family context and it is important to examine how the family environment may influence behavioral outcomes in offspring. Quality of family environment, stress and coping skills are the variables studied in the present study in the context of parental illness.

RATIONALE OF THE STUDY

There are a substantial number of studies focused on children and adolescents of parents with chronic illness. However, very few empirical studies have been conducted on their adult offspring to find out whether negative outcomes are carrying over the years. Relative inattention and lack of adequate empirical support on adult offspring of ill parents is a gap in research. Hence, present study focuses on adult unmarried offspring (18-25 yrs) of mentally ill parents, physically ill parents and normal parents with special reference to quality of family environment, stress and coping skills.

METHOD

Objective

Compare offspring of mentally ill parents, physically ill parents and normal parents with respect to quality of family environment, stress and coping skills.

Study Design

The present study has been designed to compare the offspring of parents having functional difficulties to perform their proper parenting role due to certain chronic illnesses with offspring of normal parents. The data has been analyzed to compare offspring of chronically ill parents with matched normal as well as between offspring of mentally ill and that of physically ill parents.

Study groups have been compared on the following variables:

1. Quality of family environment
2. Stress
3. Coping skills

Hypotheses

1. Offspring of normal parents have significantly better *quality of family environment* than that of offspring of mentally ill and physically ill parents.
2. Offspring of normal parents experience less *stress* compared to offspring of mentally ill and physically ill parents.
3. Offspring of normal parents have significantly better *coping skills* than that of offspring of mentally ill and physically ill parents.

Sample

The present study has been conducted at Trivandrum city, Kerala state. The research sample consist of 300 subjects from three groups- offspring of mentally ill parents (OMIP) (N=100), offspring of physically ill parents (OPIP) (N=100) and offspring of normal parents (ONP) (N=100). The offspring of ill parents has been selected from the two government hospitals namely, Mental Health Centre, Trivandrum and General Hospital, Trivandrum. Details of the parent's illness are taken from hospital records. The age of subjects range from 18-25 years and have educational qualification of 8th standard and above. They are unmarried, low socio-economic status and from both sexes.

The matched controls are selected from the normal population of the same habitat as that of the offspring of ill parents are selected. Matching is done on age, sex, education, marital status, socio-economic status, residential area and health status of parent.

General Criteria used for the selection of offspring of mentally ill parents

1. Offspring of patients having schizophrenia, bipolar affective disorder and unipolar depression.
2. Parents are admitted in the wards of Mental Health Centre, and Psychiatry wards of General Hospital, Trivandrum.
3. Parents have scores 50 and below on SF-36 Health Survey (Standard US Version) (shows severe functional limitation)
4. Minimum duration of parent's illness is 5years.

General Criteria used for the selection of offspring of physically ill parents

1. Offspring of patients having hyper tension, diabetes mellitus, asthma and coronary artery disease.
2. Parents are admitted in the medical wards of General Hospital, Trivandrum.
3. Parents have scores 50 and below on SF-36 Health Survey (Standard US Version) (shows severe functional limitation)
4. Minimum duration of parent's illness is 5 years.

General Criteria used for the selection of offspring of normal parents

1. In this group both parents of the subjects do not have any physical or mental illness, which interferes with his or her normal day to day functioning
2. Parents have scores 75 and above on SF-36 Health Survey (Standard US Version).

Tools

For the present study, following instruments have been used to measure the severity of dysfunction of parent, socio-demographic variables, quality of family environment, stress and coping skills among offspring.

- **The Short Form 36 Health Survey (SF-36)** by Ware, Snow and Kosinski (1993)

To measure severity of dysfunction in mentally parents SF-36 health survey is administered. This widely used scale is designed as a general indicator of health status. The 36 items of the SF-36 are drawn from the original Medical Outcomes Study questionnaire and the General Well Being Schedule. The reliability and validity of the SF-36 has been demonstrated in multiple studies which have surveyed more than 3000 patients with various medical and psychiatric conditions. In general, the median alpha reliability for all scales exceeds 0.80 and the two weeks test-retest correlation exceeds0.8, with the test-retest correlation after a delay of six months ranging between 0.6 and 0.9.

- **Personal Data Sheets** (developed by the researcher)

Two personal data sheets have been constructed for the present study - one for offspring of mentally ill parents (PDA-1) and one for offspring of normal parents (PDS-2).They comprising 25 items in PDS-1 and 24 items in PDS-2 and are required to be filled in by the patients before the actual administration of the scales. The items are designed to elicit the demographic information about the offspring, their residential background and the details of their parents.

- **Family Environment Scale (FES)** by Moos and Moos (1974)

FES is developed by Moos and Moos in 1974. FES is a 90 item scale, comprises of ten subscales that measure the social-environmental characteristics of all types of families. These ten subscales assess three sets of dimensions: the Relationship dimensions, the Personal Growth dimensions, and the System Maintenance dimension.

The internal consistencies of FES are all in an acceptable range, varying from moderate for Independence (.61) and Achievement Orientation (.64) to substantial for Cohesion (.78), Organization (.76), Intellectual- Cultural Orientation (.78), and Moral- Religious Emphasis (.78).

- A Questionnaire on **Stress** (developed by the researcher)

A 76-item questionnaire has been developed by present researcher to measure stress experienced by offspring of chronically ill parents as well as normal parents. The questionnaire comprises of two dimensions, namely psychological dimension as well as physical dimension of stress. The psychological dimension measures anxiety, depression, inferiority, fear and irritability among subjects. The items were initially constructed in English and translated to Malayalam (regional language) with the help of some experts. Standardization procedure has been conducted for Malayalam version of the questionnaire. Internal consistency of the Stress questionnaire was estimated using Cronbach's alpha and has been found to be .82. The alpha coefficient for traits (anxiety, depression, inferiority, fear and irritability) ranges from .66 to .79.

- **Coping Resources Inventory (CRI)** by Hammer and Marting (1988)

Coping Resources Inventory was developed by Hammer and Marting in 1988. It consists of 60 statements, measures resources in five domains namely cognitive, emotional, physical, spiritual/ philosophical and social. Internal consistency reliabilities of the CRI scales are estimated using Cronbach's alpha. Reliability scores for scales range from .56 to .88 for different samples, suggesting that the CRI scales are fairly homogeneous and are reliably tapping the constructs. The coefficients for the Total Resource Score are quite high (ranging from .89 to.93).

PROCEDURE

From the hospital records patients suffering the illness for at least 5 years were selected. The offspring of these patients were approached personally. The SF-36 Health Survey was administered to estimate the severity of dysfunction of the parent. Parent who scored below 50 (shows severe functional limitation) was selected for the study. Offspring of patients having more than one chronic illness and both parents having chronic illnesses were also excluded from the study to make the sample more homogenous. All the tests are given individually. No time limit is imposed for the completion of the tests. The matched controls are selected from the normal population of the same habitat as those of the offspring of ill parents.

RESULTS

The data of the present study was primarily analyzed to see whether there was any significant difference between offspring of mentally ill parents, physically ill parents and that of normal parents on each of the variables under study namely, quality of family environment, stress and coping skills. One-way ANOVA and Duncan's multiple comparison tests were carried out to test hypotheses from 1 to 3 framed for the study.

The results shown in Table-1 indicate that the mean differences between study groups are statistically significant for all the three dimensions of family environment namely, family relationship dimension, family personal growth dimension and family system maintenance dimension. Duncan's Multiple Comparison Tests were conducted to see mean difference between groups.

Mean values shown in Tables 1 a, 1b & 1c clearly and consistently show that family environment of normal parents is better than that of ill parents. Hence hypothesis 1 stated offspring of normal parents have significantly better **quality of family environment** than that of offspring of mentally ill and physically ill parents has been accepted. It also shows that offspring of mentally ill parents got lowest scores in all the three dimensions compared to other two groups.

One way ANOVA results also indicate that mean differences between study groups are statistically significant for both dimensions of stress (Table 1). Duncan's Multiple Comparison Tests were conducted further to see mean difference between groups.

Table 1

One way ANOVA on Dimensions of Quality of Family Environment, Stress and Coping Skills of offspring of Mentally ill, Physically ill and Normal parents

		Sum of Squares	*df*	*Mean Square*	*F*
Family Relationship Dimension	Between Groups	85.787	2	42.893	6.129**
	Within Groups	2078.400	297	6.998	
	Total	2164.187	299		
Family Personal Growth Dimension	Between Groups	2046.020	2	1023.010	44.550***
	Within Groups	6820.100	297	22.963	
	Total	8866.120	299		
Family System Maintenance Dimension	Between Groups	190.407	2	95.203	8.251***
	Within Groups	3426.980	297	11.539	
	Total	3617.387	299		
Physiological symptoms of Stress	Between Groups	2054.687	2	1027.343	4.588**
	Within Groups	66499.900	297	223.905	
	Total	68554.587	299		

(Contd...)

		Sum of Squares	*df*	*Mean Square*	*F*
Psychological symptoms of Stress	Between Groups	6612.527	2	3306.263	5.600**
	Within Groups	175360.310	297	590.439	
	Total	181972.837	299		
Coping Skills	Between Groups	805.047	2	402.523	1.074
	Within Groups	111311.790	297	374.787	
	Total	112116.837	299		

* (one-tailed).

** Significant at the 0.05 level (one-tailed).

*** Significant at the 0.005 level.

Table 1a - c

Duncan's Multiple Comparison Test for Dimensions of Family Environment

Table 1 - a

Family Relationship Dimension

Duncan[a]

Type of Parental Illness	N	Subset for alpha = .05	
		1	2
Mental Illness	100	15.64	
Physical illness	100		16.58
No illness	100		16.90
Sig.		1.000	.393

Means for groups in homogeneous subsets are displayed.

a. Uses Harmonic Mean Sample Size = 100.000.

Table 1-b

Family personal growth dimension

Duncan[a]

Type of parental illness	N	Subset for alpha = .05		
		1	2	3
Mental illness	100	21.11		
Physical illness	100		23.10	
No illness	100			27.37
Sig.		1.000	1.000	1.000

Means for groups in homogeneous subsets are displayed.

a. Uses Harmonic Mean Sample Size = 100.000.

Table 1-c

Family system maintenance dimension

Duncan[a]

Type of parental illness	N	Subset for alpha = .05	
		1	2
Mental illness	100	7.62	
Physical illness	100	8.53	
No illness	100		9.57
Sig.		.059	1.000

Means for groups in homogeneous subsets are displayed.

a. Uses Harmonic Mean Sample Size = 100.000.

Table 1 d and e

Duncan's Multiple Comparison Test for Dimensions of Stress

Table 1 d

Total Physiological Symptoms of Stress

Duncan[a]

Type of Parental Illness	N	Subset for alpha = .05	
		1	2
No illness	100	59.45	
Mental illness	100		64.44
Physical illness	100		65.43
Sig.		1.000	.640

Means for groups in homogeneous subsets are displayed.

a. Uses Harmonic Mean Sample Size = 100.000.

Table 1-e

Total psychological symptoms of stress

Duncan[a]

Type of parental illness	N	Subset for alpha = .05	
		1	2
No illness	100	112.57	
Physical illness	100		121.62
Mental illness	100		123.24
Sig.		1.000	.638

Means for groups in homogeneous subsets are displayed.

a. Uses Harmonic Mean Sample Size = 100.000.

Tables 1d and 1e shows that both psychological symptoms of stress and physiological symptoms of stress are less among offspring of normal parents. Hence hypothesis 2 stated offspring of normal parents experience less **stress** compared to offspring of mentally ill and physically ill parents has been accepted. It also shows that psychological symptoms are highest among offspring of mentally ill parents, but physiological symptoms are highest among offspring of physically ill parents.

The result of one-way ANOVA confirms the absence of significant differences between study groups on the variables coping skills (Table 1). Hence hypothesis 3 stated offspring of normal parents have significantly better **coping skills** than that of offspring of mentally ill and physically ill parents has been rejected.

DISCUSSION

The present findings related to quality of family environment of chronically ill parents are consistent with earlier studies (e.g. Keitner & Miller, 1990; Rutter & Quinton, 1984; Downey & Coyne, 1990). Chronic illness by its range and diversity, touches upon the family at every point and contributes to family problems of every description. The impact of serious illness is not only experienced by the patient, but also by those around him or her who are exposed to various forms of psychological, economic, and social stressors which may accompany the illness (Armistead, Klein & Forehand,

1995). Circumstances such as marital discord, social adversity, multiple caretakers (Oates, 1997), unemployment, and separations due to hospital admissions as a result of the illness also add to the risk (Hall, 1996).

In most cases, lack of adequate social stimulation, apathy, growing up with poor parenting models, isolation from extended family and social supports are the conditions that make it hard for persons who are living with an ill parent. Parent-child interactions of poor quality and frequent physical separations between parent and child contribute to the potential for significant disruptions in the parent-child bond (Seifer&Dickstein, 1993; Solnit&Leckman, 1984).

The results of the present study showed significant difference between offspring of chronically ill parents and of normal parents on both psychological symptoms of stress as well as on physiological symptoms of stress. Families in which a parent has a serious illness may experience impaired parenting performance due to various aspects of the illness (Minde, 1991; Nicholson, Sweeney, & Geller, 1998). This may be observed as dysfunctional parent-child interactions or increased levels of parental distress about parenting (Goodman & Brumley, 1990; Minde, 1991; Mowbray, Oyserman, & Ross, 1995; Nicholson et al., 1998).

Prevalence rates of stress disorder among children of mentally ill parents have been found to be several times higher than that observed for children from the general population (Beardslee, Bemporad, Keller, & Klerman, 1983; Rutter, Silberg, O'Connor, & Simonoff, 1999). Although this increased risk for disorder is attributable, in part, to the genetic heritability of serious forms of psychopathology (Rutter et al., 1999), children of parents with serious mental disorders are also more likely to be exposed to multiple perinatal, cognitive, familial, and psychosocial risks which impact health and well-being (Erickson, 1998; Goodman, 1984; Minde, 1991).

The present study revealed that there is no significant difference between offspring of chronically ill parents and of normal parents regarding coping skills. It shows that offspring of chronically ill parents cope with the stressful situation as well as that of normal parents. Kerala has a highly conducive physical, social and cultural environment to health facilities such as wide network of health infrastructure, medical advancements, higher literacy rate, and general health awareness. This may also help the offspring of ill parents to cope with the situation as well as that of normal parents. Medical progress has made it possible to take a more hopeful attitude toward many long-term illnesses, and to regard them with a new optimism. This may also help the offspring of ill parents to cope with the situation as that of offspring of normal parents.

Various personal factors and illness-related factors can influence the coping with parental mental illness including care given by other un affected parent, available support system, relationship with peers, personality of offspring, increased responsibilities, changes in routines, and changes in the marital relationship. These stressors vary in their controllability. Offspring's perceived controllability over the above mentioned factors have tremendous influence on his or her coping styles (Compas, Banez, Malcarne, & Worsham, 1991).

REFERENCE

1. Armistead, L., Klein, L., Forehand, R. (1995). Parental physical Illness and child functioning. *Clinical Psychology Review*, 15, 409–422.
2. Beardslee,W., Bemporad, J.,Keller, M., & Klerman, G. (1983). Children of parents with major affective disorder: A review. *American Journal of Psychiatry, 140,* 825–832.
3. Birenbaum,L.K., Yancey,D.Z., Philip,D.S., Chand,N., & Husten, G.(1999). School-age children's and adolescents' adjustment when a parent has cancer. *Oncology Nursing Forum*, 26(10), 1639-1645.
4. Compas, B. E., Banez, G. A., Malcarne, V., & Worsham, N. (1991). Perceived control and coping with stress: A developmental perspective. *Journal of Social Issues, 47,* 23-34.
5. David, K. A. (2000). *The burden of sympathy: How families cope with mental illness.* New York: Oxford University Press.
6. Davies, P., & Windle, M. (1997). Gender-specific pathways between maternal depressive symptoms, family discord, & adolescent adjustment. *Developmental Psychology*, 33(4), 657-668.
7. Downey, G., & Coyne, J.C. (1990). Children of depressed parents: An integrative review. *Psychological Bulletin*, 108, 50-76.
8. Erickson, M. T. (1998). Etiological factors. In Ollendick, T. H. & Hersen, M. (Eds.), *Handbook of child psychopathology* (pp. 37–61). (3rd ed). New York: Plenum Press.

9. Fendrich, M., Warner, V., & Wiessman, M. (1990). Family risk factors, parental depression, and psychopathology in offspring. *Developmental Psychology*, 26, 40–50.

10. Garber, J. & Little, S. (1999). Predictors of Competence among Offspring of Depressed Mothers. *Journal of Adolescent Research*, 14(1), 44-71.

11. Goodman, S.H., & Brumley, H.E. (1990). Schizophrenic and depressed mothers—relational deficits in parenting. *Developmental Psychology*, 26(1), 31–39.

12. Goodman, S. H. (1984). Children of disturbed parents: The interface between research and intervention. *American Journal of Community Psychology*, *12*, 663-687.

13. Hall, R.C.W. (1996). Global assessment of functioning: A modified scale. *Psychosomatics*, 36, 267-275.

14. Hammer,A.L., & Marting,M.S. (1988). *Manual for Coping Resources Inventory*. California: Consulting Psychologists Press.

15. Jacobsen, T., Miller, L.J., & Kirkwood, K.P. (1997). Assessing parenting competency in individuals with severe mental illness: A comprehensive service. *Journal of Mental Health Administration*, 24(2), 189-199.

16. Kelley, S.D.M., Sikka, A., & Venkatesan, S. (1997). A review of research on parental disability: implications for research and counseling practice. *Rehabilitation Counseling Bulletin*, 41, 105-121.

17. Keitner, G.I.,&Miller, I.W. (1990). Family functioning and major depression—An overview. *American Journal of Psychiatry*, 147(9), 1128-1137.

18. Korneluk Y.G., & Lee. CM. (1998). Children's adjustment to parental physical illness. *Clin Child Family Psychol Review*, 1,179-193.

19. Lewis, F. M., Woods, N. F., Hough, E. E., & Bensley, L. S. (1989). The family's functioning with chronic illness in the mother: The spouse's perspective. *Social Science Medicine, 29*, 1261- 1269.

20. Maria,G.A. & Beverly, F.I.(2003). Parental depression, parenting and family adjustment and child effortful control: Explaining externalizing behaviors for pre-school children. *Journal of Applied Developmental Psychology*, Vol. 24(2), 143-177.

21. McCue, K., & Bonn, R. (2003). Helping children through an adult's serious illness: Role of the pediatric nurse. *Pediatric Nursing*, 29(1).

22. Minde, K. (1991). The effect of disordered parenting on the development of children. In M. Lewis (Ed.), *Child and adolescent psychiatry: A comprehensive textbook* (pp. 398-410). Baltimore: Williams & Wilkins.

23. Moos,R.M., & Moos,B.S. (1974). *Manual for Family Environment Scale*. California: Consulting Psychologists Press.

24. Morgan, J., Stanford, M., & Johnson, C. (1992). The impact of a physically ill parent on adolescents: Cross-sectional findings from a clinic population. *Canadian Journal of Psychiatry*, 37, 423-427.

25. Mowbray, C.T., & Oyserman, D. (2003). Promoting the healthy development of school age children and adolescents of parents with mental illness. *Encyclopedia of Prevention*.

26. Mowbray, C.T., Oyserman, D., & Ross, S. (1995). Parenting and the significance of children for women with a serious mental illness. *Journal of Mental Health Administration*, 22(2), 189-200.

27. Mowbray, C.T., Oyserman, D., MacFarlane, P., Bybee, D., & Rueda-Riedle, A. (2001). Life circumstances of mothers with serious mental illness. *Psychiatric Rehabilitation Journal*, 25(2), 114-123.

28. Neff, J. (1994). Adult children of alcoholic or mentally ill parents: Alcohol consumption and psychological distress in a tri-ethnic community sample. *Addictive Behaviors*, 19, 185-197.

29. Nicholson, J., Sweeney, E. M., & Geller, J. L. (1998). Mothers with mental illness II: Family relationships and the context of parenting. *Psychiatric Services*, 49, 643-649.

30. Oates, M. (1997). Patients as parents: The risk to children. *British Journal of Psychiatry*, 170(32), 22-27.

31. Rolland, J. (1987). Chronic illness and the life cycle: A conceptual framework. *Family Process*, 26, 203-221.Rosenfield (1997)

32. Rutter, M., & Quinton, D. (1984). Parental psychiatric disorder: Effects on children. *Psychological Medicine*, 14, 853-80.

33. Rutter, M., & Silberg, J., O'Connor, T., & Siminoff, E. (1999). Genetics and child psychiatry: II. Empirical research findings. *Journal of Child Psychology & Psychiatry & Allied Disciplines*, 40, 19-55.

34. Seifer, R., & Dickstein, S. (1993). Parental mental illness and infant development. In Zeanah, C. H. Jr., et al. (Eds.). *Handbook of infant mental health* (pp. 120-142). New York: Guilford Press.

35. Solnit, A. J., & Leckman, J.F. (1984). On the study of children of parents with affective disorders. *American Journal of Psychiatry*, 141, 241-242.

36. Ware, J.E., Snow, K. K., & Kosinski, M. (1993). *SF-36 Health Survey: Manual and Interpretation Guide*, Boston, MA: The Health Institute, New England Medical Center.

37. Zahn-Waxler, C., Cummings, E., McKnew, D., & Radke-Yarrow, M. (1984). Altruism, aggression, and social interactions in young children with a manic-depressive parent. *Child Development*, 55(1), 112-122.

38. Zemencuk, J., Rogosch, F.A., & Mowbray, C. T. (1995). The seriously mentally ill woman in the role of parent: Characteristics, parenting sensitivity, and needs. *Psychosocial Rehabilitation Journal*, 18(3), 77–92.

16

Relationship Between Work Stress and Body Mass Index

T. Rajeswari*, T. Sandhya, P. Veerraju*****

ABSTRACT

Obesity has been recognized as a global epidemic threatening of life. Today in India obesity defined as a body mass index (BMI) greater than 27 kg/m^2. The proportion of overweight and obese people has grown rapidly, and obesity has now been widely recognized as an important public health problem. At the same time, stress has increased in working life. Stress can be one of the major underlying causes of Obesity in some people. Stress has a direct influence on metabolism, weight and the fat accumulation. We used cross-sectional questionnaire data obtained from 205 female and male employees of a private organization. In women, physical health deteriorated monotonically with increasing BMI, whereas in men, poor physical health was found among the obese only.This study shows an association between work stress and BMI.

* **Department of Human Genetics, Andhra University, Visakhapatnam, India.**

** **Department of Chemistry, G.V.P. Degree College, Visakhapatnam, India.**

*** **Professor, Department of Human Genetics, Andhra University, Visakhapatnam, India.**

INTRODUCTION

Obesity is a burgeoning problem in the developed world, and certain behaviors, such as increased portion sizes and reduced physical activity, can help explain why the obesity epidemic is spreading (Brunner EJ, et al, 2007). The World Health Organization estimates the number of obese people will almost double to at least 700 million in 2012 from 400 million in 2005. While the problem of obesity has been well publicized, clinicians should also understand that societal factors play a prominent role in obesity.

There is increasing evidence that obesity and overweight may be related, in part, to adverse work conditions. Studies with various methodologies have reported that job pressures and job strain are positively associated with BMI. Business globalization during the last 10 years has greatly affected society and the life of people. The worldwide market has prompted 24 hours operation in many companies resulting in the need for a large number of shift or night workers, which in turn has changed all of society to a 24 hours operating basis. This has imposed on changes in the lifestyle and behavior of all people. Since in the early 1950s, the prevalence of overweight and obesity has been increasing in most industrialized nations, however, this trend accelerated in the 1990s.

Obesity was associated with psychological tension and anxiety, much of which was derived from high demands and poor decision latitude at work (Nishitani N, et al, 2006). The effects of stress at work constitute a major public health issue. Stress is a fundamental experience of modern work, and several models have been used to provide a formal description of their relationship in an attempt to design company-wide programs of intervention capable of minimizing the impact of stress on organizational, economic, and health outcomes mechanisms linking work stress to cardiovascular risk are complex. Overweight or obesity may exert other significant effects on the development of various health problems in occupational populations. Osteoarthritis and neck pain, sleep apnea and consequent daytime sleepiness, adult-onset bronchial asthma, and accidents and absence from the workplace have been reported to relate to obesity.

There is a trend increasing prevalence of overweight and obesity in the adult population in INDIA. Lifestyle-related factors such as high blood pressure, drinking habits, diet, and physical inactivity are well established determinants of obesity. So-called lifestyle behaviors are themselves influenced by strategies people use to cope with stress.

An imbalance between work and associated individual factors (financial, self-esteem, marital and social) gained from work results in an increased risk of ill health Stress as a risk factor for poor health has been examined less frequently in population studies. Recent population-based research has demonstrated an association between living in an unsafe neighborhood and poor self-rated health, further supporting the theory that stress influences population health. Work stress might also contribute to the prevalence of obesity, and the current study addresses this issue in a cohort of computer workers followed over time. Although the association between current obesity and work stress is well known, the cumulative effect of obesity is unknown. Using data from the present study, we examined the association between BMI with work stress.

The aim of the present study is to report the prevalence of high levels of overweight and obesity as risk factors as defined by the WHO (WHO, 2004). The WHO has recommended that the optimal BMI for Asian populations be narrowed to 18.5-23 kg/m2.

DEFINITIONS/CUTOFF POINTS

The purpose of a BMI cutoff point is to identify the proportion of people within each population with a high risk of a health condition that warrants a public health or clinical intervention. Although the definition of obesity differs in Western populations, a BMI of 27 kg/m^2 was used as the cutoff value for the population under study, as defined by the World Health Organization for the Indian population. Asian populations typically have a different percentage of body fat related to BMI and have a high risk for type 2 diabetes and cardiovascular diseases.

According to the WHO consultation, the additional BMI cutoff points for Asian populations are 23 kg/m^2 (overweight and at increased risk for BMI-associated diseases) and 27kg/m^2 or higher (obese and at high risk for BMI-associated diseases). Because reported job strain varies between men and women, analyses were stratified by sex.

METHODS

The aim of the study was to examine the relationship between psychosocial and other working conditions and body-mass index (BMI) in a working population. Self-administered health behavior survey which also assessed socio demographic and job-related characteristics, including perception of work strain.

The study was publicized among the workers through a letter and participation in the study was on a volunteer basis. The workers answered a questionnaire with questions on demographic, occupational and lifestyle characteristics and a Standardized clinic-based assessment of BMI, self-reported functional health status assessment was collected along with the interview method to estimate overweight and obesity prevalence among computer professionals, Visakhapatnam using BMI criteria suggested by the World Health Organization for Asian populations worldwide.

The demographic characteristics are gender (male and female), age (<29, 30-39, 40-49 and > 50 years) and BMI. Other potential risk factors examined included age, prior stress symptoms marital status, marital relationship, work-related mental strain, and the social support and information about work stress was obtained by self-report in interviews and these are answered as Very satisfied, satisfied, and dissatisfied for the assessment of work stress.

RESULTS

Table 1 shows sex differences in BMI. Body Mass Index (BMI) of computer professionals, Visakhapatnam Using World Health Organization Criteria for Asian Adults, 2004 (N = 205).

Table 1

Prevalence of Overweight/Obesity by Age and Sex

Age group	*Males Nanobese (BMI≤23) (N±S.E)*	*Obese (BM≥23)*	*Females Nanobese (BMI≤23) (N±S.E)*	*Obese (BMI≥23)*	*Total Nanobese (BMI≤23) (N±S.E)*	*Obese (BMI≥23)*	X^2
20-29 yrs. (n=41)	13±0.13	03±0.33	12±0.13	13±0.12	25±0.09	16±0.11	**19.8
30-39 yrs. (n=42)	09±0.16	06±0.18	06±0.21	21±0.09	15±0.012	27±0.08	
40-49 yrs. (n=88)	36±0.06	13±0.09	24±0.07	15±0.11	60±0.04	28±0.07	
50+yrs. (n=34)	15±0.11	00	09±0.16	10±0.15	24±0.09	10±0.15	
Total=205	**73±0.04**	**22±0.10**	**51±0.06**	**59±0.05**	**124±0.02**	**81±0.04**	

** The two-tailed P value is less than 0.0001 is considered to be extremely statistically significant.

There were sex differences in workstress and other job and health characteristics central to this study. This sex difference was found in the BMI risk age groups 30-49 and 40-49. There was no difference in the younger age groups and also in elderly groups.

Table 2

The prevalence of BMI by Sex in the total population

BMI	*Women NO (%±SE) Mean ± SE*	*Men NO (%±SE) Mean ± SE*	*Total NO (%±SE) Mean ± SE*	
<23 (normal)	51(46.4±0.05) 21.2±0.10	73(76.84±0.02) 22.12±0.09	124(60.49±0.02) 21.66±0.09	* t=46.9
≥23 (overweight/ obse	59(53.6±0.04) 27.6±0.08	22(23.16±0.09) 28.3±0.08	81(39.51±0.04) 27.9±0.09	
Total	**110**	**95**	**205**	

* The two-tailed P value less than 0.0001 by conventional criteria; this difference is considered to be extremely statistically significant. (df=203).

In the present study , The population average BMI <23 is 60.49%(N=124) of the population was non obese, but the 39.51%(95) are obese people, which are very high and alarming, due to the risk factors related with overweight and obesity.

The mean BMI in non obese population is 21.66, and in overweight or obese population the mean BMI value is 27.9. In women it was higher than in men. Our study showed that women were more likely to be overweight and obese than men. This factor significantly correlates with previous studies.

We have shown that the association of with clustered individual risk factors appears to be mediated by BMI. Our results appeared not to be modified by BMI. Young adults were found to have experienced more occupational stress than the middle aged. Work strain was associated with BMI (45.6%).

Table 3

Associations with Individual Factors of BMI and sex in the total population

Variables	*Nanobese*		*Obese*		*Total nanobese N (124) (%)*	*Total obese N (81) (%)*	*Total N(205) (%)*
	F	*M*	*F*	*M*			
Marital status							
Married	49	41	33	29	90(72.5)	62(76.5)	152(74.1)
Single	21	13	11	08	34(27.4)	19(23.4)	53(25.8)
Children (N=152)							
≤ 2	22	18	09	13	40(32.2)	22(27.1)	62(30.2)
≤ 3	16	11	17	11	27(21.7)	28(34.5)	55(26.8)
None	11	12	07	05	23(18.5)	12(14.8)	35(17)
Marital relationship							
Very satisfied	06	11	08	03	17(13.7)	11(13.5)	28(13.6)
Satisfied	32	22	21	10	54(43.5)	31(38.2)	85(41.4)
Dissatisfied	11	08	04	16	19(15.3)	20(24.6)	39(19)
Work career							
Very satisfied	12	10	08	06	22(17.7)	14(17.2)	36(17.5)
Satisfied	23	25	25	05	48(38.7)	30(37)	78(38)
Dissatisfied	16	38	20	17	54(43.5)	37(45.6)	91(44.3)

(Contd...)

Variables	*Nanobese*		*Obese*		*Total nanobese N (124) (%)*	*Total obese N (81) (%)*	*Total N(205) (%)*
	F	*M*	*F*	*M*			
Social activities							
Very satisfied	19	26	22	08	45(36.2)	30(37)	75(36.5)
Satisfied	16	25	20	06	41(33)	26(32)	67(32.6)
Dissatisfied	16	22	17	08	38(30)	25(30.8)	63(30.7)

Women who were dissatisfied with combining paid work and associated life factors were more likely to have gained weight. Men with low job demands were less likely to have gained weight. All of these associations were independent of each other.

Table 4

Risk of Work stress (%) and BMI in the total population

Work stress	*Nonobese (BMI<23) N=124(%)*	*Obese (BMI>23) N=81(%)*	*Total N=205 (%)*
Unreasonable pressure	36(29)	24(29.6)	60(29.2)
Powerlessness	18(14.5)	17(21)	35(17)
Strenuous working conditions	46(37)	32(39.5)	78(38)
Responsibility for person	62(50)	44(54)	106(51.7)
Work Supervision	35(28)	19(23)	54(26.3)
Pay	54(43.5)	34(53)	88(42.9)
Shift work	28(22.5)	32(39.5)	60(29.2)
Day work	16(12.9)	12(14.8)	28(13.6)

The prevalence of obesity was higher among shift workers compared to day workers, Shift workers had higher BMI than day workers, and shift working was associated with BMI. Job demands were positively associated with BMI. Pay (53%) and Powerlessness also associated with increasing BMI (21%). The responsibility for person (54%) shows more impact on Obesity and related risk factors. This study offers some evidence that self-reported job demands, and, to a lesser degree strain, is associated with the BMI.

DISCUSSION

Studies of psychosocial working conditions and BMI have demonstrated an association between high job strain (Kouvonen A, et al, 2005), pressures on the job (House JS, etal, 1986) and a borderline association between high psychological demand and BMI .These results indicate that demands, control, or some combination of these may be associated with increased BMI but clear results from this small number, of largely cross-sectional studies, do not emerge.

Previous studies from this group have shown cross sectional and longitudinal relations of employment grade or work stress with central obesity and weight gain. (Kivimaki M, et al, 2006). Inherent in the job-strain model is the assumption that work characteristics, such as conflicting demands, time pressure, working hard, etc., are universally 'demanding' to all workers. However, individuals differ in their response to the same events and in methods for coping with work-related stress (Wendy L Hellerstedt et al, 1997).

Our population-based sample is representative of occupational groups in the general population. Therefore, our findings can be generalized to the general working population. However, some limitations must be taken into account. First, the cross-sectional design of our study cannot support causal inferences between occupational factors and BMI. Second, information on independent and dependant variables except BMI were collected using self-reports.

The present study also agrees with previous studies that the impact on the subjective health of participants is due mostly to an increased rate of associated diseases, but also by adding to the total disease load in the single individual. (Wandell PE, 2005).

Our findings suggest that psychosocial work conditions may impact BMI, particularly among men, and that largely independently of stress at work and longer working hours among men may increase BMI.

CONCLUSION

Few work-related factors were associated with weight gain. BMI was found to be a useful index for the prediction of stress. Findings extend existing evidence of the work stress consequences of obesity in this representative sample, and suggest that obesity may have long-term implications for distress in computer workers. Shift work may be directly responsible for increased body mass index

Furthermore, it has been clearly shown that urbanization affects prevalence, with higher rates in urban areas than in rural communities (Athyros VG, et al, 2005).

There are several limitations that should be considered when interpreting the .findings from this study. It is difficult to infer a causal relationship, and it is impossible to determine its direction from cross-sectional data. Although we studied for several potential confounders such as gender, age group, behaviour. However, we did not observe any association and It is difficult to assess the validity of these self-reports.

REFERENCES

1. Athyros VG, Bouloukos VI, Pehlivanidis AN, Papageorgiou AA, Dionysopoulou SG, Symeonidis AN, Petridis DI, Kapousouzi MI, Satsoglou EA, Mikhailidis DP. The prevalence of the metabolic syndrome in Greece: The MetS-Greece Multicentre Study. *Diabetes Obes Metab.* 2005; **7: 397**-405. doi: 10.1111/j.1463-1326.2004.00409.x.

2. Brunner EJ, Chandola T, Marmot MG. Prospective effect of job strain on general and central obesity in the Whitehall II Study. Am J Epidemiol. 2007; 165: 828-837.

3. Georges E, Wear M: **Body fat distribution and job stress in Mexican-American men of the Hispanic Health and Nutrition Examination Study.** *American Journal of Human Biology* 1992, **4:** 657-667.

4. House JS, Strecher V, Metzner HL, Robbins CA: **Occupational stress and health among men and women in the Tecumseh Community Health Study.** *Journal of health and social behavior* 1986, **27:** 62-77.

5. Kouvonen A, Kivimaki M, Cox SJ, Cox T, Vahtera J: **Relationship between work stress and body mass index among 45,810 female and male employees.** *Psychosom Med* 2005, **67:** 577-583.

6. Kivimaki M, Head J, Ferrie JE, Shipley MJ, Brunner E, Vahtera J, et al. Work stress, weight gain and weight loss: evidence for bidirectional effects of job strain on body mass index in the Whitehall II study. *Int J Obes* advance online publication, 17 January 2006; doi:10.1038/sj.ijo.0803229.

7. Nishitani N, Sakakibara H. Relationship of obesity to job stress and eating behavior in male Japanese workers. *Int J Obes* (Lond). 2006; 30:528-533.

8. Wandell PE. Quality of life of patients with diabetes mellitus. An overview of research in primary health care in the Nordic countries. *Scand J Prim Health Care.* 2005; **23:68**–74. doi: 10.1080/02813430510015296.

9. Wendy L Hellerstedt and Robert W Jeffery The Association of Job Strain and Health Behaviours in Men and Women. *International Journal of Epidemiology,* 1997.

10. World Health Organization Expert Consultation. Appropriate body-mass index for Asian populations and its implications for policy and intervention strategies. *Lancet*. 2004; 363: 157-163.

SECTION—2
HEALTH AND LIFE STYLE

17

Prevalence of Low Back Pain, Sleeplessness and Headache Towards Occupational Stress

M.V.R.Raju*, N.D.S. Naga Seema**

ABSTRACT

The study attempts to investigate the significance and influence of low back pain, sleeplessness and headache with Occupational Stress. The total sample for the study was 440 (Males 403 and Females 37). The Occupational Stress Index (A.K. Srivastava and A.P. Singh, 1981) was used. A quantitative survey method was employed using statistical procedures such as t-test, ANOVA and multiple regression. The findings of the study pointed out that sleeplessness, low back pain and headache significantly differed with Occupational Stress Factors. It was also revealed that age, number of children, monthly income, and service in present position significantly influenced occupational stress factors. Implications of the study would be discussed in line with findings.

Stress is a fundamental element that appears to adversely affect the well-being of individual employees as well as organizations as a whole (Quick, Murphy, & Hurrell, 1992; Schwartz, Pickering, & Lansbergis, 1996; Spector, Dwyer, & Jex,

* **Professor and Head, Department of Psychology, Andhra University, Visakhapatnam.**

** **Research Scholar, Department of Psychology, Andhra University, Visakhapatnam.**

1988; Wong, Cheuk, & Rosen, 2000 Salvo Lubbers, Rossi, and Lewis (1995) indicated that 50% to 80% of the diseases experienced by employees are stress-related, and that job-related stress results in organizational problems such as low job satisfaction and low productivity.

Growing concerns about the impact of occupational stress on both employee well-being and organizational effectiveness have stimulated efforts to understand the sources and consequences of stress in the workplace. Individual whose health or happiness has been ravaged by an inability to cope with the effects of job-related stress, the costs involved are only too clear. Stress-related problems exact a heavy toll on individuals' lives (Watts & Cooper, 1998).

According to Cox (1985) stress is "a complex psychological state deriving from the person's cognitive appraisal of the adaptation to the demands of the work environment".

Working conditions of jobs have been linked to physical and mental health. It was found that poor mental health related directly to unpleasant work conditions, physical effort and speed in job performance and excessive, inconvenient hours (e.g. shifts). In addition, researchers have found increasing evidence that repetitive and dehumanizing environments adversely affect physical health (Cooper & Marshall, 1978; Kornhauser, 1965; Osipow, 1998; Osipow & Davis, 1988; Sharit & Salvendy, 1982)

The total number of hours that a person works can produce strain. Numerous studies have found a significant correlation between the overall number of hours worked and various indices of health and well-being. Individuals working more than 48 hours a week are most susceptible to health problems. Deosthalee & Pravin G (2000) explored the effect of gender, age and educational qualification on occupational stress experienced by 152 male and 46 female engineers working in different organizations.

Srivasthava (2002) examined the relationship between job and life stress and health outcomes of management personnel. As compared to Job stress, life stress was found to be a stronger predictor of health outcomes life stress was significantly related to higher systolic BP, PHC, and PHH. Aminabhavi (2002) compared Occupational stress among 78 employees of Nationalized and Non-

Nationalized banks. Analysis revealed that nationalized bank employees reported significantly higher occupational stress than the non-nationalized bank employees.

Misra (1997) examined the differences were found between reported occupational stress among public & private sector public relation officers. Higher stress was reported by public sector public relation officers. Elovainio et al. (2003) found that sleeping problems and health behaviors (alcohol consumption) mediate the association between organizational justice and employee health. Spector (2002) identified that occupational stress has been recognized as a major health issue for modern work organizations. The study highlighted the condition of the workplace that have been shown to lead to negative emotional reactions (e.g., anxiety), physical health problems in both the short term (e.g., headache or stomach distress) and the long term (e.g., cardio vascular disorders), and counter productive behavior at work.

METHOD

Objectives

- To examine the significant difference between Biographical variables with Occupational Stress.
- To identify the influence and interaction between Occupational Stress and Sleeplessness, Low back pain and Headache.

Method

Sample

The sample for the present study consisted of 440 employees working in Visakhapatnam Steel Plant. The male were 403 and female 37. Their age ranged from below 30 years to above 50 years.

Independent variables were age group, number of children, monthly income, and years of service in present position, physical health problems, sleeplessness, low back pain, headache.

Experimental Design

A Quantitative study utilizing survey research methods. Random sampling technique was employed. The data were analyzed using both descriptive and inferential statistical techniques according to the objectives of the study and nature of the data.

Statistical Analysis

Various statistical techniques were employed as deemed appropriate in view of the objectives of the study and as dictated by the nature of the data. Inferential statistics ANOVA, t-test and multiple regression.

The results and discussions are presented as follows:

1. Biographical Variables and Occupational Stress
2. Physical Health Factors and Occupational Stress
3. Multiple regression analysis by taking each Physical health variable as dependent variable and Occupational stress dimension as Independent variable.

The table 1 indicates that the age of the employees has a significant influence on occupational stress dimensions like role conflict (m=15.71) and unreasonable group/political pressures (m=12.57). Employees aged below 30 years have significantly higher mean scores on these dimensions as compared to their older counterparts (aged 31-40 years, 41-50 years and above 50 years). It is possible that due to less age employees with less work experience new to the job, experience role conflict and unreasonable group/political pressures.

Employees below 30 years are young, enthusiastic with fresh and creative thoughts. They want to work enthusiastically but experiences role conflict due to contradictory instruction given by their immediate boss or senior/top level management for which they find difficult to fulfill. Role conflict is least experienced by employees with above 50 years age group when compared to below 30 years. This is possible due to good amount of experience in the job, elder age group i.e. above 50 years are less frequent to experience role conflict.

Biographical Variables and Occupational Stress

Table 1

Descriptive statistics of occupational stress scores by Age group

Occupational Stress Factors		*Age in years*				F
		Below 30 N=7	*31-40* N=176	*41-50* N=195	*Above50* N=62	
Role Over load	Mean	18.00	16.66	16.88	16.63	0.394
	SD	4.47	3.41	3.95	3.58	
Role Ambiguity	Mean	10.00	9.80	9.88	9.60	0.221
	SD	4.24	2.53	2.33	2.65	
Role Conflict	Mean	15.71	13.78	13.42	13.13	2.371*
	SD	3.68	2.87	2.55	3.40	
Unreasonable group/political pressure	Mean	12.57	11.09	11.00	11.85	2.176*
	SD	3.78	2.80	2.52	3.21	
Responsibility for persons	Mean	11.43	10.17	10.14	10.52	1.476
	SD	3.15	1.88	1.90	2.32	

(Contd...)

Occupational Stress Factors		*Age in years*				*F*
		Below 30 N=7	*31-40* N=176	*41-50* N=195	*Above50* N=62	
Under participation	Mean	12.57	11.65	11.72	11.19	1.125
	SD	1.13	2.37	2.41	2.58	
Powerlessness	Mean	9.71	9.27	9.06	8.82	1.116
	SD	0.76	1.96	1.87	2.07	
Poor peer relations	Mean	13.71	12.68	12.81	12.53	0.665
	SD	2.56	2.06	2.44	2.65	
Intrinsic impoverishment	Mean	10.86	10.59	10.71	10.32	0.420
	SD	2.41	2.32	2.47	2.90	
Low status	Mean	7.71	7.70	7.98	8.24	1.233
	SD	2.75	2.00	2.00	2.30	
Strenuous working condition	Mean	12.43	10.42	10.75	10.44	2.024
	SD	2.07	2.46	2.36	2.48	
Un-profitability	Mean	5.29	5.22	5.35	5.40	0.326
	SD	0.95	1.54	1.43	1.66	

Significant $^*p<0.05$ level.

Unreasonable group and political pressure is also experienced by the younger age group of employees below 30years. It is possible as they are young, new to the job role with less work experience, experiences with groups which are not directly important but hinders the working by its interference such as making adjustments between group pressures and formulate rules and instruction, working unwillingly due to certain group/political pressures in the order to maintain group conformity.

Employees above 50 years are second highest to experience unreasonable group/political pressure. It is possible due to their age factor, experience they are all prone to unreasonable group pressure in order to maintain group conformity.

The table-2 indicates that employees number of children has a significant influence on occupational stress dimensions like responsibility for persons, powerlessness, poor peer relations, low stress and un-profitability.

Employees having two children have significantly higher mean score (10.42) on the dimension responsibility for persons as compared to other groups of no. of children (one, three & above and none). Employees having more than three children have significantly higher mean scores on the dimension powerlessness (m = 10.03), poor peer relations (m = 12.87) and low status (m = 8.74) employees having no children (none) are significantly high on un-profitability (m =5.55).

Responsibility for persons is high among employees having two children. It refers to the improvement and development of the people which can consequently head to the prosperity of the organization. This applies to the family setting as well. Employees with two children are interested to develop their children in all aspects which lead to the overall development of their children.

Employees having children 3 and above are significant on the occupational stress dimension powerlessness. Feelings of powerlessness exist among employees having children 3 and above when suggestions or orders are not paid much attention concerning distribution of assignments, it indicates the employees having children 3 and above feel that they are unable to hold control over their children, fulfil the child's needs and other requirements to make them satisfied.

Table 2

Descriptive statistics of occupational stress scores by Number of Children

Occupational Stress Factors		No. of Children				
		One N=106	*Two* N=92	*Thee and above* N=31	*None* N=11	*F*
Role Over load	Mean	17.01	16.80	16.03	16.09	0.689
	SD	3.55	3.70	4.09	3.75	
Role Ambiguity	Mean	9.50	9.86	10.13	10.55	1.079
	SD	2.23	2.55	2.64	2.70	
Role Conflict	Mean	13.57	13.57	13.42	13.73	0.038
	SD	2.73	2.86	2.92	3.47	
Unreasonable group/political pressure	Mean	11.26	11.19	10.55	11.91	0.824
	SD	2.51	2.77	3.55	2.77	
Responsibility for persons	Mean	9.92	10.42	9.61	9.64	3.112*
	SD	1.88	1.95	2.50	1.75	

(Contd…)

Poor Peer relations is also experienced by employees having children 3 and above are frustrated due to their children's education and future plans as a result worry a lot about their children. They cannot facilitate but hinders the proceedings of the tasks in the work situation.

Low status is experienced by employees having children 3 and above. It is possible because the status of the employee has in the society due to the nature and position of the job is affected by the number of children.

Un-profitability is experienced by employees having no children at all. This is possible because, there are less or no reward is being benefited in comparison to the input in the job is high among the employees. Employees having no children, feel less rewarded in the society as well as feels insecure in the organization.

Table 3 indicates that monthly income of employees have significant influence on occupational stress dimensions like unreasonable group/political pressure, responsibility for persons, powerlessness and poor peer relations, employees monthly income 20,000/- to 25,000/- are highly significant on unreasonable group/political pressure (m =11.65) and responsibility for persons (m=10.69) employees monthly income ranged 15,000/- – 20,000/- are significant on the factor powerlessness (m = 9.46) and poor peer relations (m = 12.79) was significant on employees monthly income (25,000/- and above).

Employees monthly incomes (20,000/- to 25,000/-) are significant on the Occupational Stress dimension unreasonable group and political pressure. It is possible as there employees belong to middle level management as a result experience interference or group pressure from the superiors as a result they experience highly unreasonable group/political pressure.

Responsibility for persons is also high among employees whose monthly income is (20,000/- to 25,000/-). Employees of this group are satisfied with their job as a result feel responsible to the improvement and development of the people which can consequently lead to the prosperity of the organization.

Table 3

Descriptive statistics of occupational stress scores by Monthly Income

Occupational Stress Factors		*Monthly income (in thousands)* 15,000/- to 20,000/-N = 81	20,000/- to 25,000 N = 101	Above 25,000/- N = 258	*F*
Role Over load	Mean	16.27	17.16	16.79	1.301
	SD	3.42	3.05	3.99	
Role Ambiguity	Mean	9.62	9.79	9.88	0.336
	SD	2.08	2.34	2.66	
Role Conflict	Mean	13.70	13.56	13.51	0.140
	SD	2.53	2.92	2.91	
Unreasonable group/political pressure	Mean	10.02	11.65	11.36	9.389**
	SD	3.00	2.78	2.60	
Responsibility for persons	Mean	9.65	10.69	10.22	6.309**
	SD	2.10	1.92	1.93	

(Contd...)

Occupational Stress Factors		*Monthly income (in thousands)*			
		15,000/- to 20,000/-N = 81	*20,000/- to 25,000 N = 101*	*Above 25,000/- N = 258*	*F*
Under participation	Mean	11.84	11.36	11.67	0.994
	SD	2.30	2.24	2.50	
Powerlessness	Mean	9.46	8.68	9.19	4.038*
	SD	2.12	1.72	1.92	
Poor peer relations	Mean	12.79	12.22	12.91	3.290*
	SD	2.53	2.22	2.28	
Intrinsic impoverishment	Mean	10.49	10.61	10.64	0.113
	SD	2.26	2.47	2.54	
Low status	Mean	7.51	7.90	8.03	2.020
	SD	1.78	1.93	2.17	
Strenuous working condition	Mean	10.37	10.46	10.73	0.930
	SD	2.55	2.14	2.48	
Un-profitability	Mean	5.22	5.43	5.28	0.479
	SD	1.55	1.42	1.51	

Significant *$p<0.05$ level

Significant**$p<0.01$level

Employees monthly income being (15,000/- to 20,000/-) are significant on powerlessness. It indicates that employees under lower level management feels that their suggestion or orders in the job are not paid much attention concerning appointments, training programmes at higher levels, as a result feelings of powerlessness exist. Sometimes the employees feel that the organization is not utilizing their skills, opinions, suggestion, decision in making important appointments, training programme.

Employees with monthly income above 25,000/- are significant on poor peer relations due to lack of mutual poor peer relations. An employee drawing monthly income 25,000/- above feels that some of their colleagues and subordinates try to defame and malign them as unsuccessful; this is possible according to their position, seniority and high salary.

Table 4 indicates that employees years of service in the present position has a significant influence on occupational stress dimensions like role overload, powerlessness, poor peer relations, intrinsic impoverishment, low status and strenuous working condition.

Employees service in present position (11-15 years) have significantly higher mean score on role overload (m=21.00), powerlessness (m = 11.00), intrinsic impoverishment (m= 11.30), low status (m=9.20) and strenuous working condition (m = 13.00) and the employees whose service in present position was below 5 years significantly have higher mean score on the dimension poor peer relation (m = 12.89).

Employees working for number of years in current position (11-15 years) are highly significant on role overload. It is possible due to working in the same department and in the same position for more number of years they feel that there are too many expectation from the significant roles in their role set and as a result experience role overload.

Table 4

Descriptive statistics of occupational stress scores by Service in present position

Occupational Stress Factors		*Service in present position (in years)*					
		Below 5 N=328	*5-10* N=68	*11-15* N=10	*16-20* N=22	*Above 20* N=12	*F*
Role Over load	Mean	16.71	16.84	21.00	15.64	16.92	3.936**
	SD	3.58	3.66	5.72	3.72	2.97	
Role Ambiguity	Mean	9.72	10.38	9.80	9.41	9.67	1.157
	SD	2.48	2.60	2.15	2.36	2.31	
Role Conflict	Mean	13.48	13.79	15.20	12.86	14.33	1.575
	SD	2.89	2.69	1.40	2.61	3.34	
Unreasonable group/political pressure	Mean	11.02	11.62	11.50	11.18	12.83	1.819
	SD	2.79	2.87	1.72	2.34	2.59	
Responsibility for persons	Mean	10.13	10.43	10.90	10.18	11.17	1.330
	SD	2.07	1.61	0.74	1.82	2.29	

(Contd...)

Occupational Stress Factors		*Service in present position (in years)*					F
		Below 5 N=328	*5-10* N=68	*11-15* N=10	*16-20* N=22	*Above 20* N=12	
Under participation	Mean	11.61	11.94	12.30	11.55	10.08	1.739
	SD	2.45	2.12	2.00	2.91	1.83	
Powerlessness	Mean	9.07	9.32	11.00	8.59	8.67	3.263*
	SD	1.86	1.94	2.49	2.20	1.92	
Poor peer relations	Mean	12.89	12.21	12.70	11.86	12.83	2.057*
	SD	2.36	2.27	2.02	1.78	1.11	
Intrinsic impoverishment	Mean	10.58	11.12	11.30	9.77	9.42	2.282*
	SD	2.47	2.61	2.26	2.29	1.51	
Low status	Mean	7.81	8.31	9.20	7.91	7.08	2.328*
	SD	1.98	2.04	4.13	1.74	1.78	
Strenuous working condition	Mean	10.55	10.62	13.00	9.77	11.58	3.723**
	SD	2.35	2.48	3.13	2.62	1.98	
Un-profitability	Mean	5.22	5.53	5.90	5.27	5.83	1.408
	SD	1.46	1.66	0.74	1.83	1.03	

Significant *p<0.05 level.

Significant **p<0.01 level.

Employees working in present position (11-15 years) are significant on powerlessness. It is possible due to the level of designation, difference in educational qualification and seniority level and also number of years of experience. They experience that they are not paid much attention concerning distribution of assignment, appointments and training programme therefore feelings of powerlessness exist.

Employees working in the present position for below 5 years are significant of poor peer relations. This is possible because employees in the present position are high on their job role, filled with creative and enthusiasm as a result they experience that their colleague do not cooperate with these voluntarily in solving administration problems, tries to defame them and lack sufficient mutual co-operation.

Employees working in the present position between 11-15 years are significant on intrinsic impoverishment. Due to monotonous assignments, lack of opportunity in utilizing abilities, employees experience deficiency within the job due to working in the same position for many years.

Employees working in the present position 11-15years are significant of low status. There is a feeling that their job did not enhanced their social statues, and also feels that working so long higher authorities did not give due significance to their post and work.

Employees working in the present position 11-15 years are significant on strenuous working condition. Employees working in the present position for so many years continuous to work under these circumstances, risky and complicated as a result their job involved either psychological or physical risk.

PHYSICAL HEALTH FACTORS AND OCCUPATIONAL STRESS

Table 5

Sleeplessness and Occupational stress

Occupational Stress Factors	*Sleeplessness N=19*		*No sleeplessness N=421*		*'t' Value*
	Mean	*SD*	*Mean*	*SD*	
Role Overload	17.84	3.89	16.73	3.68	1.2862
Role Ambiguity	11.89	3.07	9.71	2.42	3.7946**
Role Conflict	15.42	3.91	13.48	2.76	2.9446**
Unreasonable group/ political pressure	13.74	3.00	11.06	2.71	4.1906**
Responsibility for Persons	10.68	1.38	10.20	2.01	1.0313
Under participation	11.95	2.50	11.62	2.41	0.5874
Powerlessness	9.89	1.97	9.09	1.92	1.7948
Poor Peer Relations	13.79	2.68	12.68	2.30	2.0380*
Intrinsic Impoverishment	11.58	2.27	10.57	2.47	1.7537
Low Status	8.26	2.56	7.89	2.03	0.7773
Strenuous Working Condition	12.95	2.88	10.50	2.35	4.4040**
Un-profitability	5.00	1.73	5.32	1.49	0.9066

Significant *p<0.05 level, Significant **p<0.01 level

Table 5 indicates that employees who suffer with Sleeplessness experience Role Ambiguity (m = 11.89), Role Conflict (m = 15.42), Unreasonable group/political pressure (m = 13.74), Poor Peer Relations (m = 13.79) and Strenuous Working Condition (m = 12.95).

It is possible because insufficient sleep leads to poor performance as a result employees are not clear about the various expectations of people, faces contradictory instructions, and experiences unreasonable group/political pressure, poor peer relation and strenuous working conditions.

Table 6

Low back pain and occupational stress

Occupational Stress Factors	*low back pain N=61*		*No low back pain N=379*		*'t' Value*
	Mean	*SD*	*Mean*	*SD*	
Role Overload	17.95	3.89	16.59	3.63	2.6939**
Role Ambiguity	10.89	3.12	9.64	2.33	3.6944**
Role Conflict	14.28	3.14	13.44	2.78	2.1392*
Unreasonable group/political pressure	11.67	3.20	11.10	2.69	1.4985
Responsibility for Persons	10.28	1.84	10.22	2.01	0.2274
Under participation	12.38	2.11	11.51	2.44	2.6283**
Powerlessness	9.05	1.70	9.13	1.96	0.3109
Poor Peer Relations	12.80	2.15	12.72	2.36	0.2665
Intrinsic Impoverishment	11.46	2.88	10.47	2.37	2.9202**
Low Status	8.15	2.11	7.87	2.05	0.9950
Strenuous Working Condition	10.67	2.32	10.59	2.44	0.2425
Un-profitability	5.36	1.24	5.30	1.54	0.3152

Significant *p<0.05 level, Significant **p<0.01 level.

Table 6 indicates a highly significant difference between low back pain and Occupational Stress variable. It is observed that employees who experience Role Overload (m = 17.95), Role Ambiguity (10.89), Role Conflict (m = 14.25=8), Under Participation (m = 12.38) and intrinsic impoverishment suffer with low back pain. Employees suffering with low back pain experience Role Ambiguity, Role Conflict, Under Participation and intrinsic impoverishment.

Employees with low back pain experience role overload. When there are too many expectations from the significant role in the job they continuously work on these expectation and accomplishes the tasks as a result they are both physically and mentally involved during meeting too many expectations and accomplishments for which they significantly suffer with low back pain and experience role load.

Role Ambiguity is high on employees suffering with low back pain. This is because when employees confront too many jobs at once they experience physical and mental stress as a result they are unclear of the job and suffers with physical ailments as low back pain and experience role ambiguity.

Similarly role conflict significantly contributes to low back pain. Job involves not only mental strain but also physically the body is involved in accomplishing tasks. Therefore, employees suffering with low back pain experience role conflict.

Low back pain is highly significant on the occupational stress factor under participation. This is because due to serious physical illness like low back pain, employees feel that they lack opportunities to participate in important issues of the organization. Hence, employees experience under participation.

Low back pain is highly significant on the occupational stress factor intrinsic impoverishment. This is possible because employees with low back pain work continuously and feel their assignments as monotonous in nature and considers deficiency with in the job.

Table 7

Headache and occupational stress

Occupational Stress Factors	*Headache N = 51*		*No headache N = 389*		*'t' Value*
	Mean	*SD*	*Mean*	*SD*	
Role Overload	17.63	3.79	16.67	3.67	1.7531
Role Ambiguity	10.41	2.76	9.73	2.44	1.8460
Role Conflict	14.27	3.45	13.47	2.74	1.9176
Unreasonable group/ political pressure	12.45	3.29	11.01	2.65	3.5312**
Responsibility for Persons	10.41	2.03	10.20	1.98	0.7144
Under participation	12.24	2.25	11.55	2.42	1.9152
Powerlessness	9.65	2.05	9.05	1.90	2.0832*
Poor Peer Relations	13.00	2.31	12.69	2.33	0.8830
Intrinsic Impoverishment	11.24	2.91	10.53	2.40	1.9314
Low Status	7.96	2.15	7.90	2.04	0.2076
Strenuous Working Condition	11.71	2.32	10.46	2.40	3.5049**
Un-profitability	5.67	1.58	5.26	1.48	1.8428

Significant *$p<0.05$ level, Significant **$p<0.01$ level.

Table 7 indicates that Headache is highly significant (m = 12.45) with regard to unreasonable group/political pressure, powerlessness (m=9.65) and strenuous working condition (m = 11.71).

Employee's suffering with headache is highly significant on occupational stress dimension unreasonable group/political pressure. It is possible as employees have to do some work unwillingly owing to certain group/political pressures to maintain group conformity.

Employees suffering with headache are significant on powerlessness. Headaches are common among people but the reason varies from person to person. Therefore, feelings of powerlessness exist among the employees with headache, or orders are not paid much attention concerning distribution of assignments, making appointments for important posts.

Employees suffering with headache are highly significant on strenuous working condition. Employees with headaches are involved in jobs related psychological or physical risk. Hence, headaches contribute to experience strenuous working condition among the employees.

Multiple regression analysis by taking each Physical health variable as dependent variable and Occupational stress dimension independent variable.

Table 8 the dependent variable 'Sleeplessness' influences the occupational stress factors role ambiguity, unreasonable group/ political pressure, strenuous working condition and un-profitability and the t-value for role ambiguity is 2.35, un-profitability is 2.36 which is significant at 0.05 level. The t-value for unreasonable group/political pressure is 2.95 and strenuous working condition is 3.04 which are significant at 0.01 level.

Sleeplessness increases with role ambiguity. This is because sufficient amount of sleep is required, if sufficient sleep is not met then the physiological, personal and work life gets disturbed as a result employees suffer with unclear job role. When employees are not clear about the various expectations people have from their role, they faces the conflict known as role ambiguity.

Table 8

Regression Summary for Dependent Variable: Sleeplessness

Occupational Stress Factors	*BETA*	*St. Err. of BETA*	*B*	*St. Err. of B*	*t(427)*	*plevel*
Intercept			99.8012	0.0960	1040.0405	0.0000
Role Over load	0.0716	0.0603	0.0039	0.0033	1.1880	0.2355
Role Ambiguity	0.1409	0.0599	0.0115	0.0049	2.3534*	0.0191
Role Conflict	0.0310	0.0654	0.0022	0.0047	0.4745	0.6354
Unreasonable group pressure	0.1685	0.0570	0.0124	0.0042	2.9556**	0.0033
Responsibility for persons	0.0031	0.0512	0.0003	0.0052	0.0603	0.9520
Under participation	0.0299	0.0543	0.0025	0.0046	0.5511	0.5818
Powerlessness	0.0755	0.0563	0.0080	0.0059	1.3405	0.1808
Poor pear relations	0.0544	0.0514	0.0048	0.0045	1.0565	0.2913
Intrinsic impoverishment	0.0468	0.0553	0.0039	0.0046	0.8467	0.3976
Low status	0.0704	0.0518	0.0070	0.0051	1.3592	0.1748
Strenuous working condition	0.1807	0.0594	0.0152	0.0050	3.0415**	0.0025
Un-profitability	0.1181	0.0500	0.0161	0.0068	2.3613*	0.0187

Sleeplessness increases with unreasonable group/political pressure this is because employees are expected to do some work unwillingly owing to certain group/political pressure. Sometimes employees are compelled to violate the formal and administrative procedures and policies as a result found everything on top of them, feel constantly under strain hence suffers sleeplessness.

Sleeplessness increases with strenuous working conditions this can be due to employees being busy and occupied more, they take longer over the things they do as a result they experience their job under tense circumstances as a result sleeplessness increases.

Sleeplessness increases with un-profitability, when employees are not provided with any financial or non-financial benefits as reward in comparison to the input in the job as a result their morale comes down and results in sleeplessness.

Table 9

Regression Summary for Dependent Variable: Low back pain

Occupational Stress Factors	*BETA*	*St. Err. of BETA*	*B*	*St. Err. of B*	*t(427)*	*p level*
Intercept			101.2962	0.1650	613.8640	0.0000
Role Over load	0.1757	0.0610	0.0165	0.0057	2.8811**	0.0042
Role Ambiguity	0.1279	0.0606	0.0178	0.0084	2.1112*	0.0353
Role Conflict	0.0282	0.0662	0.0034	0.0081	0.4268	0.6697
Unreasonable groups	0.0129	0.0577	0.0016	0.0072	0.2229	0.8237
Responsibility for persons	0.0146	0.0518	0.0026	0.0090	0.2829	0.7774
Under participation	0.1557	0.0549	0.0224	0.0079	2.8356**	0.0048
Powerlessness	0.1156	0.0570	0.0207	0.0102	2.0289*	0.0431
Poor pear relations	0.0184	0.0520	0.0027	0.0077	0.3533	0.7240
Intrinsic impoverishment	0.1020	0.0560	0.0143	0.0078	1.8220	0.0691
Low status	0.0167	0.0524	0.0028	0.0088	0.3195	0.7495
Strenuous working condition	0.1358	0.0601	0.0194	0.0086	2.2597*	0.0243
Un-profitability	0.0347	0.0506	0.0080	0.0117	0.6859	0.4932

Table 9 shows that the dependent variable 'low back pain'

influences the occupational stress factors such as role overload, role ambiguity, under participation, powerlessness and strenuous working condition. The t-value for role overload is 2.88 and under participation is 2.83 which is significant at 0.01 level. The t-value for role ambiguity is 2.11, powerlessness is 2.02 and strenuous working condition is 2.25 which is significant at 0.05 level.

'Low back pain' influences the occupational stress factors such as role overload, low back pain increases and contributes to employees being unable to carry out their assignments to their satisfaction due to excessive work load and lack of time as a result experience constantly under stain.

Low back pain contributes to employees experiencing role ambiguity. When the employees are unclear about the various expectations people have from his role, they face the conflict known as role ambiguity which increases the physical health problem such as low back pain. Low back pain is experienced by employees and also contributes to the occupational stress factor under participation, this refers to lack of opportunities to participate in important issues of the organization. When employees suggestions are not paid much attention to, feelings of powerlessness exist and increases low back pain among the employees. Employees assignments are quite risky and complicated. Hence, low back pain increases with strenuous working conditions involving psychological and physical risk.

The present study highlighted the prevalence, influence and significance between physical health problems and occupational stress factors. Significant factors resulted in health problems and occupational stress where in employees below 30 years experiences role conflict and unreasonable group/political pressures. Employees having two children are significant on responsibility for persons. Employees having children 3 and above are significant on powerlessness, Poor Peer relations, Low status. Employees having no children experiences un-profitability. Employees monthly income in between 15,000/- to 20,000/- are significant on powerlessness.Employees monthly income 25,000/- and above are significant on poor peer relations. Employees whose service in present position is below 5 years are significant on poor peer relation. Employees whose service in present position is in between 11-15 years are significant on role overload, powerlessness intrinsic impoverishment, low status and strenuous working condition.

Table 10

Regression Summary for Dependent Variable: Headache

Occupational stress factors	*BETA*	*St. Err. of BETA*	*B*	*St. Err. of B*	*t(427)*	*p level*
Intercept			99.6477	0.1542	646.3399	0.0000
Role Over load	0.0188	0.0615	0.0016	0.0053	0.3058	0.7599
Role Ambiguity	0.0033	0.0611	0.0004	0.0079	0.0542	0.9568
Role Conflict	0.0661	0.0668	0.0074	0.0075	0.9895	0.3230
Unreasonable groups	0.1575	0.0582	0.0182	0.0067	2.7086**	0.0070
Responsibility for persons	0.0015	0.0522	0.0002	0.0084	0.0293	0.9767
Under participation	0.0836	0.0554	0.0111	0.0074	1.5102	0.1317
Powerlessness	0.0658	0.0574	0.0109	0.0096	1.1463	0.2523
Poor peer relations	0.0023	0.0525	0.0003	0.0072	0.0431	0.9657
Intrinsic impoverishment	0.0183	0.0564	0.0024	0.0073	0.3248	0.7455
Low status	0.0757	0.0528	0.0118	0.0082	1.4330	0.1526
Strenuous working condition	0.1333	0.0606	0.0176	0.0080	2.2000*	0.0283
Un-profitability	0.0413	0.0510	0.0088	0.0109	0.8092	0.4189

Table 10 shows that the dependent variable 'Headache' is influencing the occupational stress factors unreasonable group/political pressure and strenuous working conditions. The t-value for unreasonable group/political pressure is 2.70 which is significant at 0.01 level and the t-value for strenuous working condition is 2.20 which is significant at 0.05 level.

Increase in headache leads to unreasonable group/political pressure among employees. Employees are expected to do some work unwillingly owing to certain group/political pressure. Sometimes employees are compelled to violate the formal and administrative procedures and policies as a result found everything on top of them, feel constantly under strain and suffer with headache.

CONCLUSION

Sleeplessness contributes to role ambiguity, unreasonable group/political pressure, strenuous working condition and un-profitability. Employees suffering with sleeplessness experiences role ambiguity, role conflict, unreasonable group and political pressure, poor peer relations and strenuous working condition and also employees. Low back pain increases with role overload, role ambiguity, under participation, powerlessness and strenuous working condition. Employees suffering with low back pain experiences role overload and role conflict. Headache increases unreasonable group/political pressures and strenuous working condition. Employees suffering with headache experiences unreasonable group/political pressure, strenuous working conditions.

REFERENCES

Aminabhavi, Vijayalaxmi A., and Triveni (2000). Variables causing occupational stress in nationalized and non-nationalized bank employees. *Journal of community Guidance and Research*,17(1), 20-29.

Cooper, C.L. & Marshall, J. (1978). Sources of managerial and white-collar stress. In C.L. Cooper & R. Payne (Eds), *Stress at Work* (pp. 81-106). Chichester, UK: Wiley.

Cox, t. (1985). Stress (2nd Ed.). New York: Macmillan

Deosthalee, Pravin, G. (2000) Effect of Gender, age, and educational maturity on Job stress. Psycho-Lingura, 30(1), 57-60.

Elovainio, Markp; Kivim, Mika; Vahtera, Jussi; Keltikangas, Liisa; Virtanen, (2003) Sleeping problems and health behaviors as mediators between organizational justice and health *Marianna Health psychology*. 22(3), 287-293.

Kornhauser, A. (1965). Mental health of the industrial worker. New York, NY: Wiley.

Misra, M. (1997) Role stress in special groups. In D.M. Pestonjee (Ed), Stress and Coping. *The India Experience* (2nd ed.) P.P 137-215)New Delhi publications.

Osipow, S.H. (1998). *Occupational Stress Inventory - Revised Edition* (OS *I-R*). *Professional Manual*. Odessa, FL: Psychological Assessment Resources.

Osipow, S.H. & Davis, A. (1988). The Relationship of coping resources to occupational stress and strain. *Journal of Vocational Behaviour*, 32, 1-15.

Quick, J., Murphy, L., & Hurrell, J. (Eds.) (1992). Stress & well-being at work. Washington, DC: APA.

Salvo, V., Lubbers, C., Rossi, A., & Lewis, J. (1995). Unstructured perceptions of work□ related stress: An exploratory qualitative study. In R. Crandall & P. Perrewe (Eds.), *Occupational stress: A handbook* (pp.3950). Washington, DC: Taylor & Francis.

Schwartz, J., Pickering, T., & Landsbergis, P (1996). Work-related stress and blood pressure: Current theoretical models and considerations from a behavioral medicine perspective. *Journal of Occupational Health Psychology*, 1, 287-310.

Sharit, J. & Salvendy, G. (1982). Occupational stress: Review and reappraisal. *Human Factors*, 24(2), 129-162.

Spector, P., Dwyer, D., & Jex, S. (1988). Relation of job stressors to affective, health, and performance outcomes: A comparison of multiple data sources. *Journal of Applied Psychology*, 73, 11-19.

Spector, Paul E. (2002). Employee control and occupational stress, *Current directions in psychological science*, Vol. 11 (4), 133-136

Srivastava. A.K., & Singh, A.P. (1981) Construction and Standardization of an occupational stress index; a pilot study, *Indian journal of clinical psychology*. 133-136

Srivsthava, Urmila R., and Singh, Ashok P. (2002) Relationship of Job and life stress to health outcomes among Indian managerial personnel. *Social science international*, 18(1), 47-57.

Watts, M., & Cooper, C.L. (1998). *Stop the world: Finding the way through the pressures of life. London: Hodder & Stoughton.*

Wong, K.S., Cheuk, W.H., & Rosen, S. (2000). The influences of job stress and supervisor support on negative affects and job satisfaction in kindergarten principals. *Journal of Social Behavior and Personality*, 15, 85-98.

18

Reproductive Health Education for Adolescents

Findings of An Intervention Study

Sibnath Deb*

ABSTRACT

Adolescence is a transition period from childhood to adulthood. A lot of physiological and psychological changes occur during this phase and they tend to become curious about the various aspects of reproductive health especially the issues related to sexuality, friendship with opposite gender etc. Some of them involve in high-risk behavior sometime under the influence of peer group members without knowing the consequences of the same. After the advancement of the HIV / AIDS the issue of adolescent reproductive and sexual health has become the primary concern for the researchers and policy makers to save adolescents from risk taking behaviour. With this background the ICMR has taken up a multi-centric intervention program with a view to developing and testing suitable reproductive and sexual health care educational modules on the same issue for the school going adolescent boys and girls. Altogether six modules were developed for the same purpose through a series of discussions and meetings among the multidisciplinary group of professionals covering six broad dimensions of reproductive health.

* **Faculty Member, Department of Applied Psychology, Calcutta University, Council Member, The International Society for Prevention of Child Abuse and Neglect, e-mail: sibnath23@rediffmail.com/sibnath23@gmail.com**

First the baseline study was conducted covering four selected schools in Kolkata with a view to understanding the current knowledge, perceptions and behaviors of adolescents among various aspects of the reproductive health. Afterwards during the intervention phase adolescents were provided correct and complete information on various aspects of the reproductive health by the subject specific experts on the basis of six modules developed through lecture session approach. Other approaches adopted to communicate the information on the issue and clarify the confusions if any included question box, special sessions for the clarification of confusion, exhibition, displaying different charts and diagrams, explaining the various aspects of the issue, teen-clubs, distribution of templates (short form of the modules) etc.

After a period of six months the same information were provided to the adolescents on the basis of six modules and thereafter the end line data were collected from all the adolescent boys and girls of four schools. During the baseline study a group of 864 adolescent boys and girls from class IX and XI were covered using a semi-structured questionnaire. During the end line study 777 adolescent boys and girls from class IX and XI were available for providing the information in the semi-structured questionnaire. It is relevant to mention here that during the end line study a few additional questions were added for understanding the views of the adolescents about the method of implementation of the program and its efficacy.

Findings reveal that the adolescents, irrespective of gender and classes have a curiosity about the various aspects of reproductive health. The major areas of curiosity were changes during puberty, pregnancy, family planning methods, abortion, sexual activities, career, gender relations, friendship with the opposite sex etc and a good number of them have misconception and/or incomplete knowledge about some of the aspects of reproductive health. Over all analysis of baseline and end line data indicates that there were positive changes in the knowledge and behaviour of the adolescent about most of the aspects of reproductive and sexual health addressed during the intervention phase and six modules were found to be very effective in disseminating correct and complete knowledge among adolescents about various aspects of reproductive health. On the basis of the findings a number of steps have been proposed at the end of the discussion.

INTRODUCTION

With an estimated 1 billion adolescent population, the world is experiencing the largest number of adolescent population in the history. As a result, adolescent reproductive health has become an increasingly important component of global health. In addition, the following issues emerged from different studies necessitated the emergence of the concept of reproductive health and thereby implementation of the same concept in India.

- Lack and/or incomplete knowledge among adolescents about various aspects of reproductive health.
- General inhibition of the parents as well as teachers to talk about the matters related to physiological changes during adolescence.
- Inadequate, inter-generational or inter-sibling communication on such matters.
- Negative influence of media and/or unreliable source of information.
- Peer group influence, which generally inculcates wrong notions among adolescents about various aspects of reproductive health.

Emergence of the Concept of Reproductive and Child Health

In order to meet the challenges of various social and health problems like over population, teen-age pregnancy, infant mortality, maternal mortality, morbidity, and STDs including HIV/AIDS, various measures have been undertaken by the Government of India.

During the 8th plan, an integrated Child Survival and Safe Motherhood (CSSM) programme was adapted by the Government of India. The process of integration of related programmes initiated with the implementation of the CSSM Programme was pushed a step further in 1994 when the International Conference on Population and Development in Cairo recommended that the participant countries should implement unified programmes for Reproductive and Child Health (RCH).

Hence, after Cairo's International Conference on Population and Development in 1994, the Government of India integrated all the health related programmes of the 8th plan under one banner entitled *'Reproductive and Child Health (RCH)'* in the 9th plan with a view to providing need-based, client-centered, demand-driven, high quality and integrated RCH services to the beneficiaries. The RCH approach has been defined as:

"People have the ability to reproduce and regulate their fertility, women are able to go through pregnancy and child birth safely, the outcome of pregnancies is successful in terms of maternal and infant survival and well-being and couples are able to have sexual relations free of fear of pregnancy and of contracting diseases".

This concept is in keeping with the evolution of an integrated approach to the programmes aimed at improving the health status of young women and children, which has been going on in the country. During the 9th Plan, the RCH Programme, accordingly, integrates all the related programmes of the 8th Plan. The concept of RCH is to provide to the beneficiaries need-based, client-centered, demand-driven, high quality and integrated RCH services (Source: Reproductive and Child Health Programme, Govt. of India, 1997). The components, which are covered under the RCH, include adolescent care, antenatal, natal, post-natal care, respiratory track infection, immunization and child care, family planning, and STDs including HIV/AIDS.

Several factors are there which make adolescents vulnerable to HIV infection and teen-age pregnancy. Adolescents are an age of transition of experimentation and risk taking. Personal development, especially with regard to self-esteem and identity is hampered due to inadequate knowledge (Boyer and Kegeles, 1991). In some cases, however, they may not be informed about the mode of transmission of HIV/AIDS and its preventive measures. Thus, their behavioural risk persists and many adolescents remain ignorant or confused about causes and prevention of HIV/AIDS and teen-age pregnancy. Furthermore, they often share distorted views of their own vulnerability of HIV/AIDS caused by the long latent period between HIV infection and AIDS. Even after being exposed to valid information via mass media, they are not keen on changing their risk behaviour (Sugerman et al., 1991).

It is essential to encourage adolescents to learn how they might be at risk and how this risk can be avoided. But this simple provision of information is hardly sufficient to change their ingrained behaviour. Information needs to be presented in a personally relevant way so that adolescents can clarify their own values and attitudes and can start understanding how the information is essential to them as individuals (Bury, 1991). Nowadays more adolescents begin to participate in sexual activity at an earlier age than they did before (Cate and Rauh, 1985; O'Reilly and Aral; 1985). On average, first sexual intercourse occurs at age 16 and begins as early as age 12 in some urban settings (Rodrigues et al., 1998). Obviously, education aimed at modifying behaviour needs to begin before sexual activity normally begins, and needs to be repeated or revised at regular intervals (Vanichseni and Choopunya, 1990). It is therefore much easier to teach them positive behaviour at an earlier age than to try to change negative behaviour later. In an impact evaluation study on HIV/STD educational programme for middle school students, it has been observed that it significantly increased students' knowledge about STDs and condom use, and increased their communication with parents. The impact on knowledge was statistically significant for both boys and girls (Middlestadt et al., 1998). In another study conducted in rural Uganda on promotion of open discussions of sexuality to enable behaviour change among the youth revealed that youth have shown positive responses to receiving sex education (Kharim et al., 1998).

NATIONAL STUDY FINDINGS

In India, few studies have been carried out on adolescents with regard to patterns and determinants of sexual behaviour and their vulnerability to HIV infection. In a study authors' found that adolescents' vulnerability to HIV is determined by societal factors. The controlling family structures and values while seeking to protect adolescents may paradoxically increase their vulnerability (Sodh, 1998). Findings of another study revealed that adolescents in low income community are at risk of STDs and HIV owing to lack of understanding of sex and sexuality, unprotected sexual activity, and presence of non-commercial context of sex. It is suggested that AIDS intervention programmes in India need to be broadened to include aspects of sexuality and gender roles and relationships

(Bharat, 1998). Sharma et al suggests that school in an ideal setting for educating students regarding HIV/AIDS transmission and safer sex education (Sharma, 1997). In an experimental study it shows that students have good power to participate in the prevention and control of HIV/AIDS. If properly guided and trained they could be the most potent force to fight the disease within their area of residence (Angeles, 1998).

The population foundation of India (PFI) commissioned a study through operations research group covering 17185 male and female students of 9th to 11th standards in the urban and rural areas of Delhi, Haryana, Rajathan and Uttar Pradesh (Source: ICMR Study (1989) Estimating Illegal Abortions at 13.3 per 1000 pregnancies). Main findings of the study are as follows:

- There was a communication gap between parents and children on matters related to sex, physiology of pregnancy, reproductive health, etc.
- There was not much interaction between parents and children as well as among teachers and students on issues related to marriage, carrier and guidance. The students reported to accept the wisdom of their parents.
- Main sources of information on sex and related matters were the class- mates, peers and chap literature. Thus, many students developed wrong notion s about marriage and sex.
- Majority of the students were inclined to accept marriages arranged by their parents. However, around 25.0% among them did not mind casual pre-marital sex.
- Because of the prevalent beliefs and values, gender bias was very much evident in their responses.

LOCAL STUDY FINDINGS

In order to understand the risk behaviour among adolescents very few studies were carried out locally. The findings of those studies have been presented below:

Deb et al., (2006) carried out a study in Kolkata with a view to understanding the knowledge, attitude and perception of adolescent boys and girls of Kolkata about different aspects of reproductive health. A group of 141 adolescent boys and girls studying in class

XI standard were selected randomly from eight English medium schools, four each from north and south Kolkata. Data were collected by a specially designed structured questionnaire after pre-testing. Although most of the students were aware of HIV/AIDS (97.2%) and family planning methods (82.3%), a large number of them had some misconceptions and incomplete knowledge about the said issues. Only 16.8 and 29.2% of them could correctly state the full form of HIV and AIDS respectively. Regarding the sequence of pathogenicity of the disease, only 36.8% possessed correct knowledge i.e., *HIV comes first*. Condom is the most common family planning method as recalled by majority of the students (80.2%), followed by IUD/Copper T (69.8%) and oral pill (55.2%). The awareness level about other family planning methods was quite low. Regarding the sex determination of a baby, only 30.5% students possessed correct knowledge i.e., *father is the main determinant of sex of a baby*. About 74.5 and 79.4% of the students had correct knowledge about minimum age of marriage for boys and girls respectively. Parent-child relationship was found to be strain in case of 40.0% students. As a result only 39 and 12% of the students share personal issues with the mothers and fathers respectively. The rest of the students either share it with peer groups or suppress it. Findings speak volumes in favour of reproductive health education for adolescents.

In order to understand the knowledge, attitude and perception of adolescents about different aspects of reproductive health, a cross-sectional study was carried out by Deb (2005) in two cities of Orissa, India. Data were collected from 407 randomly selected students (201 males and 206 females). Broadly, the areas, which were covered in the study, included reproductive organs and their functions, menstruation, family planning methods, gender determination of a baby, STDs and back-street abortion. The findings revealed certain knowledge gaps and misconceptions on these issues. In general, the students' performance in regard to identification of reproductive organs was poor. However, their knowledge about the functions of both male and female reproductive organs was found to be better and this indicates that they have got good theoretical knowledge about the physiological functions of different reproductive organs. This gap between knowledge about the reproductive organs and its functions clearly indicates defective teaching methodology.

Although, the perception of majority of the students (73.1% males and 91.3% females) about menstruation was correct, about 38.7% males and 51.3% females had some misconceptions of biological determination of sex of a baby. It is suggested to assess the teaching methodology in use in schools and colleges for teaching reproductive biology to understand the existing gap between anatomical and theoretical knowledge of reproductive organs. The findings of this study would help to take corrective measures.

CINI-Adolescent Resource Centre, an NGO carried out a study in Jharkhand in 2003 with a view to assessing and understanding the needs of the adolescents and exploring the opinions of the stakeholders on various issues pertaining to reproductive and sexual health. The study covered a total sample of 479 adolescents and 46 stakeholders. The average age of the participants was 15 years. The study employed a range of participatory methods to put the adolescents at ease. Focused group discussions, Venn diagrams, mapping, listing, ranking were some of the commonly used methods. A sizeable percentage of the adolescents (48.0%), most of them boys expressed positive attitude towards heterosexual friendship. But girls were scared owing to social stigma. The adolescents were ill informed about pubertal changes, their reproductive and sexual health, use of contraceptives and regarding pregnancy and childbirth. They were of the opinion that early marriage hampered physical and mental development Awareness about HIV/AIDS was very low as well among the adolescents attending the workshops. And, they were very keen on sex education and felt that ideally it should be imparted before marriage, to boys and girls separately. The stakeholders were in favor of sex education being imparted.

In another study Deb (2000) found that most of the head of educational institutions in Bhubaneswar, Orissa were in favour of implementation of reproductive health education despite cultural barriers.

Broad Objective of ICMR Task Force Study on Reproductive Health Education for Adolescents

The broad objective of the study was to develop feasible modules for providing reproductive and sexual health education to school going adolescents in different parts of India.

There were four specific objectives of the study. This was a multi-centric study covering six centers in India viz., Kolkata, Delhi, Jaipur, Pune, Lucknow and Kerala. This report has been developed based on findings of Kolkata study. One Structured Questionnaire was developed and pre-tested for collection of data from the students. The Questionnaire consists of eight broad sections as follows:

Section I: Profile of Adolescents

Section II: Adolescents' Needs and Practices

Section III: Knowledge and Practice

Section IV: Sexuality

Section V: Interpersonal Relationship

Section VI: Understanding RTIs, STIs and HIV/AIDS

Section VII: Life Skill Development, Risk Taking Behaviour and Substance Abuse

Section VIII: Efficacy of Intervention Program as Perceived by the Adolescents

In order to achieve the objectives first a baseline study was conducted in the four selected schools, three of which located in the urban area and one in the rural area, following the criteria of the present study. In the baseline study a group of 480 adolescents from class IX and 384 from class XI were selected purposively and data was collected using a Structured Questionnaire developed by the ICMR Task Force Team. During the baseline study data were collected from a group of 864 adolescents, 480 from class IX and 384 from class XI. Afterwards inputs were given to adolescent boys and girls following classroom lecture approach on the basis of the six modules developed.

The classroom lecture was followed by question answer session. In addition, brief educational materials were distributed among the adolescent boys and girls, which were developed on the basis of six modules. Other approaches adopted for clarification of queries of adolescents included teen-clubs, question box and exhibition.

After two rounds of the intervention end line data were collected from a group of 777 adolescents, 401 from class IX students and 376 from class IX students, using the same questionnaire. It is of relevance to mention here the some additional information were collected during the end line study in order to understand the views of the students about the method of implementation of intervention of program, utility of educational materials and its efficacy.

INTERPRETATION OF RESULTS

Some of the important findings of the ICMR Task Force study have been provided below for giving some idea about the impact of intervention programme and its efficacy. Data provided in Table 1 and 2 shows that majority of the adolescents, irrespective of gender were aware of male and female reproductive organs and further their knowledge had increased significantly after the intervention programme except of girls of class IX.

Table 1

Reproductive Organs for Male

(% of correct responses)

Male Reproductive Organs	*Class IX*				*Class XI*			
	Boys		*Girls*		*Boys*		*Girls*	
	BL	*EL*	*BL*	*EL*	*BL*	*EL*	*BL*	*EL*
Significance Level: 95%	a	b	c	d	e	f	g	h
Significance Level: 99%	A	B	C	D	E	F	G	H
Base: All	300	238	180	163	174	195	210	181
1. Testis	72.0	85.0	58.0	53.0	82.0	95.0	54.0	93.0
		A				E		G
2. Vas deferens/ spermatic cord	49.0	71.0	39.0	42.0	56.0	68.0	43.0	84.0
		A				e		G
No response	20.0	14.0	36.0	47.0	15.0	3.0	40.0	7.0
				c	F		H	

Note: *(i)* Decimal places rounded to nearest full number;

(ii) Columns Tested for Significant Test: A:B, C:D, E:F, G:H;

(iii) *Symbol in place of percentage indicates the value below 0.5%.

Table 2

Reproductive Organs for Female

(% of correct responses)

Female Reproductive Organs	*Class IX*				*Class XI*			
	Boys		*Girls*		*Boys*		*Girls*	
	BL	*EL*	*BL*	*EL*	*BL*	*EL*	*BL*	*EL*
Significance Level: 95%	a	b	c	d	e	f	g	h
Significance Level: 99%	A	B	C	D	E	F	G	H
Base: All	300	238	180	163	174	195	210	181
Female								
1. Uterus	53.0	81.0	62.0	63.0	68.0	92.0	63.0	97.0
		A				E		G
2. Ovary	67.0	79.0	72.0	63.0	79.0	89.0	68.0	96.0
		A				E		G
3. Vagina	66.0	76.0	56.0	44.0	76.0	94.0	53.0	96.0
		A	d			E		G
No response	22.0	13.0	19.0	36.0	15.0	4.0	28.0	3.0
	b			C	F		H	

Note: *(i)* Decimal places rounded to nearest full number;

(ii) Columns Tested for Significant Test: A:B, C:D, E:F, G:H;

(iii) *Symbol in place of percentage indicates the value below 0.5%.

So far as functions of reproductive organs of both male and female are concerned, majority of the adolescents, irrespective of gender had poor knowledge before the intervention programme. Their knowledge level had increased significantly after the intervention programme (Table 3).

Table 3

Functions of Reproductive Organs

(% of correct responses)

Functions of Reproductive Organs	*Class IX*				*Class XI*			
	Boys		*Girls*		*Boys*		*Girls*	
	BL	*EL*	*BL*	*EL*	*BL*	*EL*	*BL*	*EL*
Significance Level: 95%	a	b	c	d	e	f	g	h
Significance Level: 99%	A	B	C	D	E	F	G	H
Base: All	300	238	180	163	174	195	210	181
1. Uterus	48.0	63.0	39.0	44.0	48.0	84.0	31.0	93.0
		A				E		G
2. Ovary	20.0	50.0	21.0	39.0	26.0	63.0	19.0	92.0
		A		C		E		G
3. Testis	44.0	63.0	37.0	44.0	44.0	71.0	34.0	85.0
		A				E		G
4. Vagina	18.0	47.0	16.0	38.0	20.0	51.0	17.0	88.0
		A		C		E		G
5. Vas deferens/ spermatic cord	37.0	58.0	29.0	45.0	35.0	59.0	28.0	87.0
		A		C		E		G

Note: *(i)* Decimal places rounded to nearest full number;

(ii) Columns Tested for Significant Test: A:B, C:D, E:F, G:H;

(iii) *Symbol in place of percentage indicates the value below 0.5%.

Previous study findings indicated that there was a wrong perception among the people about the gender determination of the child. This particular issue was also explained to them. Data in table 19 indicates that a large number of adolescent boys and girls have a wrong perception about the issue. However after the intervention a significantly higher number of them reported that father is responsible for determining the gender of the child (Table 4).

Table 4

Knowledge of Adolescents about Gender (Sex)

Determination of the Child

Determining the Gender (Sex) of the Child	*Class IX*				*Class XI*			
	Boys		*Girls*		*Boys*		*Girls*	
	BL	*EL*	*BL*	*EL*	*BL*	*EL*	*BL*	*EL*
Significance Level: 95%	a	b	c	d	e	f	g	h
Significance Level: 99%	A	B	C	D	E	F	G	H
Base: All	300	238	180	163	174	195	210	181
1. Mother	11.0	1.0	7.0	1.0	5.0	7.0	2.0	27.0
	B		D					G
2. Father	16.0	25.0	22.0	48.0	26.0	59.0	50.0	45.0
		a		C		E		
3. Both	37.0	33.0	20.0	20.0	36.0	19.0	19.0	14.0
					F			
99. Don't know	32.0	38.0	48.0	26.0	30.0	13.0	16.0	7.0
			D		F		H	
No response	4.0	3.0	3.0	5.0	3.0	2.0	13.0	7.0
							h	

Note: *(i)* Decimal places rounded to nearest full number;

(ii) Columns Tested for Significant Test: A:B, C:D, E:F, G:H;

(iii) *Symbol in place of percentage indicates the value below 0.5%.

Data from the above table indicates that adolescents irrespective of the gender or class prefer to discuss issues like friendship with opposite sex, marriage, adult movies etc, mainly with friends followed by classmates and cousins (Table 5).

Table 5
With Whom Do Adolescents Normally Discuss Issues Like Boy/ Girl Friend, Marriage, Adult Movies, Etc.

Personal Issues Discussed With	*Class IX*				*Class XI*			
	Boys		*Girls*		*Boys*		*Girls*	
	BL	*EL*	*BL*	*EL*	*BL*	*EL*	*BL*	*EL*
Significance Level: 95%	a	b	c	d	e	f	g	h
Significance Level: 99%	A	B	C	D	E	F	G	H
Base: All	300	238	180	163	174	195	210	181
1. Father	6.0	5.0	4.0	1.0	4.0	2.0	1.0	18.0
								G
2. Mother	5.0	5.0	8.0	10.0	3.0	2.0	16.0	7.0
							H	
3. Class mate	26.0	34.0	20.0	15.0	32.0	22.0	25.0	25.0
		a			f			
4. Cousin	10.0	6.0	12.0	7.0	8.0	11.0	12.0	11.0
5. Friend	51.0	54.0	51.0	50.0	68.0	62.0	45.0	89.0
								G
6. Don't discuss	18.0	25.0	21.0	20.0	13.0	12.0	16.0	8.0
							h	
77. Others	4.0	1.0	2.0	1.0	3.0	2:0	*	-
No response	5.0	7.0	6.0	18.0	4.0	5.0	13.0	2.0
				C			H	

Note: (i) Decimal places rounded to nearest full number;

(ii) Columns Tested for Significant Test: A:B, C:D, E:F, G:H;

(iii) *Symbol in place of percentage indicates the value below 0.5%.

The study further attempted to understand whether adolescent boys and girls felt stressed and reasons for the same. About one-third of adolescents were found to be stressed solely because of study load, irrespective of gender and class followed by poor academic performance, loneliness, strained relationship, physiological changes, reproductive and sexual health etc. However, the stress was found to be decreased after the intervention program (Table 6).

Table 6
Stress of Adolescents

Causes of Stress	*Class IX*				*Class XI*			
	Boys		*Girls*		*Boys*		*Girls*	
	BL	*EL*	*BL*	*EL*	*BL*	*EL*	*BL*	*EL*
Significance Level: 95%	a	b	c	d	e	f	g	h
Significance Level: 99%	A	B	C	D	E	F	G	H
Base: All	300	238	180	163	174	195	210	181
1. Studies	41.0	53.0	41.0	32.0	36.0	43.0	35.0	35.0
		A						
2. Career	18.0	10.0	13.0	12.0	20.0	19.0	10.0	19.0
	B							G
3. Strained relationship with parents	9.0	5.0	18.0	6.0	8.0	3.0	9.0	26.0
			D		f			G
4. Strained relationship with the boy/girl friend	10.0	6.0	11.0	3.0	6.0	2.0	6.0	1.0
			D		f		H	
5. Sexual relation with some one	4.0	2.0	2.0	1.0	2.0	1.0	2.0	-
							h	
6. Poor academic performance	18.0	29.0	28.0	29.0	17.0	21.0	20.0	6.0
		A					H	
7. Loneliness	13.0	13.0.	17.0	28.0	18.0	21.0	20.0	33.0
				c				G
8. Physiological changes	5.0	13.0	4.0	1.0	4.0	-	3.0	1.0
		A			F			
9. Reproductive health problem	1.0	2.0	3.0	-	1.0	1.0	2.0	-
			d				h	
10. Sexual health problem	2.0	11.0	2.0	1.0	2.0	-	-	-
		A			f			
11. Not stressed at all	26.0	23.0	17.0	10.0	28.0	32.0	26.0	39.0
								G
12. Others	*	2.0	1.0	2.0	2.0	2.0	-	1.0
No response	5.0	10.0	9.0	12.0	9.0	8.0	9.0	3.0
		a					h	

Note: *(i)* Decimal places rounded to nearest full number;

(ii) Columns Tested for Significant Test: A:B, C:D, E:F, G:H;

(iii) *Symbol in place of percentage indicates the value below 0.5%

The two most common coping strategies adopted by the adolescents irrespective of gender and class were discussion of the issue with someone close to them and through counselling and care extended by parents followed by counseling by teachers, meditation and exercise which was most practiced by boys then girls, studies some literature/spiritual books and finally very few of them became dependent upon alcohol or drug and did something for which they felt scared and/or ashamed (Table 7).

Table 7

Coping Mechanism of Adolescents

Coping Strategy Adopted	*Class IX*				*Class XI*			
	Boys		*Girls*		*Boys*		*Girls*	
	BL	*EL*	*BL*	*EL*	*BL*	*EL*	*BL*	*EL*
Significance Level: 95%	a	b	c	d	e	f	g	h
Significance Level: 99%	A	B	C	D	E	F	G	H
Base: Those came across any serious crisis in life (Q120)	132	100	89	47	76	78	86	43
1. Discussed the issue with someone close to me	39.0	36.0	44.0	32.0	45.0	49.0	36.0	81.0
								G
2. Studied some literature/ spiritual books	8.0	11.0	10.0	15.0	13.0	8.0	9.0	-
							h	
3. Through meditation and/or exercise	23.0	29.0	7.0	4.0	18.0	5.0	7.0	2.0
					f			
4. Became dependent on drug/alcohol	1.0	4.0	2.0	-	1.0	-	1.0	-
5. Through counseling and care by teacher/counseler	12.0	25.0	16.0	23.0	14.0	27.0	19.0	5.0
		a					h	
6. Through counseling and care by parents	39.0	36.0	42.0	40.0	36.0	21.0	48.0	7.0
					f		H	

(Contd...)

Coping Strategy Adopted	*Class IX*				*Class XI*			
	Boys		*Girls*		*Boys*		*Girls*	
	BL	*EL*	*BL*	*EL*	*BL*	*EL*	*BL*	*EL*
7. Through counseling and medical treatment	18.0	8.0	13.0	6.0	16.0	1.0	10.0	7.0
	b				F			
8. Did something of which I feel scared or ashamed	5.0	-	1.0	2.0	1.0	-	-	-
	b							
No response	10.0	17.0	8.0	23.0	13.0	31.0	6.0	7.0
				c		E		

Note: *(i)* Decimal places rounded to nearest full number;

(ii) Columns Tested for Significant Test: A:B, C:D, E:F, G:H.

The information pertaining to the knowledge of adolescent boys and girls about sexually transmitted diseases are provided in Table 8. Data indicates that more than 65% of them were aware of the diseases and awareness level has increased significantly after the intervention among all the categories and girls of class IX.

Table 8
Awareness of Sexually Transmitted Diseases (STDs) among Adolescents

Awareness about STDs	*Class IX*				*Class XI*			
	Boys		*Girls*		*Boys*		*Girls*	
	BL	*EL*	*BL*	*EL*	*BL*	*EL*	*BL*	*EL*
Significance Level: 95%	a	b	c	d	e	f	g	h
Significance Level: 99%	A	B	C	D	E	F	G	H
Base: All	300	238	180	163	174	195	210	181
1. Yes	66.0	89.0	67.0	70.0	68.0	94.0	75.0	98.0
		A				E		G
2. No	29.0	4.0	29.0	21.0	25.0	3.0	18.0	-
	B				F		H	
No response	5.0	8.0	4.0	9.0	7.0	3.0	8.0	2.0
				c	f		H	

Note: *(i)* Decimal places rounded to nearest full number;

(ii) Columns Tested for Significant Test: A:B, C:D, E:F, G:H.

So far as the symptoms of STDs are concerned, findings reveal that about one-fourth to one-third of them irrespective of gender and class were aware of the symptoms. In this regard the intervention had a positive impact for increasing the knowledge of the symptoms and related issue (Table 9).

Table 9

Awareness about the Symptoms of STDs

Awareness about Symptoms of STDs	*Class IX*				*Class XI*			
	Boys		*Girls*		*Boys*		*Girls*	
	BL	*EL*	*BL*	*EL*	*BL*	*EL*	*BL*	*EL*
Significance Level: 95%	a	b	c	d	e	f	g	h
Significance Level: 99%	A	B	C	D	E	F	G	H
Base: Those who heard about STDs (Q103)	198	211	120	114	118	184	157	178
1. Yes	31.0	50.0	34.0	64.0	28.0	72.0	26.0	82.0
		A		C		E		G
2. No	63.0	37.0	58.0	32.0	61.0	20.0	66.0	8.0
	B		D		F		H	
No response	6.0	13.0	8.0	4.0	11.0	9.0	8.0	10.0

Note: *(i)* Decimal places rounded to nearest full number;

(ii) Columns Tested for Significant Test: A:B, C:D, E:F, G:H.

Replying to a question whether aids were a curable disease data indicates that more than one-fourth of them irrespective of gender and class said it was curable. End line results reveal contradictory finding that the after the intervention the misconception has increased. It may be because of two reasons. Firstly, either the adolescents did not read the educational materials provided to them during the intervention program or the resource person did not explain the issue properly or over looked the issue (Table 10).

Table 10
Is HIV/AIDS A Curable Disease?

Knowledge about Prognosis of the Disease	*Class IX*				*Class XI*			
	Boys		*Girls*		*Boys*		*Girls*	
	BL	*EL*	*BL*	*EL*	*BL*	*EL*	*BL*	*EL*
Significance Level: 95%	a	b	c	d	e	f	g	h
Significance Level: 99%	A	B	C	D	E	F	G	H
Base: Those who are aware of AIDS (Q107)	241	194	154	110	155	179	175	123
1. Yes	28.0	37.0	27.0	56.0	36.0	14.0	30.0	19.0
				C	F		h	
2. No	37.0	44.0	34.0	16.0	38.0	68.0	38.0	54.0
			D			E		G
3. Don't Know	31.0	12.0	37.0	16.0	25.0	11.0	29.0	24.0
	B		D		F			
No response	3.0	7.0	3.0	11.0	1.0	7.0	3.0	3.0
				C		E		

Note: *(i)* Decimal places rounded to nearest full number;

(ii) Columns Tested for Significant Test: A:B, C:D, E:F, G:H.

In order to understand the views of adolescent boys and girls about the method of implementation of the intervention programme and its efficacy, 15 questions were asked to adolescents. First, an attempt was made to understand their views about the topics covered during class-room discussion. Data in table 113 indicates that an over whelming number of the respondents except for girls for class IX stated that all the topics as mentioned in the table were covered in the class room discussion. It could be that about 30-40% of the adolescent girls did not attend all the intervention related sessions and/or discussion (Table 11).

Table 11

Topics Covered During Class Room Discussions as Stated by the Adolescents

	Topics Covered	*Class IX*		*Class XI*	
		Boys	*Girls*	*Boys*	*Girls*
		EL	*EL*	*EL*	*EL*
	Base: All	238	163	195	181
1.	Physiological changes which occur during adolescence	100.0	61.0	98.0	97.0
2.	Reproductive organs and functions and hygiene	100.0	61.0	98.0	97.0
3.	Nutrition	98.0	61.0	98.0	97.0
4.	Self-concept/image/ sexuality and risky behaviours	97.0	60.0	98.0	97.0
5.	Decision-making/ communication	73.0	37.0	91.0	87.0
6.	Equal role of male and female in society	93.0	56.0	56.0	69.0
7.	RTI/STI	97.0	61.0	97.0	96.0
8	HIV/AIDS	98.0	60.0	97.0	97.0
9	Scholastic achievements	87.0	56.0	70.0	76.0
10	Others	3.0	4.0	-	-
	No response	-	39.0	2.0	3.0

Note: *(i)* Decimal places rounded to nearest full number.

Majority of the respondents especially boys about 705 stated that educational materials were useful while 49-56% girls were of the same view (Table 12).

Table 12

Was Educational Material Useful?

Was Educational Materials Useful?	*Class IX*		*Class XI*	
	Boys	*Girls*	*Boys*	*Girls*
Base: All	238	163	195	181
1. Yes	78.0	56.0	71.0	49.0
2. Can't say	11.0	1.0	2.0	1.0
No response	11.0	43.0	28.0	51.0

Note: *(i)* Decimal places rounded to nearest full number.

DISCUSSION

Previous study findings reveal that adolescents lack knowledge about different aspects of reproductive health (Deb 2005a, 2005b). It happens mainly because of social and cultural barrier within their family and in their educational institutions to discuss about these issues, especially about the physiological changes. In fact, there is no scope for them to share their personal problems especially regarding reproductive health, which becomes a cause of anxiety and stress. And in turn it affects their interpersonal relationship and/or academic career. Feeling of guilt and embarrassment is common among adolescents due to onset of physiological and/or pubertal changes. Literature also suggests that today's adolescents are involved in various types of high-risk behaviors, which is a prime cause of early pregnancy and/or getting the HIV/AIDS infection (O'Reilly and Aral, 1985; Rodrigues et al., 1998 and Çollins et al., 1998). Rate of unwanted pregnancy among the late teenagers is also on the rise in the city of Calcutta (Times of India, May 26, 2000). The nature of high-risk behavior among the adolescents has been thoroughly investigated by experts in different parts of the world (Meheus, 2000). Comparatively less number of studies was conducted in developing countries like India on the issue of adolescent reproductive and sexual health. It is relevant to mention here that the planet is experiencing the highest number of the adolescents in the history of human civilization. Hence it is believed that if they are properly channelized and guided they could contribute significantly to the overall economic development of the nation as well as they can bring peace, harmony and stability in the society. This issue of adolescent reproductive health has come into the limelight after the international conference on Population And Development held in Cairo (1994) where the international health policy makers unanimously felt the need to bring all the health related programs under one umbrella called Reproductive And Child Health (RCH).

Findings reveal that the adolescents, irrespective of gender and classes have a curiosity about the various aspects of reproductive health. However, the major areas are puberty, pregnancy, family planning methods, abortion, sexual activities, career, gender relations, friendship with the opposite sex etc. It may have been that these areas were not much discussed in their environment and thus made them curious. Strangely, very few of them discuss or share information about reproductive health issues with the parents and some of them also indulge themselves in sexual activities at this age. This may be a reflection of the social scenario in India where such issues are not encouraged usually by parents/ elders. The class IX students prefer to discuss reproductive and health care with friends followed by doctors while the class XI students prefer to consult doctors for the said purpose followed by parents/guardians and friends. For sexual health they mostly consulted doctors followed by parents. Thus in this matter also parents are not much preferred. A communication gap regarding these issues may be an operative factor in this regard. So far as the issue of friendship is concerned the friends are the first choice followed by parents and guardians and teachers.

In the real life situation they think that they should consult teacher for studies and for general health, nutrition, reproductive and sexual health they should consult a doctor followed by parents and/or guardians. They also feel that their friends are the best person to discuss issues related to friendship followed by parents and guardians. Here also parents are kept as a second preference for the discussion of various issues reflecting once again the scenario that some gap either in communication or other areas exist between the parents and the adolescents as a result of which they fail to discuss various issues so freely. More than half of the adolescents reported consulting somebody regarding the above-mentioned matters. However, a large number of them (19-37%) never consulted anybody. It may be because of their personality (submissiveness, withdrawn nature) and/or social environment. In this regard, it is relevant to mention that significantly more number of class XI students consulted somebody for the above matters and issues like pregnancy etc and the consulting person was a parent.

The knowledge of the adolescents, irrespective of gender was comparatively better about the male and female reproductive organs as compared to their knowledge about the functions of the same. It clearly indicates that the biology teacher do not discuss the issue clearly in the classroom because of feeling of embarrassment. However, the intervention had a significant impact in increasing the knowledge level of adolescents about the male and female reproductive organs and their functions.

Regarding pregnancy a large number of adolescents had misconceptions. After the intervention, knowledge level had increased significantly among adolescent girls only. A large number of adolescents had misconception about the gender determines of the child. This reflects the prevailing knowledge gap in a large section of the adolescent population regarding the basic facts of life. In the Indian education system information about this sort of issues are not provided in the schools. However, the intervention was found to increase the knowledge of the adolescents.

About half of the adolescents read magazines related to romance. This was more common among the girls of class IX (70.0%). In addition, they view blue films, visit internet sites and view pornographic materials, which are perhaps normal. Surprisingly, a significantly less number of girls of class XI reported that they viewed such materials. It could be because of the lack of social permissiveness for girls.

Adolescent boys and girls have different understanding about the term 'sex'. Majority of them, irrespective of gender and class, interpret the word 'sex' as distinction between male and female gender, followed by other understanding arranged chronologically like intercourse, reproduction, hugging or kissing the opposite sex/ boy or girl/man or woman, love between opposite sex, something pleasurable and so on. This interpretation of the term 'sex' by different adolescents is reflective of their wide perception about the issue and it is related to personality of an individual.

Further an attempt was done to determine their knowledge about the kind of reproductive health care available in the health centers. The areas of knowledge were about pregnancy, family planning methods, STDs, HIV, MTP, etc. The findings clearly indicate about the efficacy of the intervention program i.e., the knowledge of the adolescent increased after the intervention. It is of relevance to mention here that about one-third of the respondents couldn't state the type of reproductive services provided in the government and private clinics.

The knowledge of the adolescents about female family planning methods for both male and female was found to be poor except one male family welfare method i.e., condom since this issue is neither discussed within family nor in the educational institution. In this regard also the intervention had a positive impact in increasing the knowledge of adolescent boys and girls about the family welfare methods.

About one-third of the adolescents are not aware of meaning of abortion. This may be attributed to the fact that in the Indian context not much of the children or adolescents are given adequate information regarding these issues. After the intervention, knowledge level among class XI girls has increased significantly. However, more than half of the adolescents feel that a qualified and/or authorized doctor should perform abortions. The knowledge level among class IX boys and girls has increased significantly after the intervention programme. Although majority of the adolescents had correct knowledge about the safe period for abortion, a large number of them either had no knowledge or misconception about the issue. Adolescents aware of safe period for abortion were asked as to what problems an unsafe abortion could cause. Fatal incidence followed by bleeding/hemorrhage, the adolescents report perforation of uterus and sepsis. After the intervention, significant changes in knowledge concerning two major problems had observed in case of adolescent girls of class XI. This may be attributed to the fact that the girls are more aware because they will have to bear a child. Moreover culturally these issues are discussed more openly in front of girls than boys.

Over all analysis of baseline and end line data indicates that there is a positive change in the knowledge and behaviour of the adolescent about most of the aspects of reproductive and sexual health addressed during the intervention phase which has been discussed issue-wise in the following section.

Efficacy of the Intervention Programme As Perceived by the Adolescents

Regarding efficacy of the intervention program, most of the adolescents feel it was very helpful and they displayed a very positive attitude towards the program.

An overwhelming number of the adolescents stated that the information, which was provided during the intervention phase, was clearly understandable and benefitted them immensely. They also think that each topic was given adequate and appropriate time. Vast majority of the adolescent further remarked that their doubts were clarified clearly during the intervention.

Question box was one of the strategies of the intervention programme to know the questions of adolescent boys and girls. More than half of the adolescent boys and girls did put up questions in the question box, which was more among adolescent boys of class IX (Table 122).

Dissemination of information is one of the long-term objectives of any intervention programme and/or awareness campaign. Hence adolescent were asked whether they talked about the issues, which were discussed in the classroom with class mates, parents, friends and other people. Classmates were the persons with whom adolescents mostly shared the issues, which they attended in the intervention programme. Very few of them especially boys shared the same with other friends or parents (Table 123).

Distribution of educational materials developed on the basis of six educational modules was one of the activities of the project to disseminate correct information among adolescent boys and girls. More than 90.0% of boys and girls of class IX and XI stated that they received educational materials except of girls of class IX.

Regarding behaviour change, a lot of positive things have been observed among adolescent boys and girls like increased self-confidence, followed by more interest in studies, comfortable with the bodily changes, talking with boys and girls easily, understanding and appreciating gender relationship.

CONCLUSION AND RECOMMENDATIONS

The present study revealed host of interesting findings. The adolescence is an age of stress and storm. The adolescent boys and girls were curious about a lot of things related especially to the relations with opposite sex. Although a common notion is that the girls are more vulnerable at this age, boys are equally at risk. Adolescent boys are found to share things less with family members and more with peers as compared to the girls. In general the awareness level regarding various important facts of life were found to be quite low in both class IX students as well as class XI students, thereby increasing their risk manifold. The intervention program was found to be highly effective in many cases in elevation of the knowledge level except in some areas of nutrition. The adolescent themselves felt that they needed knowledge regarding various aspects of reproductive and sexual health. In a nutshell, it may be stated that the current intervention program yielded success in achieving the broad objective of the study i.e., development of six educational modules on various aspects of reproductive and sexual health and ascertaining its efficacy on school going adolescent boys and girls.

Finally, the ICMR Task Force Study has come out with six experimented modules for imparting reproductive and sexual health education among adolescents, which is going to be a part of existing curriculum programme for the secondary level students. The modules, which were developed and used, are as follows:

- *Module I:* Growing Up Concerns And Nutrition
- *Module II:* Reproductive And Sexual Health & Hygiene
- *Module III:* Body Image, Sexuality & Risk Taking Behaviour
- *Module IV:* Interpersonal & Gender Relationships
- *Module V:* Understanding RTIS/ STIS &HIV / AIDS
- *Module VI:* Life Skill Development & Scholastic Achievement

The intervention program was found to be highly effective in many cases in increasing knowledge level except in some areas of nutrition. The adolescent themselves felt that they needed knowledge regarding various aspects of reproductive and sexual health. In a nutshell, it may be stated that the current intervention program yielded success in achieving the broad objective of the study.

SOME CHALLENGES

- Getting permission from the school authorities
- Reluctance in allotment of classes
- Coeducational Schools' unwillingness to involve into sex related issues
- Managing the session within the time limit.
- Multiple number of sections for e.g., 9 sections in one of the participating schools
- Matching the time of Resource Persons with that of Schools

LEARNING EXPERIENCES FROM THE INTERVENTIONS

- Enthusiastic Participation of the Students
- Students pool of questions
- Teachers Participation in some schools
- Initial Reluctance on the part of the Schools
- Non Participation of Teachers in some schools
- Infrastructure Difficulties

ENCOURAGING PICTURE

- Interventions provided a platform for interaction of the school adolescents with an outside resource person
- It provided the ice-breaking tool for the school adolescents.

Recommendations

- On the basis of the findings of the present study, the followings steps are recommended for effective implementation of future intervention program.
- Taking proper steps to ensure the full cooperation from the school authorities for effective implementation of the intervention program so that they provide minimum class for disseminating information among the adolescents.

- Small handouts to be developed for the adolescent boys and girls describing the key information on various aspects of reproductive and sexual health.
- Parents should be involved in the intervention program for improving their skills in dealing with curiosities of adolescents and in developing healthy parent-child relationship.
- During the Parent-Teachers meeting, problems faced by the adolescents on these issues should be dealt with by holding discussions regarding the same.
- So far as modules are concerned, much emphasis should be given on nutrition issue followed by sexuality and HIV/AIDS.

REFERENCES

Angeles R.E. (1998). The Development of Students as HIV/AIDS Educators Reaching Out To Their Peers in School, Members of Their Family, Relatives, Friends and Neighbours. Paper Presented In The *12th World AIDS Conference* Held In Jeneva, 295.

Boyer B. And Kegeles S. (1991). AIDS Risk And Prevention Among Adolescents. *Social Science & Medicine*, 33, 11-23.

Bury K. J. (1991). Teenage Sexual Behaviour And The Impact Of AIDS. *Health Education Journal*, 50, 43-48.

Deb, Sibnath (2005). Knowledge, Attitude And Perception of Adolescents About Different Aspects of Reproductive Health: A Cross-Sectional Study, *Social Science International*, 21, 1, 70-92.

Deb, Sibnath (2006). Adolescents Perceived Reproductive Health: A Cross-sectional Study in Kolkata, *Social Science International*, Vol.22, No.1, pp. 38-58.

Deb, Sibnath (2000). Attitude And Perception of Heads of Educational And Industrial Institutions Towards Introduction of Reproductive Health Education. *Indian Journal of Psychological Issues, Vol. 8(2) December, pp. 37-47.*

Kharim H., Asuzi S., Tani S., Waka P., Idoro J.W. And Homsy J. (1998). Promoting Open Discussions About Sexuality To Enable Behaviour Change Among The Youth In Rural Uganda. Paper Presented In the *12th World AIDS Conference* Held In Jeneva, 245.

Middlestadt S.E., Kaiser J., Hirsch L., Simkin L., Radosh A., Santelli J., Banspach S., And Collins J. (1998). Impact of An HIV/STD Prevention Intervention on Urban Middle School Students. Paper Presented in the *12th World AIDS Conference* Held In Jeneva, 239.

O'Reilly K.R. and Aral S.O. (1985). Adolescence and Sexual Behaviour: Trends and Implication for STD. *Journal Of Adolescent Health Care*, 6, 298-310.

Report of A Study Entitled 'Adolescent Speak'. The Study Was Carried out by CINI-Adolescent Resource Centre In Jharkhand In 2003 (Unpublished).

Reproductive and Child Health Programme: Schemes For Implementation, Department of Family Welfare, Ministry of Health And Family Welfare, Government of India, Oct.1997.

Rodrigues A, Kerr-Pontes L and Mota RM (1998). Sexual Behavior and AIDS Transmission Among High School Students in A Megacity from the North-Eastern of Brazil. Paper Presented in *The 12th World AIDS Conference* Held In Geneva, 244.

Sodh G., Zoysa De I., Sen A., and Varma M. (1998). Patterns and Determinants of Sexual Behaviour of Adolescents in A Slum of New Delhi, India. Paper Presented in the *12th World AIDS Conference* Held In Jeneva, 246.

Sharma A.K., Sehgal V.N., Kant S., Choubey D., and Bharadwaj A. (1997). Knowledge, Attitude, Belief and Practice Study on AIDS Among Senior Secondary Students. *Indian Journal of Community Medicine*, XXII, 4, 168171.

Vanichseni S. and Choopunya K (1990). AIDS KAP Survey Among Secondary School Boys. *Thai AIDS Journal*, 2, 76-80.

19

A Cross Cultural Study of the Effects of Spirituality on Life Satisfaction and Explanatory Styles of Afghani and Pakistani Students

Alay Ahmad*

ABSTRACT

Earlier studies suggest impact of spirituality on human behaviour (for example, Anderson and Worthey, 1997; Wulff, 1996).Spirituality is distinct from religion (e.g.; Zinnabauer, Pargament and Scott, 1999).It acts as norm that guides and directs our behavior. No research on this issue has been carried out in Pakistan. Keeping in view its significance we planned to study impact of spirituality on two variables of our subjects namely life satisfaction and explanatory life styles. In the present investigation twenty-six Afghani and thirty - seven Pakistani unmarried male, ranging in ages from 20 to 25 years, students of BBA of a local university participated in the study. Subjects did not significantly differ on their parents' socio-economic status .They were living in a middle-class residential area. All of them could read, write and speak English and Urdu languages. Afghan students rarely interact with their Pakistani class-fellows. Afghan students are fashionable

* **Professor and Head, Department of Applied Psychology and Mass Communication, Dean Faculty of Social Sciences, Preston University Kohat-Peshawar campuses Email kuju7@yahoo.cm, alayahmad@hotmail.com**

than their counterparts .Afghan students are living in Pakistan since their birth and most of them frequently visit their homes in Afghanistan.

Before the main study a pilot study was made. Before administration of questionnaires, rapport with the subjects was developed. Complete instructions were given to them .They were assured that the study was not connected with their examinations as well as their responses would be confidential. As a first step demographic information on a pre-tested closed-ended questionnaire was administered. In order to measure spirituality, Howden's (1992) Spiritual Assessment Scale (SAS) consisted of 28 items to measure purpose and meaning in life, innerness, inter connectedness and transcendence on 6 point Likert Scale was administered on all subjects . After completion of SAS, a seven-point Life Satisfaction Scale, (Warr, 1979) was given to all subjects to measure their satisfaction with salient features of their daily life and activities .Similarly, Michael and Carver (1985) 12 item True/ False scale to measure respondents' pessimism and optimism was given to them . After administration of above instruments, subjects were debriefed.

Mean, SD, SD Error, t and correlation were computed on all variables. Major results are mentioned below .Our study shows a significant difference between Afghani and Pakistani subjects on SPS ($t=3.224$, $df= 61$, $p<.01$).There is significant correlation between Afghani and Pakistani subjects on Life Orientation and Spirituality($r =.274$, $df=61$, $p< .05$). There is also significant correlation between Afghani and Pakistani subjects on Life Orientation and Spirituality($r= .298$, $df=61$, $p<05$). Above results are explained in terms of relevant theories. There is a need to undertake a larger cross-cultural study with a more extensive sample, the findings the findings of which would have implications for psychologists.

A cursory review of literature on spirituality and organization reveals that earlier no serious attempt on this issue was made by researchers. One would agree with several authors and investigators that earlier researchers and managements did not pay attention to towards role of spirituality in organizations. Multiple possible reasons may be cited in this regard in particular no scientific work was done on formulation of concepts and operationalization of spirituality, applied significance in organizations with special reference to their employees as well as clients . Spirituality and human behavior are interrelated with each other. Spirituality in my opinion is analogous to frame of reference that guides, directs, resocilisesd individuals about values, norms, and ethics.

Spirituality recently has been defined in many ways by investigators. If one is aware about his/her environment and able to link it with related aspects of environment like clients, their native cities, country, planet and universe, it will be called spirituality as connectedness that is feeling of relatedness with others (Zumeta, 1993), and harmonious interconnectedness with environment (Burkhardt,1989) . In summary, spirituality refers to relationships to four dimensions .Relationship with others such as honesty, positive thinking .Second, relationships with forgiving, and finally relationships with high power e.g.; self evaluation.

Burkhardt (1989) defines spirituality as, "Spiriting is the unfolding of mystery through harmonious interconnectedness that springs from inner strength"(p. 74).Titone(1991) defines " Spirituality may or may not include belief in God. It is one's personalized experience and identity pertaining to a sense of worth, meaning, vitality, and connectedness to others and Universe ... It pertains to ones' relationship with ultimate sources of inspiration, energy, and motivation: it pertains to an object of worship and reverence; it pertains to the natural human tendency toward healing and growth" (p 8). It is the first aspect of present study.

A large number of scholars conducted studies on spirituality. Spirituality consist of love, power, and freedom (Emed, 1995), clients' behavior is influenced by spirituality (Lindgren and Coursey, 1995). Several studies support positive role of spirituality reducing ethnicity (Bowmen and Harrell, 2002); spirituality based coping techniques play a very significant role in social and health psychological issues in particular. For example, it improves interactional processes between members of the groups and teachers'-students' adjustment aspects (Rogers and Dantley, 2002), HIV (Simoni *et al*, 2002).

Recently, researchers have also paid serious attention towards spirituality and religious aspects .For example, Walker and Dixon (2002) positive relationship between higher levels of spirituality belief and religious participation with academic achievement.

Life Satisfaction is second aspect of the present study. Life satisfaction is hypothetical construct. It may be explained in terms of hedonistic calculus. .One of the main aims of persons may be to maximize pleasure and minimize pain. That is pain-pleasure principal is the basis of life satisfaction. One of the most important contributions in this regard is made by Diener (1984) who emphasized on feeling of subjective-well-being (SWB). Diener's concepts include positive and negative emotions (affective component) and life satisfaction (that is cognitive-judgmental aspect). Lack of self-confidence create several problems in satisfaction such as unsuccessful, pessimistic, and negative feeling .Earlier researches found several factors leading to satisfaction. For example, income, high status, social factors (Blishen and Atkinson, 1980; Argyle, 1987), economic factor does not influence happiness (Kaman and Campbell, 1982) unmarried people's life is aimless (Argyle, 1991), married Taiwanese couple were satisfied with their jobs as well as they had satisfactory marital life (Tsou and Lik, 2001), mothers express aggression (Harding, 1985). Relationships with others and sense of belongingness have direct impact on happiness (Argyle, 1987).

Criteria of satisfaction are one's own judgment (Shin and Johnson, 1978). Several studies show relationship between life satisfaction and religiosity. In one study, it was found that life satisfaction is related with religiosity and women were more religious than males (Bergan and Conatha, 2002)Life satisfaction Researches carried out by earlier experts in this field (eg; Mastekassa, 1984) can be reviewed in literature cited elsewhere.

EXPLANATORY LIFE STYLES

Explanatory life styles refer to one's personality trait those events as good or bad (Peterson and Seligman, 1984).We are concerned with optimism and pessimism aspects of explanatory life styles .Let us briefly define both dimensions of explanatory life styles. According to Scheier and Carver(1985) optimism refers to ' a generalized expectancy that good, as opposed to bad, outcomes will generally occur when confronted with problems across important life domains,, Optimistic people is logical and his/her activities are planned (Franken, 1994) .They see positive picture of the world . Optimism is a learned process(1991), dispositional optimism helps in coping techniques and individuals continue their efforts to achieve their goals (Schier and Carver,1987;Reker and Wrong, 1985;Cousins, 1977).

Pessimistic exploratory life style is dominated by dark and negative side of the picture .Such people always belief in negative aspect of one's life. They have depressive dispositional life style and they consider harmful situations are developed because of stable cause e.g.; it is never going to go away, global eg; it is going to ruin everything do), and one's own internal facto e.g. it's me and external factor refers environmental factor (Seligman, 1991) .Pessimistic explanatory life styles can also discussed in terms poorer immune functions (Kamen-Siegal *et al*, 1991).

In summary, explanatory life styles of optimistic is characterized as futurist – bright aspects of life while explanatory life styles of pessimistic is based on gloomy side of situation.

METHOD

Sample

As a first step demographic information on pretested closed ended questionnaire in English language was obtained. Sixty-three unmarried male enrolled Muslim students of BBA (8th and 9th semesters) of a local university at Peshawar randomly selected as volunteer subjects of whom 26 Afghani (Refugees or Mahajirs) and thirty-seven were Pakistani nationals. Afghani students were residing in Peshawar since their birth and frequently visit their native cities while most of the Pakistani students never visited Afghanistan. Afghani students are fashionable and wear fast colored dresses as compared to their class fellows. All subjects could write, read, speak English, and Urdu languages easily. There were no significant differences on socioeconomic factors and educational levels of subject's parents of both the groups. Subjects were residents of middle class residential area of Peshawar. Afghan subjects live in over crowded houses as compared to their counter parts .The results of pilot study are not included in the present study.

INSTRUMENTS

Following instruments were employed in the present study:

SPIRITUALITY ASSESSMENT SCALE (SAS)

Howden's (1992) SAS was employed to assess subjects' spiritual orientation on a 6 point Likert Scale from Strongly Agree (SA-6) to Strongly Disagree (SD-1).The internal consistency reliability for the SAS is equal to 0.70. This scale consists of 28 items with the following four aspects of spirituality: Purpose and Meaning in Life, Innerness (or Inner Resources), Inter connectedness and Transcendence. Examples of SAS are given below:

Item number 1. I have a general sense of belonging.

Item number 2. I enjoy being of service to others

LIFE SATISFACTION SCALE (LSS)

Warr's (1979) 10 items scale was used to measure LSS. This 7 point Scale measures daily style of life of the person from 1(*I am extremely dissatisfied*), to 7 point (*I am extremely satisfied*) .A high score indicates high satisfaction while low score shows extremely low satisfaction . Test-retest of LSS is very high: r=0.87.

Examples of items used in LSS:

Item number 4. Your social life

Item number 7.What the future seems to hold you.

LIFE ORIENTATION SCALE (LOT)

In order to measure optimism and pessimisms, a 12 item scale of Scheier and Carver (1985) was used. The split half reliability was 0.69.

Optimistic Direction Items

Items 1, 4, 5, and 11 measure optimistic direction. Items 2, 6, 7, and 10 were dropped .A score of I was assigned to each True answer and a score of I was subtracted for each False answer.

Pessimistic Direction Items

Items 3, 8, 9, and 11 measure pessimistic direction. I score was given for each False answer and I score was subtracted from the total for each True answer.

Total score shows level of optimism .The higher the total scores out of a possible maximum of 8, the greater the subjects' optimism.

Examples of LOT as follows:

Item number 5. I am always optimistic about my future

Item number 10. I don't get upset too easily

METHOD

Before the main study a pilot study was made on 20 male subjects of BBA in order to refine Personal Information Schedule (PSI) .On a fixed date and time, participant assembled in a comfortable room and complete instructions were given in English language. They were also directed to read carefully instructions printed on each Scales. Rapport was developed with them and they were assured that their responses would not be disclosed and this study was not related to their university. After administration of PSI, Spiritual Assessment Scale (SAS) was given to the subjects. Because they were naïve and never experienced psychological test, free trail of each scale was given to them. Life Satisfaction Scale (LSS) followed by Life Orientation Test (LOT) and were administered .Debriefing was made in order to eliminate possible effects of the study .All subjects were offered teas after each session.

RESULTS

Table 1

Correlation between Spirituality and Optimism among Afghan and Pakistani (N=63)

Group	*Scales*	*N*	*Mean*	*SD*	*r*	*p*
Afghan	Spirituality	26	51.23	9.425		
	Optimism	26	3.38	.752	.021	n.s
Pakistani	Spirituality	37	47.19	12.523		
	Optimism	37	2.97	.897	.381*	.02

*p < .05; **p <.01

Table-1 shows correlation between the scores of spirituality and optimism of Afghans and Pakistanis. The result reveals that there is no correlation between optimism and Spirituality among

Afghans while the scores of Pakistanis show that there is a positive correlation between spirituality and optimism (p<.05).

Table 2

Correlation between Spirituality and Pessimism among Afghan and Pakistani (N=63)

Group	*Scales*	*N*	*Mean*	*SD*	*r*	*p*
Afghan	Spirituality	26	51.23	9.425		
	Pessimism	26	1.50	1.105	.031	n.s
Pakistani	Spirituality	37	47.19	12.523		
	Pessimism	37	1.59	1.142	.215	n.s

*p < .05; **p <.01.

Table-2 shows correlation between the scores of spirituality and pessimism of Afghans and Pakistanis. The result reveals that there is no significantly positive correlation between Spirituality and Pessimism among Afghans and Pakistanis.

Table 3

Correlation between Spirituality and Life Orientation Scale among Afghan and Pakistani (N=63)

Group	*Scales*	*N*	*Mean*	*SD*	*r*	*p*
Afghan	Spirituality	26	51.23	9.425		
	LOS	26	4.88	1.451	.034	n.s
Pakistani	Spirituality	37	47.19	12.523		
	LOS	37	4.59	1.607	.349*	.03

*p < .05; **p <.01

Table-3 shows correlation between the scores of spirituality and Life Orientation Scale of Afghans and Pakistanis. The result reveals that there is no correlation or negligible correlation between Spirituality and Life Orientation Scale among Afghans while the scores of Pakistanis show that there is a low degree of positive correlation between spirituality and optimism.

Table 4

Correlation between Spirituality and Life Satisfaction among Afghan and Pakistani (N=63)

Group	*Scales*	*N*	*Mean*	*SD*	*r*	*p*
Afghan	Spirituality	26	51.23	9.425		
	Life Satis	26	133.27	11.127	.346	n.s
Pakistani	Spirituality	37	47.19	12.523		
	Life Satis	37	120.05	18.674	.226	n.s

*p < .05; **p <.01

Table-4 shows correlation between the scores of spirituality and Life Satisfaction of Afghans and Pakistanis. The result reveals that there is no significant positive correlation or negligible correlation between Spirituality and Life Satisfaction among Afghans and Pakistanis show that there is an insignificant low degree of positive correlation between spirituality and Life Satisfaction.

Table 5

Mean difference and t-value of Afghan and Pakistani on scores of optimism (N=63)

Group	*N*	*Mean*	*SD*	*t*	*p*
Afghan	26	3.38	.752	-1.913	.06
Pakistani	37	2.97	.897		

df=61

Table-5 shows the mean difference among Afghans and Pakistanis on the scores of Optimism. The result reveals that there is no significant difference between scores of Afghans and Pakistanis on Optimism p>.05, p>.01.

Table 6

Mean difference and t-value of Afghan and Pakistani on scores of pessimism (N=63)

Group	*N*	*Mean*	*SD*	*t*	*p*
Afghan	26	1.50	1.105	.328	.744
Pakistani	37	1.59	1.142		

df=61

Table-6 shows the mean difference among Afghans and Pakistanis on the scores of Pessimism. The result reveals that there is no significant difference between scores of Afghans and Pakistanis on Pessimism p>.05, p>.01.

Table 7

Mean difference and t-value of Afghan and Pakistani on scores of life orientation scale (N=63)

Group	N	*Mean*	SD	t	p
Afghan	26	4.88	1.451	-.734	.466
Pakistani	37	4.59	1.607		

df=61.

Table-7 shows the mean difference among Afghans and Pakistanis on the scores of Life Orientation Scale. The result reveals that there is no significant difference between scores of Afghans and Pakistanis on Life Orientation Scale p>.05, p>.01.

Table 8

Mean difference and t-value of Afghan and Pakistani on scores of life satisfaction scale (N=63)

Group	N	*Mean*	SD	t	p
Afghan	26	51.23	9.425	-1.391	.169
Pakistani	37	47.19	12.523		

df=61

Table-8 shows the mean difference among Afghans and Pakistanis on the scores of Life Satisfaction scale. The result reveals that there is no significant difference between scores of Afghans and Pakistanis on Life Satisfaction p>.05, p>.01.

Table 9

Mean difference and t-value of Afghan and Pakistani on scores of spirituality scale (N=63)

Group	N	*Mean*	SD	t	p
Afghan	26	51.23	9.425	-3.224	.002
Pakistani	37	47.19	12.523		

df=61

Table-9 shows the mean difference between the scores of spirituality and Life Satisfaction of Afghans and Pakistanis. The result reveals that Pakistanis scored higher than Afghans on Spirituality scale and the results are significant at $p<.05$.

Table 10

Correlation between Spirituality, Optimism, Pessimism, Life Orientation and Life Satisfaction on the total sample (N=63)

Scale	*Mean*	*SD*	*r*	*p*
Optimism	3.14	.859	.347**	.005
Pessimism	1.56	1.118	.130	.309
Life Orien	4.71	1.539	.274*	.030
Life Satis	48.86	11.441	.298*	.018

*p<.05;

**p<.01.

Table-10 shows correlation between the scores of Spirituality, Optimism, Pessimism, Life Orientation and Life Satisfaction on the total sample of Afghans and Pakistanis. The result reveals that Spirituality is positively correlated with Optimism, Life orientation, and Life satisfaction on the other hand Spirituality is poorly correlated with Pessimism.

DISCUSSION

Our study shows that spirituality is a prime variable that has impact on life orientation and life satisfaction important components of explanatory life styles. Afghan subjects since their birth facing many problems like education, housing, employment, health, marriage, and absence of father or mother or in some cases of both. One of the most important factors that emerged during interview after completion of the study was identity loss; by and large they are in search of identity that developed negative attitude towards optimism and life satisfaction. Our Afghan subjects are not confident about their future .We cannot and should not underestimate personality aspect of our Afghan subjects that made the in a particular direction. One should also consider Pakistani subjects' general tendency .They have better environment as compared with their counterparts. Pakistani subjects have also same conditions of a lesser intensity. At a global level, probably one may agree that peoples of developing and in particular under developing nations may have this dilemma.

Researchers have paid serious attention to examine applied significance of spirituality in the daily activities of individuals of different walks of life .Our study has been supported by a larger numbers of earlier studies that there is a positive relationship between spirituality and mental health, and life satisfaction (Payne *et al*,1991) .On the opposite side pessimism as a negative personality trait is poorly correlated with spirituality .One may conclude from the present study that spirituality improves life satisfaction and reduces the chances of pessimistic: negative thinking.

There is a need to undertake a larger cross-cultural study with a more extensive sample, the findings of which would have implications for social and health scientists in general and psychologists in particular.

REFERENCES

Anderson, D.A &Worthy (1997), Exploring a fourth dimension: Sprituality as a resource a for the couple therapist. *Journal of Marital and Family Therapy*. 23(1), 3-12

Argyle, M (1987), *The Psychology of Happiness*. London: Methuen

Argyle, M (1991), Cooperation: The basis of sociability. London: Routledge.

Bowen, R.T.L; & Harrell, J.P (2002), Racist experience and health outcomes: An Examination of spirituality as a buffer. *Journal of Black Psychology*, 28(1), 18-36.

Burkhardt, M.A (1989), Spirituality: An analysis of a concept, *Helistic Nursing Practice*, 3(3), 69-76.

Diener, E (1984), Subjective well-being. *Psychology Bulletin*, 95, 542-575.

Emed, Y (1995), Control Theory and Spirituality, *Journal of Reality Therapy*, 14(2), 63-66.

Frankl, V.E (1963), Man's search for meaning, New York: Washington Square.

Howden, W (1992), Development and psychometric characteristics of the Spirituality Assessment Scale: PhD Dissertation (unpublished), Texas University.

Kamen-Siegal (1991), Explanatory style and cell-mediated immunity in elderly men and women, *Health Psychology*, 10, 29-235.

Lindgren, K.N; and Coursey, R. D (1995), Spirituality and serious mental illness: A two-part Study, *Psychological Rehabilitation Journal, 18*(3), 93-117.

Mastekaasa, A (1984), Multiplicative and additive models of job and life satisfaction, *Social Indicators Research*, 14, 141-163.

Payne, I. R; Bergin, A .E; Biellena, K. A; and Jenkins, P.H (1991) Review of religion and mental Health: Prevention and the enhancement of psychological functioning, *Prevention in Human Services*, 9, 11-40.

Reker, G.T; and Wong, P.T.P (1983), Coping with stress: Divergent strategies of optimists and Pessimists, *Journal of Personality and Social Psychology,* 51 (6), 1257-1264.

Scheier, M.F; and Carver, C.S (1985), Optimism, coping, and health: assessment and implications of generalized outcome expectancies on health, *Journal of Personality,* 55, 169-210.

Seligman, M.E.P (1991), learned optimism, New York: Knopf.

Simoni, J. M; Martone, M.G; and Kerwin, J.F (2002), Spirituality and psychological adaptation among women with HIV/AIDS: Implications for counseling, *Journal of Counseling Psychology,* 49 (2), 139-147.

Tson, M .W; and Lin, J.T (2001), Happiness and domain satisfaction in Taiwan, *Journal of Happiness Studies,* 2 (3), 208-213.

Warr, P (1979), Scales for the assessment of some work attitudes and aspects of psychological well–Being, *Journal of Occupational Psychology,* 52, 129-148.

Wulff, D. M (1996). The psychology of religion: An overview. In E .P .Shapraspe (Eds), Religion and t*he clinical practice of psychology,* Washington, D.C: American psychological Association.

Zinnbauer, B.J; Pargament, K.I; and Scott, A. B (1999), The emerging meaning of religious and spirituality: Problems and prospects, *Journal of Personality,* 67, 889-919.

Zumeta, Z .D (1993), Spirituality and meditation. The soul of family meditation, *Meditation Quarterly,* 11 (1), 25-38.

20

Addictive Behaviour and Common Mental Disorders
A General Hospital Based Study

Nalini Bikkina*, U. Vindhya**

ABSTRACT

Common Mental disorders was a term coined by Goldberg and Huxley to describe "disorders which are commonly encountered in community settings, and whose occurrence signals a breakdown in normal functioning". Epidemiological studies have linked mental disorder to social malaise and economic recession. From the socio-pathological perspective, over the past few decades many maladies like crime, mental disorders, family disorganization, juvenile delinquency, alcoholism and drug abuse and much that now passes as the result of pathological processes have been considered as indicative of sick societies implying thereby the inadequacies or failures of social controls or social norms in given societies. Thus the importance of the role of social factors in many mental health problems becomes clear. The objectives of this study therefore were to examine the distribution of addictive behaviour and to study the association between addictive behaviour and common mental disorders. The study used a cross-sectional survey design. The tools used were the GHQ-28 and a socio-demographic

* Research Scholar, Department of Psychology & Parapsychology, Andhra University.

** Professor, Department of Psychology & Parapsychology, Andhra University.

data sheet. Results showed a significant association between addictive behaviour and several dimensions of Common Mental Disorders as measured by GHQ-28.

Common Mental Disorders was a term coined by Goldberg and Huxley (1992) to describe "disorders which are commonly encountered in community settings, and whose occurrence signals a breakdown in normal functioning".

The revolution in public health with its impact on the preventive and promotive aspects of mental health and the revolution in psychiatry recognizing the socio-cultural factors in mental health problems have led to certain researches which attempt to examine individuals with potential mental health risks and the role of psychosocial factors associated with mental health problems (Satyavathi, 1988).

Epidemiological studies have linked mental disorder to social malaise and economic recession (Cockerham, 1989). From the socio-pathological perspective, over the past few decades many maladies like crime, mental disorders, family disorganization, juvenile delinquency, alcoholism and drug abuse and much that now passes as the result of pathological processes (Frank, 1936) have been considered as indicative of sick societies implying thereby the inadequacies or failures of social controls or social norms in given societies. Thus the importance of the role of social factors in many mental health problems becomes clear (Satyavathi, 1988).

These disorders manifest with a mixture of somatic, anxiety and depressive symptoms. However, undue partitioning of these categories of disorders ignores their commonalities (Kroenke, 2000). Several studies have described the clinical presentations of these disorders in general health care settings. The commonest complaints are somatic, in particular tiredness and weakness, multiple aches and pains, dizziness, palpitations and sleep disturbances (Chaturvedi, Upadhyaya & Rao, 1988; Ebigbo, Janakiramaiah & Kumaraswamy, 1989; Patel, Pereira & Mann, 1998; Srinivasan & Suresh, 1990). However, these are distress states with non-somatic aetiology (Patel et al., 1997).

Common Mental Disorders are the third most frequent causes of morbidity in adults (prevalence rates) worldwide (World Health

Organization, 1995). They are an important cause of disability and pose a significant public health problem (Ormel et al., 1994). The warning of a mounting crisis of unmet needs for the countless millions with such disorders have been building up over the past 20 years.

The WHO Multinational Study of the prevalence, nature and determinants of common mental disorders in general medical care settings was conducted in 14 countries (Ustun et al., 1995). The study showed that though the prevalence of mental disorders across the sites varied considerably, the results clearly demonstrate that a substantial proportion (about 24%) of all patients in these settings had a mental disorder. The most common diagnoses in primary care settings are depression, anxiety and substance abuse disorders. These disorders are present either alone or in addition to one or more physical disorders. There are no consistent differences in prevalence between developed and developing countries. Indeed, the only similarities across centers were the general observations of the ubiquity of common mental disorders, the comorbidity of anxiety and depression, and the association of common mental disorders and disability even after adjustment for physical disease severity. On the other hand, specific variables showed substantial variations; thus the prevalence rates of common mental disorders ranged from 7% to 52% of attenders; physician recognition of common mental disorders varied from 5% to nearly 60% and the association of key variables such as gender, physical ill-health and education with common mental disorders were in opposite directions in different centers. These findings demonstrate the need for locally relevant studies with locally validated methodologies whose aim is to identify local needs and inform local health services (Patel & Winston, 1994).

Substance abuse is emerging as a serious public health concern in India. In today's context what is even more alarming is the fact that the first-time users belong to a much younger age group. Also, our society's traditional prohibition-oriented attitude that once frowned upon alcohol use has been replaced by a newfound acceptance. The social, psychological and economic implications of substance abuse are enormous. Crime rates ranging from assault to murder are also known to increase with addiction. The loss to the family is difficult to quantify. The emotional trauma, shame and grief resulting therefrom and the frequent threat of violence and subsequent separation destroys the family system. Addiction impacts children's lives too, often leaving them to bear its consequences till late into their adulthood (Thirumagal & Ranganathan, 2003).

A review of studies in India showed that the levels of depression and social dysfunction were reportedly high among drug addicts (Ganju, 2000; Mitra & Mukhopadhyay, 2000). Non-psychotic psychiatric illness may occur due to poverty caused by alcohol consumption (Patel, Pereira & Mann, 1998).

The alcohol consumption rate in Kerala has increased manifold and is today one of the highest in the country. Kerala stands first in the per capita consumption of alcohol (Krishnakumar, 2000b). Kerala has also shown an increase in crimes registered under the Narcotic Drugs and Psychotropic Substances Act. There is now a fast expanding market for narcotics in the State. The State Mental Health Authority (SMHA) identified drug addicts as another group at risk (Krishnakumar, 2000a). Depression together with alcohol or drug use can be lethal.

Aggressive marketing is playing a substantial role in the globalization of alcohol and tobacco use among young people, thus increasing the risk of disorders related to substance use and associated physical conditions (Klein, 1999).

Alcohol use is rising rapidly in some of the developing regions of the world (Jernigan et al., 2000; Riley & Marshall, 1999; World Health Organization, 1999) and this is likely to escalate alcohol related problems. Alcohol use is also a major reason for concern among the indigenous people around the world, who show a higher prevalence of use and associated problems. Also, the risk of having a non-psychotic disorder was associated with having abused alcohol (Hintikka et al., 2000).

Point prevalence of alcohol use disorders (harmful use and dependence) in adults has been estimated to be around 1.7% globally according to Global Burden of Disease 2000 analysis. The rates are 2.8% for men and 0.5% for women. The prevalence of alcohol use disorders varies widely across different regions of the world, ranging from very low levels in some Middle Eastern countries to over 5% in North America and parts of Eastern Europe (World Health Organization, 2001). Alcohol intoxication seems to be an important risk factor for major depression (Hamalainen et al., 2001).

The link between tobacco use and mental disorders is a complex one. People with mental disorders are about twice as likely to smoke as others. Epidemiological studies have revealed associations between cigarette smoking and psychiatric disorders (Glassman, 1993). Never- and ex- smokers had relatively low rates of psychiatric disorder, whereas, among current smokers, risk of psychiatric disorder, increased with the number of cigarettes smoked (Rasul et al., 2001). Associations between cigarette smoking and psychological symptoms have been observed for affective and anxiety disorders (Jorm, 1999), symptoms of depression (Hamalainen et al., 2001; Son et al., 1997; Tamburrino et al., 1994) and risk of suicide (Davey-Smith, Phillips & Neaton, 1992; Hemenway, Solnick & Colditz, 1993; Tanskanen, Viinamaki, Hintikaa, Koivumaa-Honkanen & Lehtonen, 1998).

Individuals with current mental disorders had a smoking rate of 41% compared with 22.5% in the general population, and it is estimated that 44% of all cigarettes smoked in the US are consumed by people with mental disorders (Lasser et al, 2000). Individuals with depression are also more likely to be smokers (Pornerleau et al., 1995). Though the traditional thinking has been that depressed individuals tend to smoke more because of their symptoms, new evidence reveals that it may be the other way round. A study of teenagers showed that those who became depressed had a higher prevalence of smoking beforehand – suggesting that smoking actually resulted in depression in this age group (Goodman & Capitman, 2000).

Besides tobacco and alcohol, a large number of other substances – generally grouped under the broad category of drugs – are also abused. These include illicit drugs such as heroin, cocaine and cannabis. The period prevalence of drug abuse and dependence ranges from 0.4% to 4% (World Health Organization, 2001).

The implication of these studies is that substance abuse is a crucial factor in the prevalence and maintenance of non-psychotic psychiatric illnéss.

METHODOLOGY

The study was conducted in Kannur, a district in north Kerala. The study used a cross-sectional survey design. The sample consisted of 190 patients who visited the outpatient wards of three general hospitals. A socio-demographic data-sheet was prepared by the investigator and translated into Malayalam for the purpose of the study. The General Health Questionnaire - 28 (GHQ 28), used as a screening device measures the dimensions of somatic symptoms, anxiety and insomnia, social dysfunction and depression. It was translated into Malayalam for the purpose of the present study. Addictive behaviour was categorized into None, Smoking, Drinking and Drugs and measured as part of a semi-structured interview.

The objectives of the study were:

- To examine the distribution of addictive behaviour across the sample based on the scores obtained on the General Health Questionnaire – 28 by the respondents.
- To study the association between addictive behaviour and common mental disorders in the sample.

For the purpose of this study, the cut-off score between cases and normals was taken as between 5 and 6 so that respondents with 5 or fewer symptoms are considered normal and those with 6 or more are considered *cases*. The responses on the General Health Questionnaire were individually analyzed to arrive at an estimate of the patterns of psychological morbidity and its association with addictive behaviour.

For analysis, the Statistical Package for Social Sciences (version 10.0) was used. Frequencies were used to note the distribution of the sample and the cases among the sample across addictive behaviour. The *F* test was done along with the *t* test to examine the relationship between GHQ-28 totals and addictive behaviour and between individual dimensions of the GHQ-28 and addictive behaviour.

RESULTS

On the variables related to addictive behaviour, it was found that those who were significantly affected were those addicted to alcohol as shown in Table 1. Aggressive marketing is playing a substantial role in the globalization of alcohol use among young people, thus increasing the risk of disorders related to substance use and associated conditions (Klein, 1999., Jernigan et al.,, 2000., Riley & Marshall, 1999., World Health Organization, 1999). Also, the risk of having a non-psychotic disorder was associated with having abused alcohol (Hintikka et al., 2000). Non-psychotic psychiatric illness may also occur due to poverty caused by alcohol consumption (Patel, Pereira & Mann, 1998).

Table 1

Distribution of non-cases and cases on Addictive behaviour

Variables	*Non-cases*		*Cases*		*Total*		*Chi-Square*
	n	%	*n*	%	*n*	%	
Addictive behaviour							
None	104	69.3%	46	30.7%	150	100%	df = 2
Smoking	6	60.0%	4	40.0%	10	100%	13.970**
Drinking	10	33.3%	20	66.7%	30	100%	

** Significant at 0.01 level.

To understand the relationship between addictive behaviour and the four dimensions of the GHQ-28, an ANOVA was done. The GHQ-28 has four sub-scales measuring four dimensions of psychological distress. The sub scales are: A-Scale consisting of items on somatic symptoms; B-Scale dealing with anxiety and insomnia; C-Scale consisting of items on social dysfunction; and D-Scale comprising items on severe depression.

Table 2

Mean scores on somatic symptoms across addictive behaviour

Variables	*n*	*Mean*	*Standard deviation*	*F*
Addictive behaviour				
None	150	0.69	1.33	
Smoking	10	1.80	1.81	7.446**
Drinking	30	1.60	1.59	

** Significant at 0.01 level.

On the variables related to addictive behaviour those who scored significantly higher on somatic symptoms were from the group that reported smoking as shown in Table 2. People with mental disorders are about twice as likely to smoke as others. Epidemiological studies have revealed associations between cigarette smoking and psychiatric disorders (Glassman, 1993). Never- and ex- smokers had relatively low rates of psychiatric disorder, whereas, among current smokers, risk of psychiatric disorder, increased with the number of cigarettes smoked (Rasul et al., 2001). Associations between cigarette smoking and psychological symptoms have been observed for affective and anxiety disorders (Jorm, 1999), symptoms of depression (Hamalainen et al., 2001; Son et al., 1997; Tamburrino et al., 1994) and risk of suicide (Davey-Smith, Phillips & Neaton, 1992; Hemenway, Solnick & Colditz, 1993; Tanskanen et al., 1998).

Individuals with depression are also more likely to be smokers (Pornerleau et al., 1995). Though the traditional thinking has been that depressed individuals tend to smoke more because of their symptoms, new evidence reveals that it may be the other way round.

Table 3

Mean scores on Anxiety and Insomnia across Addictive behaviour

Variables	*n*	*Mean*	*Standard deviation*	*F*
Addictive behaviour				
None	150	0.82	1.18	
Smoking	10	1.20	1.48	3.522*
Drinking	30	1.43	1.22	

* Significant at 0.05 level.

Of the variables related to addictive behaviour, those who scored significantly higher mean scores on anxiety and insomnia were found to be addicted to drinking alcohol as shown in Table 3. The risk of having a non-psychotic disorder was found to be associated with having abused alcohol (Hintikka et al., 2000). The alcohol consumption rate in Kerala has increased manifold and is today one of the highest in the country (Krishnakumar, 2000b) and this is likely to escalate alcohol related problems including anxiety and insomnia.

Table 4

Mean scores on Social dysfunction across Addictive behaviour

Variables	*n*	*Mean*	*Standard deviation*	*F*
Addictive behaviour				
None	150	3.23	1.09	
Smoking	10	2.10	1.10	**4.932****
Drinking	30	3.30	1.29	

** Significant at 0.01 level.

It was found that the highest mean score on social dysfunction was obtained by those who were drinking alcohol as shown in Table 4. It is not surprising that those who were dependent on alcohol scored significantly higher on social dysfunction. As the person with addictive drinking becomes more and more concerned with the need to obtain alcohol, interpersonal skills and attendance to usual interests and responsibilities may deteriorate. Excessive drinking may also induce persistent anxiety, which might further result in social dysfunction. Excessive drinking is also liable to cause profound social disruption particularly in the family. Marital and family tension and conflicts are virtually inevitable, which may even lead to long-lasting consequences such as separation and/or divorce.

Table 5

Mean scores on depression across Addictive behaviour

Variables	*n*	*Mean*	*Standard deviation*	*F*
Addictive behaviour				
None	150	0.50	1.13	
Smoking	10	0.00	0.00	**1.490**
Drinking	30	0.70	1.21	

No significant differences were found in the mean scores on depression across the variables related to addictive behaviour as shown in Table 5.

Table 6

Mean GHQ-28 totals across Addictive behaviour

Variables	*n*	*Mean*	*Standard deviation*	*F*
Addictive behaviour				
None	150	5.22	2.67	
Smoking	10	5.00	1.76	**5.383****
Drinking	30	7.03	3.61	

Those who scored significantly higher on GHQ-28 were people who had drinking as a regular habit as shown in Table 6. Alcohol abuse has emerged as a major health concern, with both physical and psychological manifestations (WHO, 1999). The risk of having a non-psychotic disorder has been associated with having abused alcohol (Hintikka et al., 2000). The alcohol consumption rate in Kerala has increased manifold and is today one of the highest in the country. Kerala stands first in the per capita consumption of alcohol (Krishnakumar, 2000b).

CONCLUSION

Somatization was found to be associated with smoking behaviour. Anxiety and insomnia, social dysfunction and overall mental morbidity, as measured by GHQ-28 were significantly associated with addiction to alcohol.

Estimates of the prevalence of harmful substance abuse among general hospital populations vary with the medical problems addressed. Several efforts to combine medical care and substance abuse treatment in medical settings are limited by time in medical settings. Most of these efforts can provide patients with rapid substance abuse assessment and brief interventions. A brief intervention usually involves a short counseling session during which the counselor or medical provider assesses the patient's substance use, gives the patient feedback on the assessment results, and then negotiates a plan of action with the patient to change his or her behavior.

Brief substance abuse interventions can potentially reduce health-care costs. Certainly, many patients need intensive substance abuse treatment such as inpatient or outpatient programs. In these cases, brief interventions serve to help the patient become motivated to seek this intensive treatment sooner than he or she might without help.

REFERENCES

Chaturvedi, S.K., Upadhyaya, M.P., & Rao, S. (1988). Somatic symptoms in a community clinic. *Indian Journal of Psychiatry,* 30, 369-374.

Cockerham, W.C. (1989). *Sociology of Mental Disorder.* (2nd ed.). Englewood Cliffs: Prentice Hall.

Davey-Smith, G., Phillips, A.N., & Neaton, J.D. (1992). Smoking as independent risk factor for suicide: Illustration of an artifact from observational epidemiology? *Lancet, 340,* 709-712.

Ebigbo, P.O., Janakiramaiah, N., & Kumaraswamy, N. (1989). Somatization in cross-cultural perspective. In. K. Peltzer, & P. Ebigbo (Eds.), *Clinical Psychology in Africa* (pp. 233 - 250). Enugu, Nigeria: Chuka Printing Company.

Frank, L.K. (1936). Society as the patient. *American Journal of Sociology,* 42, 335-344.

Ganju, V. (2000). Depression, social anxiety and approval motive patterns of narcotic drug addicts in comparison with relapsed and abstinent. *Journal of the Indian Academy of Applied Psychology,* 26 (1-2), 41-45.

Glassman, A.H. (1993). Cigarette smoking: Implications for psychiatric illness. *American Journal of Psychiatry,* 150 (4), 546-553.

Goldberg, D.P. & Huxley, P. (1992). *Common Mental Disorders.* London: Routledge & Kegan Paul.

Goodman, E., & Capitman, J. (2000). Depressive symptoms and cigarette smoking among teens. *Pediatrics,* 106 (4), 748-755.

Hamalainen, J., Kaprio, J., Isometsa, E., Heikkinen, M., Poikolainen, K., Lindeman, S., & Aro, H. (2001). Cigarette smoking, alcohol intoxication and major depressive episode in a representative population sample. *Journal of Epidemiology and Community Health,* 55, 573-576.

Hemenway, D., Solnick, D.J., & Colditz, G.A. (1993). Smoking and suicide among nurses. *American Journal of Public Health,* 83 (2), 249-251.

Hintikka, J., Hintikka, U., Lehtonen, J., Viinamaeki, H., Koskela, K., & Kontula, O. (2000). Common mental disorders, suicidality and use of health care services during late adolescence in Finland. *Journal of Adolescent Health,* 26 (1), 2-3.

Jernigan, D.H., Monteiro, M., Room, R., & Saxena, S. (2000). Towards a global alcohol policy: Alcohol, public health and the role of WHO. *Bulletin of the World Health Organization,* 78, 491-499.

Jorm, A.F. (1999). Association between smoking and mental disorders: Results from an Australian National Prevalence Survey. *Australian and New Zealand Journal of Public Health,* 23 (3), 245 - 248.

Klein, N. (1999). *No logo: Taking on the brand bullies.* New York: Picador.

Krishnakumar, R. (2000a, April 28). State of Despair. *Frontline,* 97-100.

Krishnakumar, R. (2000b, November 24). The lure of the brew. *Frontline,* 36-39.

Kroenke, K. (2000). Somatization in primary care: It's time for parity. *General Hospital Psychiatry,* 22 (3), 141-143.

Lasser, K., Wesley, B.J., Woolhandler, S., Himmelstein, D.U., McCormick, D., & Bor, D.H. (2000). Smoking and mental illness: A population-based prevalence study. *Journal of the American Medical Association, 284,* 2606-2610.

Mitra, G., & Mukhopadhyay, A. (2000). Psychological factors in drug addicts and normals: A comparative study. *Journal of Projective Psychology and Mental Health,* 7 (1), 53-78.

Ormel, J., Von Korff, M., Ustun, T., Pini, S., Korten, A., & Oldehinkel, T. (1994). Common mental disorders and disability across cultures. Journal of American Medical Association, 272, *1741-1748.*

Patel, V., Pereira, J., Coutinho, L., & Fernandes, R. (1997). Is the labeling of common mental disorders as psychiatric illness clinically useful in primary care? *Indian Journal of Psychiatry, 39* (3), 239-246.

Patel, V., Pereira, J., & Mann, A.H. (1998). Somatic and psychological models of common mental disorder in primary care in India. Psychological Medicine, 28 *(1), 135-143.*

Patel, V., & Winston, M. (1994). The universality of mental illness revisited: Assumptions, artifacts and new directions. *British Journal of Psychiatry, 165,* 437-440.

Pornerleau, O.F., Downey, K.K., Stelson, F.W., & Polerleau, C.S. (1995). Cigarette smoking in adult patients diagnosed with attention deficit hyperactivity disorder. *Journal of Substance Abuse, 7* (3), 373-378.

Rasul, F., Stansfeld, S.A., Davey-Smith, G., Hart, C.L., & Gillis, C. (2001). Sociodemographic Factors, Smoking and Common Mental Disorder in the Renfrew and Paisley (MIDSPAN) Study. *Journal of Health Psychology, 6* (2), 149-158.

Riley, L., & Marshall, M. (Eds.). (1999). *Alcohol and public health in eight developing countries.* Geneva: World Health Organization. (Unpublished document WHO/HSC/SAB/99.9).

Satyavathi, K. (1988). Mental health. In J. Pandey (Ed.), *Psychology in India: The State-of-the-Art. Volume 3: Organizational Behaviour and Mental Health* (pp. 217-287), New Delhi: Sage Publications.

Son, B.K., Markovitz, J.H., Winders, S., & Smith, D. (1997). Smoking, nicotine dependence and depressive symptoms in the CARDIA study. Effects of educational status. *American Journal of Epidemiology,* 145 (2), 110-116.

Srinivasan, T.N., & Suresh, T.R. (1990). Non-specific symptoms and screening of non-psychotic morbidity in primary care. *Indian Journal of Psychiatry.* 32 (1), 77-82.

Tamburrino, M.B., Lynch, D.J., Nagel, R.W., Stadler, N., & Pauling, T. (1994). Screening women in family practice settings: Associations between depression and smoking cigarettes. *Family Practice Research Journal, 14* (4), 333-337.

Tanskanen, A., Viinamaki, H., Hintikaa, J., Koivumaa-Honkanen, H.T., & Lehtonen, J. (1998). Smoking and suicidality among psychiatric patients. *American Journal of Psychiatry,* 155 (1), 129-130.

Thirumagal, V., & Ranganathan, S. (2003). Meeting challenges in the field of addiction. In. V. Patel, & R. Thara (Eds.), *Meeting the Mental Health Needs of Developing Countries. NGO Innovations in India* (pp. 289-308). New Delhi: Sage Publications.

Ustun, T., Sartorius, N., Costa e Silva, J., Goldberg, D., Lecrubier, Y., Ormel, J., Von Korff, M., & Wittchen, H., (1995). Conclusions. In. T.B. Ustun, & N. Sartorius. (Eds.), *Mental illness in general health care: An international study* (pp. 371-375). Chichester: John Wiley and Sons.

World Health Organization (1995). *The World Health Report 1995: Bridging the Gaps.* World Health Organization: Geneva.

World Health Organization. (1999). *Global status report on alcohol.* Geneva: World Health Organization. (Unpublished document WHO/HSC/SAB/ 99.11).

World Health Organization. (2001). *The World Health Report 2001. Mental Health: New Understanding, New Hope.* Geneva: Author.

21

Need Saliency and Human Happiness

F.M. Sahoo*

ABSTRACT

The present investigation is directed towards examining the proposition that human happiness is significantly associated with satisfaction of their *salient needs,* and it is unrelated to the satisfaction of nonsalient needs. Males and females from highly urbanized, moderately urbanized and less urbanized areas were asked to rank-order their needs. This was helpful in identifying their salient and nonsalient needs. They were further asked to indicate the extent each of the needs was satisfied. Moreover, their happiness was assessed with the help of a standardized measure of human happiness. The examination of the relationship between salient needs satisfaction and happiness supported the prediction. Similarly, the relationship was found between nonsalient need satisfaction and happiness. There was no sex difference on happiness. The results were explained in light of contemporary theories of happiness. The major implications were also discussed.

Human happiness refers to inner harmony – a state of tranquility of ones own mind. Philosophers down the ages have tried to unravel how this inner harmony is achieved. Some great scholars weighed happiness with the quality of life of society. David

* Professor, Centre of Advanced Study in Psychology, Utkal University, Bhubaneswar, Orissa.

Hartley, Joseph Priestly and Jeremy Bentham construed a good society as that which allows greatest happiness for the greatest number. A good society ensuring better quality of life breeds happiness. Highlighting this aspect, Confucius stressed the relationship between individuals. Great thinkers of the ranks of David Hume and Baron de Montesquieu had aptly made a fundamental conclusion that the pursuit of happiness is the basis for both social well being and individual motivation. A modern-day scientist judges the quality of life of a society by measuring the amount of goods and services produced by a society, low crime rate, a long life expectancy, respect for human rights and an equitable distribution of resources.

Though influenced by external factors, happiness is not solely dependent on them. Thomas Aquinas had defined the quality of human life in terms of virtue, closeness to God and other personal qualities of an individual. Aristotle, the Greek philosopher had remarked "although human kind values a great many things such as health, fame and possessions because we think that they will make us happy, we value happiness for itself." Happiness is the only intrinsic goal that people seek for its own sake, it is the bottomline of all desires. Many have opined that the prerequisite of happiness is the ability to get fully involved in life. So happiness is both a product and a process in itself.

The contemporary approach to defining and measuring quality of life is directly in terms of subjective well-being (SWB)-how individuals evaluate their lives, both in terms of satisfaction judgements and in terms of affective reactions (moods and emotions). The areas of SWB has three hall-marks. First, it is subjective. According to Campbell, it resides within the experience of the individual. Objective conditions are seen as potential influences on SWB. Second, SWB includes positive measures. Third, a SWB measure typically includes a global assessment of all aspects of a persons life.

In defining happiness, it is common sense to combine the frequency and intensity of pleasant emotions. That is, the people considered to be the happiest are those who are intensely happy more of the time. Ed Diener et al (1995) however opine that how much of the time a person experiences pleasant emotions is a better predictor than positive emotional intensity of how the person reports being.

Further, emotional intensity forms a factor that is independent of SWB. Thus feeling pleasant emotions most of the time and infrequently experiencing unpleasant emotions, even if the pleasant emotions are only mild, is sufficient for high reports of happiness.

Although most people report being above neutral in mood, the majority of the time intense positive moments are rare even among the happiest individuals. Instead happy people report mild to moderate pleasant emotions most of the time when alone or with others and when working or at leisure.

PREDICTORS OF HAPPINESS

It seems likely that the variables that influence people's evaluations of their lives do vary across cultures. Predictors of life satisfaction are systematically related to characteristics of societies: individualism vs collectivism, income per person and cultural homogeneity.

Self-reported happiness predicts other indicators of well-being compared with those who are depressed. Happy people are less self-focused, less hostile and abusive, and less vulnerable to disease. They also are more loving, forgiving, trusting, energetic, decisive, creative, sociable and helpful.

Causes of SWB may differ across cultures. Veenhoven (1991) showed that the influence of income on SWB differs across nations. Diener and Fukita found that the predictors of individual SQB differed in an analogous manner. Based on a persons goals, different resources predicted his/her happiness. Taken together, these results clearly indicate that there are different predictors of happiness for different people and in different societies.

Among the several theories four central theories related to happiness are activity theories, judgement theories, topdown versus bottom up theories, and telic theories.

Activity theories maintain that happiness is a by product of human activity. The most explicit formulation about activity and subjective well being is the theory of flow. Activities are seen as pleasurable when the challenge is matched to the persons skill level. If an activity is too easy, boredom will develop. If it is too difficult, anxiety will result.

Judgement theories maintain that happiness results from a comparison between some standard and actual conditions. In social comparison theory one uses other people as a standard. If a person is better than others, that person will be satisfied and happy.

Bottom-up theories maintain that happiness is simply the sum of many small pleasures. In contrast, the *top down approach* assumes that a person enjoys pleasures because he or she is happy and not vice versa.

Telic theories of subjective well being maintain that happiness is gained when some state, such as goal or need, is reached. One theoretical postulate offered by Wilson (1960) is that the "satisfaction of needs causes happiness and conversely, persistence of unfulfilled needs causes unhappiness."

Needs are deficiencies and are created wherever there is a physiological or psychological imbalance. It is the unsatisfied need that creates tension, therefore, unsatisfied needs are the starting points for under-standing of motivation.

MOTIVATIONAL FORMULATION

Maslow, the father of humanistic psychology (1954) deserves credit for analyzing human needs and suggesting their break-up in hierarchical order. According to him, man's needs are arranged in a hierarchy or importance ranging from the lowest need (physiological) to safely, love, self-esteem (ego), and finally self actualizations. This hierarchy of prepotency of urgency of satisfaction means that the most urgent needs will be monopolized. Man is continuously wanting. Therefore all needs are never fully-satisfied. As soon as one's need is satisfied, its prepotency diminishes and the next higher unsatisfied need emerges to replace it. This is a never ending process which serves to motivate man to strive to satisfy his or her needs. Finally, the needs are interdependent and overlapping.

Herzberg's (1959) theory of motivation has been referred to as the motivator-hygiene theory. It has same basis assumptions. First, the factors that are present when job satisfaction is produced are separate and distinct from factors that lead to job dissatisfaction. The satisfier relates to the content or nature of the job and dissatisfier describes the employee's relationship to the context of environment in which they engage their work. Therefore, satisfier relates to what employee does, dissatisfier to the environment in which they do it. So it is the hygiene factor that affects job dissatisfaction, whereas motivational factors make people happy with their job by serving need for psychological growth.

Alderfer (1972) advocated the ERG theory which is basically a reworking of Maslow's theory. There are three groups of core needs; existence, relatedness, and growth. The existence of group provides our basic material existence requirements. This is the counterpart of the physiological and safety needs of Maslow. Relatedness refers to the desire for maintaining important interpersonal relationships and tally with Maslow's love needs and external component of esteem need. Growth needs denote an intrinsic desire for personal development. This includes the intrinsic component of esteem and characteristic of self-actualisation. This theory does not assume a rigid hierarchy and all the three categories can operate at the same time. This theory also contends that when a higher-order-need level is frustrated, the individuals desire to increase a low level needs takes place. This theory is more sensitive to individual difference.

McClelland (1961) proposed the three need theory which opines that these needs are important in organizational setting to understand motivation. The three needs are the needs for achievement, power and affiliation.

If all the theories of motivation are compared, we find that they emphasize similar sets of relationships. Maslow views the rarely satisfied higher level needs as motivating force. Herzberg sees satisfiers as motivating force. Alderfer considers growth needs to be the most important and McClelland views power needs as motivators.

In recent time, most of the organizational theories are influenced by Maslows conceptualization. His identification of the basic individual needs find an important place in present day management literature.

However most of theories discussed earlier are based on their observation of individualistic western societies where the need for personal achievement, control and autonomy are considered most important. In contrast, in the developing eastern societies, societal security is considered more important to life that one's freedom and control. People may find work very interesting if it guarantees such security, but may not care for freedom and control. The collective nature of Indian social system contrasts with individualistic western societies where individual is given primary importance. Consequently, the use of Maslow-type of framework which basically evolved in "me" societies of the West is inapplicable in non-western societies. It is also observed that western employees maintain a gap between norms in the family and norms in work spheres. However, as family influences are deeply ingrained in the Indian psyche, there is great deal of carry-over effect from family to work norms.

The western model assumes that protestant ethic type socialization training is the only way of bringing higher involvement. This work ethic trains people to believe that autonomy and personal achievement needs are salient and can provide opportunities for the expression of one's individuality. Countries like India promote in their members a sense of collectivism and saliency for some other needs. Indian people develop beliefs in centrality of work not because work can promote personal achievement, but because the work can fulfill the collective goals of brotherhood and sharing of life.

It was also felt that the satisfaction of intrinsic work needs does not necessarily lead to greater involvement. Most existing instruments to measure alienation reflect a cultural bias, as they include items that place emphasis only on intrinsic need satisfaction.

According to Kanungo (1982) "Empirical research on worker's alienation and involvement in both sociological and psychological literature is fought with conceptual ambiguities. In addition, instruments developed to measure work alienation and involvement often contain inherent methodological inadequacies, since they are based on constructs that are conceptually ambiguous".

The lack of cross-cultural applicability of western-based theories has led Kanungo (1982) to propose a new pancultral formulation. This represents the motivational approach termed the *need saliency model*. Therefore, concept in this model is the saliency of needs which is in contradiction to need hierarchy.

The motivational approach has universal applicability. In contrast to the humanistic approach there is no value orientation in this motivational approach. In this scheme, the distinction between extrinsic and intrinsic needs become unnecessary. Potency of each of the needs is considered in terms of its relation to a given subset of human population. The motivational approach of need saliency model offers a framework having greater cross-cultural generality.

In the context of different life conditions, individuals believe that happiness or sadness depends on whether the condition is perceived to have the potential for satisfying salient needs. The saliency or the importance of different needs for an individual is determined by his or her past experiences with the groups of which he or she was a member (socialization process). People of different groups (such as from different countries) tend to develop different need structures and set different goals and objectives for their lives. Even within a country or culture, there will be differences between groups owing to the differences in the need saliencies of the two groups. Value differences stem especially from past socialization processes and from influence of the norms of the group to which the people belong.

The importance attached to various life conditions reflect the saliency of the needs of the people. The salient needs tend to determine the central life interests of the individuals. In life, the saliency of a need in individuals may be reinforced when they find that through this they are capable of meeting their other needs.

The construct of need saliency has pan cultural elements. However, the application of this pan-cultural framework can further be extended by incorporating some cultural specific aspects relevant in Indian sociocultural system. The Indian society represents a case where resource constraints are often experienced. Consequently, the association between peoples reactions to un-controllability and their happiness is likely to be a significant aspect. The cultural matrix of specific countries has also influenced the evolution of their motivational framework.

More specially, need saliency theory of motivation explicates happiness as a function of salient need satisfaction. No distinction between intrinsic and extensive factors is recognized. This contemporary view of happiness is an important theoretical development and it needs empirical examination in various cultural systems.

The present study examines the above proposition in three subcultures of India.

As argued above, it seems plausible that human happiness is linked with satisfaction of salient needs. Although humans long for the satisfaction of all possible needs, constraints are experienced in pursuing all needs. Accordingly, humans may settle for needs that are considered most important. While this construct of need saliency has been examined and supported in the context of work motivation, it has not been investigated in the field of human happiness. The present investigation is primarily directed towards this objective. In addition, the purpose of the study is to examine the linkage between human happiness and a few other variables.

A precise formulation of the research question can be undertaken with the help of testable hypotheses. The conceptual analysis indicated above generates following hypotheses.

1. Happiness is related to salient need satisfaction.

2. Happiness is unrelated to non-salient need satisfaction.

METHOD

The primary purpose of the present investigation was to examine the role of salient criterion satisfaction of highly, moderately and less urbanized males and females respectively from Mumbai, Damanjodi and Bhubaneswar and determining their subjective well-being. Thus, the other objective was to examine the need saliency hypothesis in the context of gender and setting.

AN OVERVIEW OF THE DESIGN

The study involved 2 (males vs females) X 3 (highly, moderately and less-urbanized settings) factorial design. The males and females were categorized into six groups on the basis of gender and settings. The participants of these six subgroups were compared with respect to a number of dependent measures. The dependent measures included measures of salient criterion satisfaction score, non-salient criterion satisfaction scores, total criterion score, overall satisfaction, happiness score, graphic score, life satisfaction score, social orientation and education.

PARTICIPANTS

The participants were randomly drawn from three different settings: the highly urbanized, the moderately urbanized and the slightly urbanized. The participants for the highly urbanized setting were drawn from Mumbai (18 males and 18 females). The participants for the moderately urbanized setting were drawn from Damanjodi (40 males and 18 females). The participants for the slightly urbanized setting were drawn from Bhubaneswar (20 males and 18 females). Thus, there were in all one hundred and thirty two participants (36 from Mumbai, 58 from Damanjodi, 38 from Bhubaneswar). All the participants were married. They were all educated and their minimum qualification was high school certificate. Since more than half of the participants were working, most of them were highly educated. The age range of the respondents varied from 25 yrs to 55 yrs. The participants were active in their respective domains when the study was conducted. Almost all the participants had middle socio-economic status.

MEASURES

In the present study, a multipart questionnaire, "Personal Orientation Questionnaire" was used to measure subjective well-being. Earlier version of mental health available are heavily loaded on one or two specific negative dimensions such as anxiety, depression and stress. With recent changes in the notion of good living, more and more positive attributes such as competence, control and family relation demanded a modified scale of psychological well-being. The multipart "Personal Orientation Questionnaire" comprises of six sub-measures.

Measure of Context-Specific Importance of Needs: This consists of separate operational measures of the perceived importance of needs in the context of work, family and life in general. First, respondents are asked to rank sixteen different outcomes people seek in their lives according to their perceived importance. These are: "Abundance of leisure activities", "Material prosperity", Receiving respect and recognition in society", "Close intimate friendship", "Appreciation of your unique abilities," "Job satisfaction", "Opportunity for extended religious activities", "Smooth social relations", "Absence of physical illness", "Promising job prospects for children," "Scope for independent thought and action (autonomous activities) "Your own professional success", "A secured life", Own and children's academic achievements", "Support from the most loved person", "Opportunity for greater personal achievement". The sixteen items represent the entire spectrum of human need categories (existential, belonging and growth needs) suggested by various need theorists.

Participants are asked to think specifically in life context and give ranking to same sixteen items in order of importance. A rank of "1" represents the most important and "16" the least important one. The needs ranked 1 and 2 are termed as salient and those ranked "15" and "16" are termed non-salient needs. It may be noted that the need categories are worded in the questionnaire in generic terms to ensure operational construct equivalency in different contexts.

Measure of Need Satisfaction Potential of the Context: In this second part, a total of 16 items are given to measure need satisfaction potential. These are consistent with the measures of need importance in life as described in Part-1. these items measuring potential need satisfaction are worded to reflect how far a context has got a potential to meet a need of an individual. They include statements like, "With the kind of appreciation of my unique abilities, I feel", "With the type of support from the most lived person, I feel", etc. A 6-point ordinal scale is provided in each context. A rating of 1 indicates extreme dissatisfaction and 6 represents extreme satisfaction. Thus, from minimal satisfaction to maximal satisfaction, the total need satisfaction score is obtained by summing up scores of all sixteen items. A salient need satisfaction score is obtained by summing scores given in the satisfaction potential of salient needs identified from Part-1. Similarly, non-salient need satisfaction score is found by adding scores of non-salient needs identified from Part-1. And an overall satisfaction score is obtained from the ranking of the seventeenth item.

Measure of Happiness: In the model of Beck's Depression inventory measure, this part was developed. It measures the degree of happiness involved with different evaluation of ourselves based primarily on feelings. There are 14 groups of statements, four statement in each group. The participant is asked to pick one statement in each group that best describes the way he or she had been feeling for the past two weeks. For example (a) I do not feel happy (b) I feel happy much of the time (c) I am happy all the time (d) I am so happy I feel ecstatic. The first statement in each group is a negative statement and does not measure happiness. Hence it has no value, it is given zero while scoring. The last statement in each group is given the highest score of 3, since the statements are put in the order of increasing importance (increasing value). The happiness score is derived by adding the marks of all 14 groups of statements.

Measure of Life Satisfaction: This part consisting of 10 general statements has been adopted from the life orientation questionnaire by Sahoo(2005). The statements are "The life I live is close to my ideal", "I enjoy the respect I am given", My family members would describe me as satisfied", I wish I had more respect given to me", "I am pleased with the way I have fulfilled my duties", "I wish I were more at peace", "If could live my life once again, I would want it to be exactly the same", I feel good about my life", "My family members approve of my life", "I feel at peace". A 7-point ordinal scale is provided. Each statement has to be evaluated accordingly and then rated. A rating of 1 indicates strong disagreement and 7 represents strong agreement, while a rating of 4 indicates neutral stand. Each item is scored according to the level of agreement. The more is the agreement, the higher is the score, except for item four and six. They are "I wish I had more respect given to me", "I wish I were more at peace". Reverse scoring has been undertaken for these two items. The total life satisfaction score is obtained by summing up scores of all 10 times.

Measure of Well-Being through Graphic Scale: The graphic item portrayed a human figure (representing self) and a flower (representing happiness) with varying distances between them. The greatest distance was depicted for number one figure while at number seven the distance between the figure and the flower was minimal, depicting happiness to be central to one's life. The participant was asked to encircle the number that best represented his or her opinion as to how far he or she viewed himself or herself to be from happiness in his life. The graphic score was the number that the participant had encircled. The greater closeness to flower (happiness) indicated higher score. The highest score was 7.

Measure of Social Orientation: In this section, five specific social activities were placed like "Films", 'Talks", "Dances", "Concerts", "Sports". The participants were given a five point ordinal scale to reflect whether they attended each of these specific activities all the time, quite frequently, once in a while, rarely or never, within one's organization. Each activity was separately ranked from never to all the time. The never attend response was marked zero while highest marks were awarded to "attend all the time" response. The highest mark was 4. The total social orientation score was obtained by adding the scores of all five activities.

Life Quality Dimension: Measurement was also directed to scale other factors of the participants like the average number of hours per week they contribute to professional activity, to family in taking care of children's growth and education, in voluntary work (social work) exercise and in recreational activities.

Socio-demographic Variables: These included questions about some necessary personal factors about the participants. It included information about their sex, age, marital status, educational qualification and income.

PROCEDURE

The study continued over a period of three months. Before collecting the data, the three subcultural participants were identified and then approached at their respective work places or at their homes.

The investigator approached each respondent individually and imparted a clear description of what to do. The instruction for each part of the questionnaire was adequately explained and care was taken to ensure that they understood the instructions. The questionnaire was in English and each participant received an explanation on a face-to-face basis by the investigator. More-over, detailed written instructions were also provided on all the questionnaires for their reference and guidance. Space was provided for their responses. Care was also taken to assure them that their participation in the study was voluntary and their response would remain confidential and be used only for research purposes. It was informed to each participant that the research was concerned with the general conclusions rather than the individual responses. So each participant was requested to respond to each item in the questionnaire freely and frankly without any hesitation.

Most of the participants were asked to go through the questionnaire and fill it up in the presence of the investigator. But as the questionnaires were lengthy and respondents were busy, some of the participants also took the questionnaire to their home and returned it the next day. The participants were instructed to finish the entire questionnaire in a time period of maximum one and a half hours.

All the participants were requested to rank sixteen different outcomes people seek in their lives according to their perceived importance (Measure of Context-Specific Importance of Needs). In the second section (Measure of Need Satisfaction Potential of the Context), the participants were asked to indicate the degree of satisfaction for the same items of Part-1. This section also had an added item referring to the overall satisfaction in one's life. In the third section (Measure of Happiness), the participants were asked to select one statement out of four in each group, which closely reflected their state for the last two weeks. In the fourth selection (Measure of Life Satisfaction), the participants were asked to indicate the amount of their agreement or disagreement with each of the items. In the fifth section of graphic figures (Measure of Well-Being through Graphic Scale), the participants were asked to indicate as to how far or how close they were from happiness in their life. In the last section (Measure of Social Orientation), the participants had to indicate the activities they were actively involved with and the average number of hours they spent on them per week. They had to depict the level of involvement in social activities within their own organization. Information about some necessary personal factors was collected from all the participants.

In accordance with the design of the study, participants were categorized into three quasi-experimental subgroups within each of the groups of male and female participants.

Responses to all parts of questionnaires were scored following a scoring key and were them tabulated for analysis. The analyses were carried out to examine the hypotheses formulated earlier. The internal consistency was examined in the form of correlational analysis. Appropriate statistical tests were employed to test the major predictions. The comparison of groups was attempted.

RESULTS

The purpose of the present empirical investigation was to examine the role of need saliency in happiness. The result offers a numbers of salient features. The findings can be organized under several broad rubrics: Perceived individual difference, group difference, analysis of association.

PERCEIVED INDIVIDUAL DIFFERENCES

Prior to the statistical analysis, the salient and the non-salient need criteria indicated by participants of different groups, are recorded (see Table-1). for each group. On the basis of the priority ratings, the salient and non-salient needs are identified. The identification of salient needs vis-à-vis non-salient needs from priority rankings shows little variation across groups.

Considering the group of males, it is shown that though they come from three different urbanized settings, their non-salient needs are identical. Males attach least importance to the abundance of leisure activities and opportunity for religious activities in determining their own subjective well-being. Males of moderately urbanized setting share one of their salient needs (i.e. job satisfaction) with males of highly urbanized setting, the other salient need (i.e. of a secured life) they share with mildly urbanized males. The second salient need of males of highly urbanized setting is receiving respect and recognition in society. The males of mildly urbanized setting attach importance to receiving respect and recognition in society, along with another salient need (scope for independent thought).

Table 1

Salient and Non-salient Criteria Indicated by Participants of Different Groups

Groups	*Salient Criteria*	*Non Salient Criteria*
Highly urbanized males	1. Job satisfaction 2. Respect and recognition in society	1. Abundance of leisure activities 2. Opportunity for religious activities.
Highly urbanized females	1. Support of the most loved person. 2. Absence of physical illness	1. Abundance of leisure activities. 2. (i) Material prosperity (ii) Opportunity for religious activities.
Moderately urbanized males	1. Job satisfaction 2. A secured life	1. Abundance of leisure activities 2. Opportunity for religious activities.
Moderately urbanized females	1. A secured life 2. (i) Support of the most loved person person (ii) Smooth social relations	1. Abundance of leisure activities 2. Job satisfaction.
Mildy urbanized males	1. A Secured life 2. (i) Respect and recognition in society (ii) Scope for independent thought	1. Opportunity for religious activities 2. Abundance of leisure activities.
Mildly urbanized females.	2. A secured life 2. Absence of physical illness	1. Material prosperity 2. Abundance of leisure activities

Considering the group of females, it is found that females from different settings indicate at least one common non-salient need (i.e. abundance of leisure activities). Females of highly urbanized setting also indicate "opportunity for religious activity" along with "material prosperity" as their second non-salient need. Similarly females of mildly urbanized setting also report material prosperity as their other non-salient need.

But the females of moderately urbanized setting report job satisfaction as their second non-salient need. The females of mildly urbanized group setting share a salient need (i.e. of a secured life) with females of moderately urbanized setting while another salient need (i.e. absence of physical illness) with females from highly urbanized setting. Females of highly urbanized group rated "support of the most loved person" as their first salient need. This criterion of "support of the most loved person" along with "smooth social relations" has surfaced as the second salient need of females of moderately urbanized setting.

Interestingly as shown by Table-1, a comprehensive picture of salient and non-salient need criteria denotes the similarities and dissimilarities on the part of the six subgroups based on sex and setting.

In this study, the salient criteria include variables that are considered the most important as rated by each individual. They are specific to the concerned individuals. The present study tests the prediction that happiness is related to salient need satisfaction and is unrelated to non-salient need satisfaction.

GROUP DIFFERENCES

The examination of relationship between happiness and need satisfaction has included a number of dimensions. Accordingly analysis has been undertaken with respect to each of the dimensions as well as the overall well-being. The dimensions include salient need satisfaction, non-salient need satisfaction, total need satisfaction, overall satisfaction happiness score, graphics social orientation.

Table 2

Analysis of Variance Performed on Satisfaction Dimensions

Dimensions	*Source*	*Df*	*Ms*	*F*
Salient needs satisfaction	Setting	2	.73	.19
	Sex	1	.95	.25
	Setting X sex	2	.70	.19
	Error	126	3.80	
Non-salient needs satisfaction	Setting	2	4.39	1.29
	Sex	1	1.25	.37
	Setting X sex	2	5.61	1.65
	Error	126	3.40	
Total needs satisfaction	Setting	2	59.44	.68
	Sex	1	.142	.002
	Setting X sex	2	8.425	.10
	Error	126	87.01	
Overall satisfaction	Setting	2	1.95	3.16
	Sex	1	.08	.14
	Setting X sex	2	.16	.27
	Error	126	.62	

Table 3

Mean Satisfaction Scores of Participants

Dimensions	*Settings*	*Males*		*Females*		*Combined*	
		M	*Sd*	*M*	*Sd*	*M*	*Sd*
Salient needs satisfaction	Highly urbanized	10.39	1.91	10.44	2.04	10.42	1.95
	Moderately urbanized	10.27	1.88	10.17	1.50	10.24	1.76
	Less urbanized	10.70	1.89	10.22	2.44	10.47	2.15
	Combined	10.45	1.89	10.28	1.99		
Non-salient needs satisfaction	Highly urbanized	8.67	1.64	9.22	0.94	8.94	1.35
	Moderately urbanized	8.13	1.99	8.83	1.95	8.34	1.99
	Less urbanized	8.60	1.64	7.94	2.39	8.29	2.03
	Combined	8.47	1.76	8.66	1.76		
Total needs satisfaction	Highly urbanized	77.50	10.11	78.00	9.91	77.75	9.87
	Moderately urbanized	75.20	8.22	75.89	7.21	75.41	7.86
	Less urbanized	76.15	10.87	75.17	10.29	75.68	10.47
	Combined	76.28	9.73	76.35	9.14	76.35	
Overall satisfaction	Highly urbanized Moderately	5.17	.79	5.22	.73	5.19	.75
	Urbanized	5.08	.76	4.80	.47	5.02	.6
	Less urbanized	4.75	.78	4.72	1.07	4.74	.92
	Combined	5.00	.78	4.94	.76		

Analysis of Variance (ANOVA) performed on several forms of satisfaction does reveal neither sex nor setting difference. As shown by Table-3, Particiapnts from all three types of settings report similar levels of salient need satisfaction, nonsalient need satisfaction, total need satisfaction and overall need satisfaction. Similarly, males express as much satisfaction as do females.

Table 4

Analysis of Variance Performed on Happiness-Related Dimensions

Dimensions	*Source*	*Df*	*Ms*	*F*
Happiness	Setting	2	96.06	1.87
	Sex	1	9.82	.19
	Setting X Sex	2	92.88	1.81
	Error	126	51.43	
Graphic major of happiness	Setting	2	1910.80	1.49
	Sex	1	1679.80	1.70
	Setting X Sex	2	1767.78	1.79
	Error	126	983.41	
Life satisfaction	Setting	2	1249.56	1.39
	Sex	1	1546.41	1.66
	Setting X Sex	2	1520.15	1.63
	Error	126	930.23	
Social orientation	Setting	2	72.807.63	6.20*
	Sex	1	18.06	.65
	Setting X Sex	2	11.74	1.54
	Error	126		

* p<.01.

Table 5

Mean Happiness-Related Scores of Participants

Dimensions	*Settings*	*Males*		*Females*		*Combined*	
		M	*Sd*	*M*	*Sd*	*M*	*Sd*
Happiness	Highly urbanized	25.00	5.42	22.83	4.20	23.92	4.91
	Moderately urbanized	21.03	7.29	20.89	7.47	20.98	7.28
	Less urbanized	19.60	9.77	23.61	7.06	21.50	8.72
	Combined	21.88	7.49	22.44	6.24		
Graphic	Highly urbanized	5.5	.64	5.83	.86	5.67	.75
	Moderately urbanized	4.85	1.55	5.56	1.10	5.07	1.45
	Less urbanized	5.05	1.32	5.11	1.02	5.08	1.17
	Combined	5.10	1.17	5.50	.99		
Life Satisfaction	Highly urbanized	50.61	4.40	48.89	10.29	49.47	7.35
	Moderately urbanized	48.60	6.81	48.72	4.06	48.64	6.05
	Less urbanized	47.35	9.71	46.94	8.79	47.16	9.16
	Combined	48.85	6.97	48.48	7.71		
Social Orientation	Highly urbanized	9.28	3.29	8.33	2.70	8.81	3.00
	Moderately urbanized	9.10	3.99	10.78	3.90	9.62	4.01
	Less urbanized	6.95	3.35	7.72	2.14	7.32	2.83
	Combined	8.44	3.54	8.94	2.91		

Analysis of Variance performed on several happiness-related dimensions does not indicate significant effect for sex as well as setting on any of the variables except social orientation. There is significant setting effect for social orientation, $F(2,126)=6.20$, $p<01$ (see Table-4). As shown by Table 5, participants from moderately and highly urbanized settings show greater social orientation than do participants from the less urbanized setting (M=9.62,8.81 and 7.32 respectively). The Duncan's multiple range test shows that people in moderately and highly urbanized setting do not differ.

ANALYSIS OF ASSOCIATION

The major objective of the present investigation is to examine the hypothesized relationships between salient need satisfaction and happiness. Table 6 depicts coorelations between salient need satisfaction and various happiness related dimensions.

Table 6

Product Moment Correlation Coefficient Between Salient Need Satisfaction and Happiness Related Dimensions

Dimensions	*Group*		
	Highly urbanized (n=36)	*Moderately urbanized (n=58)*	*Less urbanized (n=38)*
1. Total need satisfaction	.82**	.57**	.69**
2. Overal satisfaction	.75**	.43**	.59**
3. Happiness	.44**	.48**	.33*
4. Graphic major of happiness	.12	.44**	.53*
5. Life satisfaction	.21	.15	.41

* p<.05.

** p<.01.

As expected, salient need satisfaction is significantly related to both total need satisfaction and overall need satisfaction in each of the three groups (see Table 6). More importantly, salient need satisfaction is significantly associated with major of happiness. In the group of highly urbanized participants, the coorelation between salient need satisfaction and happiness is highly significant, $r(34)=.44$, $p<.01$. In the groups of moderately and less urbanized settings, such coorelations are found to be also significant, r(56)=.28,p<.01 and r(36).33, p<.05, respectively. In the groups of moderately and less urbanized settings, salient need satisfaction is also significantly related to graphic major of happiness. Thus, the main prediction that happiness is significantly related to salient need satisfaction is supported.

Table 7

Product Moment Correlation Coefficient Between Nonsalient Need Satisfaction and Happiness Related Dimensions

Dimensions	*Group*		
	Highly urbanized (n=36)	*Moderately urbanized (n=58)*	*Less urbanized (n=38)*
1. Total need satisfaction	.56**	.46**	.29*
2. Overal satisfaction	.45**	.12	.12
3. Happiness	.16	.09	.08
4. Graphic major of happiness	–.01	.06	.03
5. Life satisfaction	.13	.10	.12

* p<.05.

** p<.01.

Furthermore, the examination of relationship between nonsalient need satisfaction and happiness corroborates our hypothesis. There is significant relationship between nonsalient need satisfaction and total need satisfaction as well as overall need satisfaction. But, as predicted nonsalient need satisfaction is found to be unrelated to happiness major as well as graphic major of happiness in each of the three settings. Thus, the second hypothesis is also supported

DISCUSSION

As pointed out, the results offer a number of salient futures. Each of the futures requires detailed discussion.

Need Saliency and Subjective Well-being

The present work clearly shows that salient need satisfaction is related to happiness and non-salient need satisfaction is unrelated to happiness. The perceived importance of needs is useful for identifying salient and non-salient needs. For each individual, certain needs assume greater saliency or importance than others in a particular life context. Thus the pattern of importance attached to various needs that the individual seeks to satisfy in different life contexts differ. These patterns are determined by past social and cultural influences. Again, the degree of psychological identification or involvement with given life context is a function of perceived potential of the context for satisfying the individuals specific needs.

Likewise, self-determination theory (STD) posits three basis psychological needs-autonomy, competence, and relatedness and theorizes that fulfillment of these needs is essential for psychological growth (e.g. intrinsic motivation), integrity (e.g. internalization and assimilation of cultural practices), and well-being (e.g. life satisfaction and psychological health) as well as the experiences of vitality and self-congruence). Need fulfillment is thus viewed as a natural aim of human life that delineates many of the meanings and purposes underlying human actions.

Specification of basic needs defines not only the minimum requirements of psychological health but also delineates prescriptively the nutriments that the social environment must supply for people to thrive and grow psychologically. Thus, SDT describes the conditions that facilitate versus undermine well-being within varied developmental periods and specific social contexts such as schools, workplaces, and friends. SDT does not, however, suggest that the basic needs are equally valued in all families, social groups, or cultures, but it does maintain that thwarting of these needs will result in negative psychological consequences in all social or cultural contexts. As such, contextual and cultural, as well as developmental factors continually influence the modes of expression, the means of satisfaction, and the ambient supports for these needs, and it is because of their effects on needs satisfaction that they in turn, influences growth, integrity, and well-being at both between-person and within person levels of analysis.

SDT has both important similarities and differences with Ryff and Singer's (1998) eudaimonic approach Ryan and Deci wholly concur that well-being consists in what Rogers (1963) referred to as being fully functioning, rather than as simply attaining desires.

They also are largely in agreement concerning the content of being eudaimonic (e.g. being autonomous, competent, and related). However their approach theorizes that these contents are the principal factors that foster well-being, whereas Ryff and Signer's approach uses them to define well-being.

SDT posits that satisfaction of the basic psychological needs typically fosters SWB as well as eudaimonic well-being. This results from their belief that being satisfied with one's life and feeling both relatively more positive affect and less negative affect (the typical measures of SWB) do frequently point to psychological wellness, for as Rogers (1963) suggested, emotional states are indicative of organism valuation processes. That is, the assessment of positive and negative affect useful in so far as emotions are, in part, appraisals of the relevance and valence of events and conditions of life with respect to the self. Thus, in SDT research they typically used SWB as one of several indicators of well-being. However, they have at the same time maintained that there are different types of positive experience and that some conditions that foster SWB do not promote eudaimonic well-being. For example, research by Nix et al (1999) showed that succeeding at an activity while feeling pressured to do so resulted in happiness (a positive affect closely linked to SWB) but it did not result in vitality (a positive affect more closely aligned with eudaimonic well-being). On the other hand, as predicted by SDT, succeeding at an activity while feeling autonomous resulted and both happiness and vitality. Thus, because conditions that promote SWB may not necessarily yield eudaimonic well-being, SDT research as typically supplemented SWB measures with assessments of self-actualization, vitality and mental health in an effort to assess well-being conceived of as healthy, congruent, and vital functioning.

Autonomy and Integration of Goals: Another actively researched issue concerns how autonomous one is in pursuing goals. SDT in particular has taken a strong stand on this by proposing that only self-endorsed goals will enhance well-being. So pursuit of heterogeneous goals, even when done efficaciously, will not. The relative autonomy of personal goals has accordingly, been shown repeatedly to be predictive of well-being outcomes controlling for goal efficacy at both between person and within person levels of analysis. Interestingly this pattern of findings has been supported in cross-cultural research, suggesting that the relative autonomy of one's pursuits matters whether on is collectivistic or individualistic, male or female (e.g. V. Chirkov & Ryan, 2001; Hayamizu, 1997; Vallerand, 1997).

Sheldon and Elliot (1999) developed a self-concordance model of how autonomy relates to well-being. Self concordant goals are those that fulfill basic needs and are aligned with one's true self. These goals are well-internalized and therefore autonomous and enable them from intrinsic or identified motivations. Goals that are not self-concordant encompass external or interjected motivations. Goals that are not self-concordant encompass external or interjected motivation and are either unrelated or indirectly related to need fulfillment. Scheldon and Elliot found that although goal attainment in itself was associated with greater well-being, this effect was significantly weaker when the attained goals were not self-concordant. People who attained more self concordant goals had more need-satisfying experiences and this greater need satisfaction was predictive of greater SWB. Similarly, Sheldon and Kasser (1998) studied progress toward goals in a longitudinal design finding that goal progress was associated with enhanced SWB and lower symptoms of depression. However, the impact of goal progress was again moderated by goal concordance. Goals that were poorly integrated to the self, whose focus was not related to basic psychological needs, conveyed less SWB benefits, even when achieved.

Finally, the Nix et al (1999) study showed that whereas successful goal pursuits led to happiness it was only when the pursuits were autonomous that success yielded vitality. McGregor and Little (1998) suggested that the meaningfulness of goals is a separate issue from that of goal efficiency, and in a study of personal projects they found that, whereas perceived efficiency was linked to happiness, the relative integrity of goals was linked to meaningfulness.

Sex and Subjective Well-being

The present study found subjective well being can be experienced irrespective of sex.

Sex differences found in the incidence of depression suggests potential sex difference in the role of stress and resource factors. Because fewer men than women receive treatment for depression, men and women are believed to differ in the mean levels of stressors, coping and social resources. In this regard, there is some evidence that in comparison with men, women are more exposed to environmental stressors, have lower supportive social resources and use less efficacious coping patterns. It is found that both stressful life events and social resources have a greater impact on the functioning of women than they do on that of men. Closely related to stress is the domain of depression. A large body of evidence indicates that women are more likely than men to show unipolar depression. Although the ratio of females to male depressives varies greatly from country to country, there is a consistent tendency for women to preponderate among depressives across a wide variety of nations. Women report depression at a rate twice as much as men do. All these facts made some researchers argue that women are actually more unhappy than men, but they are happy because of a need to conform to social norms.

But this study has revealed that men and women are equally likely to declare themselves "very happy" and "satisfied" with their lives. The present study was more concerned with the frequency rather than the emotional intensity of subjective well-being Ed Diener et al however opine that how much of the time a person experiences (positive) pleasant emotions is a better predictor than positive emotional intensity of how happy the person reports being. Further emotional intensity forms a factor that is independent of SWB. Thus, feeling pleasant emotions most of the time and infrequently experiencing unpleasant emotions, even if the pleasant emotions are only mild, is sufficient for high reports of happiness.

People seeking ecstasy much of the time, whether it be in a career on a love relationship, they are likely to be disappointed. Even worse, they may move to the next relationship or job seeking intense levels of happiness, which in fact are rarely long-lasting and are not necessary for happiness. Thus, feeling pleasant emotions most of the time and infrequently experiencing unpleasant emotion, even if the pleasant emotions are only mild, is sufficient for high reports of happiness. Other studies have confirmed women differ from men with respect to emotional intensity (though it be positive or even negative). Hence this paradox is found with regards to women experiencing intense sorrow at the same time being capable of experiencing happiness.

The conclusion that gender gives little clue to happiness is also found in surveys of 1,70,000 adults in 16 countries 18,000 university student in 39 countries and in meta-analysis of 146 other studies.

Setting and Subjective Well-Being

Research in subjective well-being has focused on various possible moderators such as wealth, satisfying relationships, goal attainment etc. But there has been no significant work on setting as a moderator in subjective well-being. The research on wealth and SWB by E. Diener and R. Biswas-Diener also revealed a few facts about setting like (a) people in richer nations are happier than people in poorer nations, (b) increases in national wealth within developed nations have not, over recent decades, been associated with increases in SWB. (c) within-nation differences in wealth show only small positive correlations with happiness.

Thus they stated that avoiding poverty, living in a rich country, and focusing on goals other than material wealth are associated with attaining happiness.

The meaning of well-being and the factors that facilitate it are particularly at issue in cross-cultural studies in which a principal quest is the search for systematic variants versus invariants in well-being dynamics across widely discrepant social arrangements. Christopher (1999) instructively argued that definitions of well-being are inherently culturally rooted and further that there can be no such thing as a value-free assessment of well-being. According to Christopher, all understandings of well-being are essentially moral visions based on individuals judgements about what it means to be well.

Because the very definition of well-being raise cultural questions about the meaning and equivalence of constructs, quantitatively oriented researchers have often been bereft of answers to criticisms of cultural bias. Although such concerns should continue, at least some strategies have emerged that allow statistical assessments of the cultural equivalence of psychological constructs. Illustrative is the means and covariance structure analyses, which assess the degree to which the psychometric properties of a construct can be comparable modeled across diverse populations. Cross-cultural researchers in this area will need to employ such methods as a requisite for interpretive confidence in their findings. However, because of the newness of these techniques, few studies have employed them.

Diener and colleagues have reported a number of cross-cultural factors associated with SWB. Their analyses have included both mean level differences between nations on SWB and differential correlates of well-being across nations. For example. Diener and Diener (1995) found that across nations, self-esteem was associated with well-being, but that relation was stronger in countries characterized by individualism. The strength of association of SWB to satisfaction with wealth, friends and family also varied by nation.

Such et al (1998) studied the relations of emotions and norms (social approval) to life satisfaction in 61 nations. They found that emotions were a stronger predictor of life satisfaction in nations classified as individualist, norms and emotions were equally predictive within collectivist nations. Oishi et al (1999) tested hypotheses based on Maslow's (1971) need theory and their own expectancy valence position, finding some support for each. They found that in poorer nations satisfaction with wealth was a stronger predictor of life satisfaction, whereas satisfaction with home life was more predictive in wealthier nations, suggesting to them a hierarchy of needs. They also found evidence that satisfaction with freedom was less predictive of SWB in collectivistic nations than in individualistic ones.

The Indian society is a multi-cultural society, there is wide variation with respect to languages, food habits, ceremonies, festivals, dressing habits, ethnicity etc. This diversity raises sufficient concerns about the relatively independent sources of variance in well-being owing to cultures and more proximal social contexts.

Further, Indian socio-cultural system, represents a case where resource constraints are often experienced consequently the association between peoples reactions to un-controllability and happiness is likely to be a significant aspect.

Since India is a country with varied sub-cultures which differ from each other, setting was considered as a moderator in the present study in SWB.

The result obtained in this study did not show any significant difference among the three subcultures of Mumbai, Damanjodi and Bhubaneswar with respect to SWB. This may be explained with the fact that the study had participants from middle socio-economic status. More as less middle class people in India share many common features. Their income, family structure, education level, food habits, and the knowledge of the national languages of Hindi and English, their working status, social orientation have contributed to their experience of SWB. Thus, the role of setting with proper and adequate participation of people of different socio-economic status might further reveal any setting difference in experiencing SWB.

MAJOR IMPLICATIONS

The present empirical work has produced three major implications

First, in the identification of salient needs, it has been established that salient needs differ from group to group. When the salient needs central to a group are meant the individuals of the group fell satisfied and happy and are aptly motivated to perform to the best of their capacity. In practical terms it is not always possible to fulfill all needs of an individual and moreover on group of individuals. Therefore, whenever major decisions are to be taken the salient needs of the particular group under consideration must be promptly identified. This procedure would help solve many social problems, in fact it would even save efforts in terms of money and time. The requirements of given group in its sociocultural context can be adequately met after such salient need identification.

Secondly, the finding that there is no significant gender difference in experiencing happiness can be applied in the sensitive area of women counseling. Some researchers argue that women are actually more unhappy than men, but they appear to be happy because of a need to conform to social norms. They based their argument on studies revealing consistent tendency in women to preponderate among depressives. Women report depression at a rate twice as much as men do.

The present study has emphasized on the frequency of happy episodes rather than its intensity. This rightly suggests that women experience as much happiness as men, and as often as do men. Fujita et al (1991) posit that women are only more affectively intense than men. This allows them to experience both more joy and more sorrow. The gender difference in affect intensity can explain the paradoxical presence of negative affect and to equal (or greater) overall happiness reported by women. Affect intensity is the individual difference variable that refers to one's response intensity to a given level of emotion-provoking situation. A person who interprets events in a self referential manner (personalizing) takes single event as being representative of the world at large (over generalizing), and focuses attention on emotion-provoking aspect of events (selective abstraction), will probably experience more intense emotional outcomes than a person who does not (Beck). There is some evidence that women use such maladaptive cognitive operations. Nolen-Hoeksema (1987) have shown the causal role of ruminative response style in depressive symptoms among women. Men use more active response styles.

Fujita has found that affect intensity is unitary across valence. But positive and negative hedonic level make up a bipolar affect balance dimension. This adequately explains why when researchers collected negative emotion data and the items tap both hedonic level and affect intensity they find women experiencing more negative affect than men. Whereas, if researches collect data that balances the positive affect against the negative affect, then the gender differences disappear.

Thus in helping women rise from community level depression, their ruminative response styles can be challenged and altered into an active response style. Further the women can be convinced of their potential of experiencing happiness and satisfaction as often as men and thus helping them ward off depression.

Finally, the finding that people can experience happiness irrespective to the place they belong to may be applied to people experiencing urban stress and rural stress respectively. It is found that urbanites suffer from stress due to a lot of competition for material resources. In the contemporary world urbanities often complain of dissatisfaction even amidst all comforts. They seem to envy the life of a yokel. On the other hand, people of rural India often complain of the lack of opportunities and facilities in the countryside. They feel unhappy as they see the glitter of urban areas. There is escalation of expectations among urbanities while relative deprivation among rural people in India.

The urbanities as well as rural people should be properly counseled that material advantages do not readily translate into social and emotional benefits. For a life in which one aspires for happiness energy should e invested in pursuing goals such as towards a satisfying family life, having intimate friends, and pursuing diverse interests such as art, literature, religion and philosophy etc. Eventually a person who only responds to material rewards loses the ability to derive happiness from other sources. Since material rewards at first enrich the quality of life, people tend to conclude that more must be better. What is good in small quantities becomes common place and then harmful in larger doses. Thus, a person is capable of experiencing happiness irrespective of his surrounding once he redirects his focus from material resources to social and physiological resources.

REFERENCES

Abbey, A., and Andrews, F. M. (1955). Modeling the psychological determinants at life quality *Social Indicators Research*, 16, 1-34.

Andrews, F. M., and Withey, S. B. (1976). *Social indicators of well being: Americans perceptions of life quality*. New York: Plenum press.

Cambell, A. (1981). *The sense of well-being in America*. New York: McGraw-Hill.

Csikzentmihalyi, M. (1999). If we are so rich, why are not we happy? *American Psychologist*, 54, 821-827.

Cacioppo, J. T., Gardner, W. L., and Berntson, G. G. (1999). The affect system has parallel and integrative processing components: From fallows function. *Journal of Personality and Social Psychology*, 76, 839-855.

Diener, E., and Diener, M. (1995) Cross cultural correlates of life satisfaction and self-esteem. *Journal of Personality and Social Psychology*, 68, 653-663.

Diener, E. Sandvik, E., Pavot, W. (1991). Happiness is the frequency, not the intensity, of positive versus negative affect. In F. Strack, M. Argyle, and N. Schwarz (Eds.), *Subjective Well-being: An interdisciplinary perspective* (PP. 119-139). New York: Pergamon.

Diener, E., Diener, M., and Diener, C. (1995) Factors predicting the subjective well-being of nations. *Journal of Personality and Social Psychology*, 69, 653-663.

Haring, M. J., stock, W. A., and Okun, M. A. (1984). A research syntesis of gender and Social class as correlates of subjective well-being. *Human Relations, 37,* 645-657.

Kahneman, D. (1999). Objective happiness. In D. Kahneman, E. Diever, and N. Schwarz (Eds.), Well-being: *The foundation of hedonic Psychology* (PP. 3-25). New York: Russell Sage Foundation.

Larsen, R. J. and Diener, E. (1985). A multitrait-multimethod examination of affect structure: *Hedonic level and emotional intensity. Personality and Individual Differences,* 6, 631-636.

Michalos, A. (1991). *Global report on student well-being: Life satisfaction and happiness.* Vol. 1, New York: Springer-Varlag.

Myers, D. G., and Diener, E. (1995). Who is happy? *Psychological Science,* 6, 10-19.

Myers, D. G. and Giener, E. (1996, May). The pursuit of happiness. *Scientific American,* 274, 54-56.

Suh, E. (1999). *Identity consistency, subjective well-being and culture. Unpublished doctoral dissertation,* University of Illinois at Urbana-Champaign.

Veenhoven, R. (1988). The utility of happiness. *Social Indicators Research, 20,* 333-354

22

Enhancement of Human Reproductive Behaviour with Application of Behaviour Technology

Vedagiri Ganesan*

ABSTRACT

Human Reproductive Behaviour (HRB) is governed by both Psycho-Physiological and Social- Psychological factors. Hence the management of HRB requires a comprehensive Model and Behaviour Technology. This paper presents some specific Behavioural Technologies with which the following major problems relating to HRB can be effectively managed.

1. Management of Aversion to Sex among Females.
2. Ten Pre-Requisites for Sexual Satisfaction.
3. Isolation of Human Reproduction from Sexual Satisfaction.

The application of the above Behaviour Technologies will result in:

1. Enhancement of Mental Health of Men and Women.
2. Population Control.
3. Reduction of STD and HIV Infections.
4. Empowerment of Women.

---

* **Director, Indian Institute of Behaviour Technology, P.B. No. 7301, Coimbatore, India - 641 046. Ex-Professor and Head, Dept. of Psychology, Bharathiar University, Coimbatore - 641 046, India.**

MANAGEMENT OF SEXUAL AVERSION AMONG FEMALES

Aversion towards sexual intercourse is found to be more among females than among males. The causes of sexual aversion among females are as follows:

1. Disciplinarian parenting.
2. Childhood sexual abuse.
3. Lack of Sex Education.
4. Impotence of spouse.
5. Complications during pregnancy and delivery.
6. Repeated miscarriages.

Girls with sexual aversion are keen on postponing the marriage or on avoiding the marriage. Their "sexual aversion" manifests into an "aversion towards marriage". Even when they are forced to agree for marrying, they avoid sex as much as they can. They consider sexual intercourse as something "dirty", "filthy", "nauseating" and "painful". Some are even prepared to rather die, than to participate in copulation. Many girls either before or after their marriage resort to suicide as because of their fear of sex.

These girls detest physical examination even by a female gynecologist. They avoid their body exposure to even their close female family members like their mother or sister. They detest even to touch their genitalia themselves. This may lead to hygiene problems. Their sexual aversion may influence their endocrinal, gonadal secretions, ultimately resulting in:

1. Irregular menstrual cycles;
2. Insufficient or excessive menstrual discharges;
3. Amenorhea;
4. Dysmenorhea;
5. Dysperunia;
6. Fallopian tube blocks;
7. Involuntary uterine spasms;
8. Infertility; and
9. Miscarriages.

These girls with sexual aversion also develop Hypersensitization to Males. This "Stimulus Generalization" makes them to shy away not only from unknown males, but also from their close relatives like husband, and even father and brothers. Sexual aversion sometimes turns into extreme aggressive behaviour and these girls may even violently attack their spouses. The "Possession Syndrome" often found among females, is the manifestation of sexual aversion, and it is a Self-Protective-Defensive-Behaviour to avoid sexual contact.

An innovative Behaviour Therapy Technique has been developed and used by Ganesan (1995) for the effective management of sexual aversion among females. This paper presents the findings of a study, which applied the above technique on twentythree females who had been suffering from severe sexual aversion. They aged from 18 to 35 years. Fifteen of them were married and seven of them were unmarried.

THERAPEUTIC MODULE

The clients were trained to produce Voluntary Psycho-Physiological- Relaxation-Responses as preparatory to undergoing the Touch Tolerance Therapy. The relaxation of the skeleto-muscular system, cognitive system and the respiratory system were achieved by administering the following techniques.

1. Progressive Deep Muscle Relaxation (Jacobson, 1938)
2. Mental Relaxation Response (Benson, 1984)
3. Jala Neti, Kapala Bhatti, and Bhastrika (Iyengar, 2000)

Self Defense Training Technique for Women (Ganesan, 1985) was also administered to help them acquire the self-defense skills as well as to make them feel sure that they can confidently defend themselves, as well as take to offensive action, in case of a possible sexual assault by any male in future.

TOUCH TOLERANCE DEVELOPMENT THERAPY

The client was made to lie down on her back with her eyes closed in a relaxed manner. She was asked to request the therapist to touch her fingertips one after the other finger. She was asked not to hurry up and to make further requests to touch her palm, back of the palm, wrist, fore arm, upper arm and shoulder of her right hand and later of the left hand following the same sequence.

In case she felt tense at any stage when a particular part of her body was touched, she was asked to request the therapist to stop moving up any further, and even to stop touching. This **"stimulus control"** provides a feeling of having control over the threatening-stimulus that is touching the body at a particular place. Then the client relaxed by relaxing her fingers and toes of her both hands and legs. Further she also breathed out in a prolonged manner in order to induce a relaxation response. When she felt sufficiently relaxed and comfortable, she was encouraged to proceed further.

For the lower limbs the touch was started from toes, one after the other, sole, heal, ankle, calf muscles, knee, thigh and hamstrings. Touching of upper thighs and buttocks were avoided initially. Then touch from the top of the head descended and spread all over the head in the hair distributed areas.

After this touch moves from forehead down the face to eyes, nose, cheeks, lips, chin, throat and the neck. The sexually prohibited areas from chest down to the hip were proceeded with very carefully, gradually and slowly as per the request of the client. Touching over the breast and genitalia were reserved to the conclusion of the therapy.

Both female and male therapists offered the Touch Therapy. The clients in general preferred that the therapy be administered initially by a female therapist, and later by a male therapist. The reason for preferring a female therapist in the early phase of the Touch Therapy was due to the gradual reduction in the client's inhibition to be touched by a female stranger. That is they felt more secure and less anxious to be touched by a female. But, later after acquiring sufficient desensitization to the touch by a female stranger, the clients wanted to check how far they can tolerate and handle a male stranger's touch.

CLIENT-SUPPORTED-TOUCH

The client was asked to hold the hand of the therapist, and to use the palm just like a pad, to touch the various parts of her body starting from her upper chest down to her genital.

Initially the client was asked to use the therapist's palm, just like a pad to touch her body "softly" thrice and later with "medium pressure" thrice.

The above Touch Tolerance Therapy gradually removes the aversion to sex and further develops sexual excitation as well.

The clients were also provided with information regarding the X-10: Ten Pre-Requisites for Sexual Satisfaction (Ganesan, 1980). This information prepared them cognitively, emotionally and behaviourally to develop a positive expectancy and interest in having sexual intercourse with their spouse. Further, their dysfunctional sexual behavioural patterns were replaced by compatible behavioural patterns. The married women for the first time started experiencing female orgasm. The unmarried clients could come out of their sexual aversion, and to move out of their sexual aversion, and marriage aversion. All the client felt free to move out of their house and felt happy to attend all social functions, which they were avoiding prior to therapy, due to their male aversion.

All the twenty-three clients had reported positive therapeutic outcomes and they clients were totally cured of their sexual aversion and male aversion. Follow up after a period of six months revealed that the positive therapeutic outcomes were sustained.

X-10: TEN PRE-REQUISITES FOR SEXUAL SATISFACTION:

PSYCHO-SEXUAL EMPOWERMENT OF WOMEN

Family Adjustment involves as one of its crucial and central components, the Sexual Adjustment. The quality of Sexual Adjustment and Marital Adjustment are mutually interlinked and hence, enhancing Sexual Satisfaction can effectively improve Marital Adjustment.

This paper presents some of the practical ways in which Sexual Adjustment can be significantly improved. Based on years of experience in the area of clinical practice, some ten salient and pivotal techniques have been identified and described. These techniques have proved successful in the treatment of various types of male sexual dysfunctions like impotence, pre-mature ejaculation, and performance anxiety, and female sexual dysfunctions like, frigidity, unorgasmia, vaginismus, sexual aversion, infertility, conversion reactions, etc.

The ten behavioral pre-requisites recommended for sexual satisfaction among couple are as follows:

1. Security
2. Nudity
3. Foreplay
4. Position
5. Lubrication
6. Digital Dilation
7. Slow Breathing and Slow Movements
8. Female Participation
9. Female Orgasm
10. Post-Coital Intimacy

The detailed description of the above techniques are meant to help the practitioners in the field of Marital Counseling to solve the various sex related problems among the couples and to enhance Marital Adjustment.

WEAKER SEX: MALE OR FEMALE?

The root cause of Gender Discrimination and Male Dominance has got its origin in the lack of sexual compatibility between the male and female. Though the female is said to be the **Weaker Sex** in reality, the male is the Weaker in Sexual Competence as compared to the female. As a result, the males are afraid that their inability to function effectively during sexual intercourse and this fear triggers certain defensive reactions in them. The anatomy and physiology of females makes them fit to participate in sex without much effort, where as in the case of males it requires psycho physiological balancing to initiate and maintain the erection of penis. This makes the males vulnerable to many problems, which interfere with their effective participation in copulation. A large percentage of the male population suffers from premature ejaculation because of its sexual hyper-excitability.

Hence, this group of males is unable to produce orgasm among its spouses and suffers sexual inadequacy and inferiority. The above phenomena may manifest in various types of defensive behaviors such as follows:

1. Violence towards Spouse and Women
2. Suspicion about infidelity of Spouse and Women
3. Aversion to and withdrawal from sex
4. Visiting Commercial Sex Workers
5. Becoming a Homosexual
6. Becoming a Pedophilic
7. Becoming a Fetishist
8. Becoming a Voyeur
9. Renunciation of marital life

MALE SEXUAL INHIBITION

Impotence is also a major reason why males may resort to avoidance of sexual behavior. Their inability to initiate and maintain erection at the time of copulation makes them feel sexuality inadequate.

The Male Dominance behavior is a Self-Defensive Behavior aimed at protecting their sexual vulnerability and inadequacy. Helping the male to develop sexual competence and compatibility with the spouse will go a long way in the removal of the Male's Sexual Insecurity, Gender Discrimination, Male Dominance and Male Violence.

ALCOHOLISM: A SHIELD AGAINST SEXUAL CONFRONTATION

Many males are using alcoholism as"Armour", to avoid the exposure of their sexual incompetence before their spouses. After consuming excessive alcohol men exhibit abnormal behaviors with the use of either abusive language or violent behavior towards their wives. This helps them to keep their wives "at bay" there by they can avoid the sexual intercourse, which is a highly demanding activity because of their sexual incompetence.

SUSPICION: THE GREEN EYED MONSTER

Those males who suffer from impotence or premature ejaculation know that they are not able to satisfy their spouses sexually. Hence they develop a suspicion that their wives are likely to be sexually dissatisfied and hence sexually frustrated and they may be seeking available chances to seek sexual satisfaction from other men. This paranoid suspicion about their wife's infidelity is mostly rooted in the sexual incompetence of the husbands.

Apart from the feelings of suspicion, some husbands develop sadism and hurt their wives in various ways to keep them "at bay" from copulation. This forces their wives either to get separated from their husbands for either a short period or a prolonged duration or to go and seek divorce. This results in totally relieving the husbands of their sexual responsibility to their wives.

SEXUAL DEVIATIONS

Some times the men who have an erectile dysfunction resort to non-threatening ways of satisfying their own sexual urge without caring for their wife's emotional need for an orgasmic experience. These men resort to some of the sexual deviations like Homosexuality, Bestiality, Fetishism, Pedophilia, Voyeurism or Rape. This saves them from the non-demanding nature of their partners or victims for an orgasmic experience. Sometimes the spouses of these men are forced to a resort to Lesbianism. In extreme cases, these males develop an aversion to sex and avoid marriage and stay single or resort to suicide either prior to or after they are forced to marry.

The wife's of these men, because of lack of normal sexual intercourse with their husband are likely to develop unorgasmia, frigidity, depression, suicidal tendencies and at extra marital relationships.

SUICIDE: MANIFESTATION OF SEXUAL INCOMPATIBILITY

The highest rate of suicide occurs in Finland, one of the Scandinavian countries. Majority of the suicides are committed by men, and prior to committing suicide, these men become passive and speechless and resort to violent ways of ending their lives, like jumping off high rise buildings or shooting their heads off. Finland has a significantly lower level of sub-zero temperature and this cold climate affects the sexual arousal of the males, resulting in the development of male sexual incompetence. The males who find themselves ineffective in their sexual performance develop a strong sense of self-hatred and intra-punitive aggression and a strong negative body image; this in turn makes them choose violent ways of ending their lives by hacking their bodies. Women in the Scandinavian countries are more promiscuous, may be because of the relative predominance of male sexual incompetence.

MORAL, ETHICAL, PSYCHIATRIC BREAKDOWNS AND AIDS

Apart from suicidal attempts, psychiatric breakdowns among men and women may also be triggered by sexual incompatibility between men and women. The sexual incompatibility may also encourage promiscuity and multi-partner sex, oral sex etc., resulting in a high risk of HIV infection.

X-10: TEN PRE – REQUISITES FOR SEXUAL SATISFACTION

For the successful development of sexual compatibility between men and women, both men and women can utilize the following ten steps known as X-10. These ten Prerequisites for Sexual Satisfaction will not only help in the development of sexual compatibility, but also will help in the development of Equality among the males and females and put an end to Gender Bias and Gender Dominance.

Marital Adjustment greatly influences the mental health status of not only the couples but also their children. Thus the Community Mental Health mainly depends upon the Family Mental Health and in turn of sexual health. From this point of view, for the Community Psychologists, ways of ensuring Family Mental Health and Sexual Health assume paramount importance. Marital Adjustment has as its foundation not only love, affection, and understanding between the couple, but also their compatibility for engaging satisfactorily in the act of lovemaking. Perhaps this is the reason why the laws through out the world sanction divorce when there is the establishment of sexual incompatibility among couples. Thus helping the couple to develop sexual compatibility plays a crucial role in improving Marital Adjustment, and in turn in ensuring Family Mental Health and Community Mental Health.

Based on decades of professional experience in treating number of marital problems using Family Therapy and Sex Therapy, some of the behavioral pre-requisites to be recommended by the Psychologists to the couple for enhancing their sexual satisfaction are presented below in detail.

1. SECURITY

The feeling of security is the most important requirement for satisfying sexual experience. If there is a feeling of anxiety, that will be a real "spoil-sport" for sexual satisfaction. Feelings of insecurity can stem from peculiar sources. Some example of the problem and their solutions are given below.

A. Fear of Pregnancy

Some young women are afraid of pregnancy, for they feel that it can be fatal. Mothers with grown up children, or married children, or many children are afraid that sexual intercourse will necessarily result in impregnation. This either prevents them from having sex or from enjoying sex.

All that is needed in these cases is to resort to the use of some safe and comfortable contraception. But, peculiarly, these people avoid the use of contraception and continue to suffer from insecure feelings about impregnation. They can start using condom, pill, loop, copper-T, or spermicide. The use of the method of Coitus Interruptus increases the level of anxiety during sexual intercourse, and is often dissatisfying and sexually frustrating. Best thing is not to engage in sex without the use of contraceptive.

B. Fear of Intrusion

The fear of intrusion during sexual intercourse by some one knocking at the door, a child waking up, the ring of a calling bell or the ringing of a telephone or cell phone can off set the mood. Hence, unless one is sure of no interruption for a period of one hour, one may avoid sexual intercourse. Keep the phone off the hook and switch off the cell phone. When a child or children sleep in the room, after they have slept well the couple can move to another room or area and bolt the room before having sex.

A couple was complaining that their nine-year-old daughter kept awake till late night and as a result they were to avoid sex. In such a case, they can set an alarm and wake up in the early hours, move out into another room and have sex.

Children are not to be made to sleep in between the couple. The wife and husband must sleep together, and the children can be made to sleep on either side of the couple. When the children are ten years, they can be encouraged to sleep in another area. When children sleep in between their parents, they may develop jealousy and hatred towards their father or mother. Further parents may also develop hatred towards their children as they consider them as a hindrance to their sex life.

C. Open-Door Policy to be Avoided

In some houses the "open-door policy" exists. The doors of all the rooms are kept open day in and day out. But then this is not congenial to couples when they are having sex in their bedroom. A husband felt guilty to keep his bedroom doors closed, when his widowed mother slept just outside the doorstep. A carpenter said his bedroom doors were just kept closed, without latching, for want of a latch. A couple complained that any body from their family could walk across their bedroom to go to toilet or to drink water. A couple who lived in a portion house said that unfortunately their portion was near the entrance and they have to open the gate whenever one of the neighbors entered their portion in late night.

D. In-coming and Out-going Noises to be Avoided

A young wife was allergic to the noises of others coming from the adjacent room. She felt as if her in-laws were physically present in her bedroom when she heard their voices. Some people feel that their bedroom is so transparent that the love-noises can be heard outside so that virtually others can know what is happening inside their bedroom. Such sound sensitivities can kill one's sex life. One of the best ways to solve this problem is to introduce a sound masking technique in the bedroom. That is to play some music in a radio, audiotape, CD, or TV in the bedroom on an everyday basis from 9 pm to 11 pm so that the noise of such music can mask both the in-coming and out-going noises. The Screeching of the bed or the bride also could not be heard outside.

2. NUDITY

Preparing for Nudity

When the wife is feeling hypersensitive about remaining nude in her husband's presence, the following technique can be used to prepare and to make her to remain nude. This kind of shyness toward nudity though found more among females, some males also suffer from this.

The wife is asked to strip completely and to lie down on a bed by covering her whole nude body with a bed sheet. She is told that this is a "Game" called "Open and Close Game" – where the husband will ask the wife whether she is "Ready" and then try to uncover her body by trying to pull off her bed sheet down her neck. In the beginning he is asked to apply gentle pressure in pulling the bed sheet. The wife is asked to pull the bed sheet back in position to cover her nude body up to her neck. After a little gap of time, when she announces her readiness to restart the game she is asked to say "Ready". Then once again the husband is asked to strip her bed sheet down. The pressure to pull down the bed sheet is to be gradually increased trial after trial by the husband.

When the wife is agitated about this game at any trial, just because the amount of pressure used by her husband is more threatening than what she can tolerate - the husband is asked to reduce his pressure of pulling. Twenty trials are to be done in a day. Day after day the wife is able to develop tolerance to expose more and more of her nude body to her husband. Usually within a week's time the wife is able to come out of her Hyper-sensitization to nudity and gets desensitized to remain nude before her husband.

The couple is encouraged to engage in loud laughter when the game is on. This facilitates a "Mood-Shift" on the part of the wife who feels "anxious" about exposing her nudity to her husband to a "playful mood". Further this is also a stimulus control technique, because the wife who feels that nudity is a threatening stimulus, is able to have a control over the stimulus, that is nudity, as she is made to feel that she has control over covering up her nudity.

3. FORE-PLAY

Foreplay is more satisfying for women than the sexual intercourse itself. But many men would like to skip this phase and directly go for penetration. Further men who suffer from Pre-Mature Ejaculation cannot afford to engage in foreplay, for the fear of ejaculating during foreplay itself. This they are afraid, will make them incapable of penetration.

On the contrary, when men are asked to engage in foreplay for a period of fifteen minutes prior to penetration, they gradually develop desensitization and are able to retain ejaculation for a fairly long period.

Hugging, kissing, breast-fondling etc. are to be engaged by husband and wife for a clear period of fifteen minutes prior to intromission. No compromise on this time duration is to be made by either the husband and or wife. This foreplay ensures the development and strengthening of emotional bondage between the couple. The foreplay includes sucking, licking, biting, pinching, scratching, massaging the various erotic zones like - lips, breasts, nipples, genitals, face, neck, ear-lobes, arm-pits, naval, buttocks, inner aspects of arms and thighs, and hair.

4. VENTRAL-VENTRAL LUBRICATION

Though the male and female sex organs secrete lubricant fluids prior to copulation, due to various reasons like anxiety, aging, hormonal status etc., these lubricants may be insufficient. Hence it is suggested that both the husband and wife apply some vegetable oil, like coconut oil, or scented oil or an odourless lubricant like liquid paraffin, over the penis and inside the vagina. This lubrication smoothens the copulation and reduces the faster warning up of the genitals. As a result, the period of erection of the penis can last longer, and the number of multiple orgasms experienced by the wife can be increased.

5. DIGITAL DILATION

Prior to copulation the vaginal path is to be dilated with the help of the index finger. Lubricant oil can be used while dilating. The wife herself can do the dilation. If she wishes, she can permit her husband to dilate using his index finger. The women, who suffer from "vaginismus"- where women experience pain during copulation, will stand to greatly benefit by the use of this technique. The pain will disappear within a week.

6. ASSUMPTION OF COMFORTABLE POSITIONS

I. WHAT NOT TO DO

A. Straight Knee Position is to be Avoided

The position assumed during copulation can significantly contribute to pleasure or pain, and satisfaction or dissatisfaction. A large number of couple suffers during copulation and for a period of several years by assuming the "Straight-Knee Position". In this position, the wife keeps her knees straight without bending, and keeps her legs either slightly or more wide. This position keeps her pelvis and her ventral point (vaginal path) on the horizontal-plane, which is not congenial for the penetrating penis of her husband.

B. Child-on-Chest Position is to be Avoided

Some husbands lie over their wives like a child, face flat, by transferring with almost most of their body weight on their wives. As a result of this these wives struggle to breath, suffocate and are hard pressed by their husbands' body weight. These wives can't bear their husbands' heavy weight and ask their husbands to get off as quickly as possible. This makes the husbands to feel as is their wives do not like them or sex. As a result of this Heaviness of Sex these wives develop sexual aversion sexual avoidance, unorgasmia, frigidity and in some cases sexual frustration and extra marital sexual interest and relationships. The husbands develop faster style of sexual functioning, premature ejaculation and extra-marital interest.

The husband while lying over his wife is asked to bear the weight of his trunk over both of his stretched arms with the elbows straight, which are planted on the bed. He bears his body weight on his arms, knees, forelegs, and toes.

II. WHAT TO DO

A. Bent-Knee Position

In order to move the wife's ventral point to a receptive angle, she is asked bend and draw up her knees with her feet kept away and flat on the bed. This position helps her pelvis to tilt to a 45° angle, which is congenial for the penis to enter.

This position is known as the "Missionary Position" or "Man-on-Top" Position, which is most often used through out the world.

His hip is to be just in touch with his wife's hip, but does not transfer his body weight on her. He may move his hip back and forth and in and out but the there should not be any weight bearing on his wife.

B. Knee-Lock Position or Crab-Position

The wife while lying on her back can lift her feet off the bed and lock her ankles behind the back of her husband who lies over her face down. By leveraging her ankles over her husbands lower back, she can press his hip down towards her hip as well as move her hip up and away from the bed. This position helps her to be penetrated deeper and results in the occurrence of multiple orgasms for her.

C. Jockety-Position or Woman-on-Top Position

In this female dominant position the wife sits on her husband who lies on his back. The wife joys more freedom of movement and can move her hip up and down in this position. Deeper penetration and better stimulation of the clitoris are facilitated by this position. In certain ancient cultures a rope hanging from the ceiling was held by the wife to lift her up and down against gravity to produce rhythmic copulatory movements. The husband who lies on his back is able to relax more and is able to maintain his whole attention for holding his erection for a longer duration, resulting in several multiple orgasms for his wife. Most of the body weight of the wife is borne on her feet while she squats on her husband, or on her knees and forelegs while she kneels over him. Thus the husband need not bear the weight of his wife. Men with lower back pain will find this position more comfortable.

D. Rear Entry Positions

(a) Kneeling

The wife kneels, and keeps her head down on the bed. Her hip is kept lifted up. Her husband kneels behind her and penetrates her from behind. This enables the wife to rock her hip up and down, and back and forth. The husband holds his wife's hip and moves it to and fro and up and down as required. The husband finds it comfortable to move his hip back and forth. This position facilitates deeper penetration and greater satisfaction. This also facilitates the deposition of the semen closer to the mouth of the uterus. This position adopted in conjunction with certain other conditions ensures the conception of a male baby with 80% probability.

(b) Standing

The wife stands on the floor with her knees straight and wide and bending forward, resting her head on the bed. Her husband stands behind her and penetrates her. This position permits rocking movements by the husband and wife. Further the husband can hold his wife's hip and rock it to and fro and up and down, as he wants. Deeper penetration and greater satisfaction are ensured by this position as in the previous position (Kneeling). Male progeny can be planned in this position. Compared to the previous position, this position can be adopted by pregnant women and those women who suffer from knee pain and find it painful to flex their knees.

E. Tip-of-the-Bed Position

The wife is asked to sit on the edge of the bed, and with the support of the husband, by holding one of his hand or both of his hands, his wife lies on her back. Her legs lefts hanging at the edge of the bed are lifted up and with her knees bent and kept wide, she is ready to be penetrated by her husband. Her buttocks, is to just jut out of the edge of the bed. Her husband stands on the floor and enters her. This position permits deeper penetration and results in greater satisfaction. Deeper deposition of semen closer to the mouth of the uterus and the incidence of a male child is 80% probable. Men and women with obesity can find this position more suitable. This position enables a face-to-face contact, kissing, and fondling or sucking the breasts.

7. SLOW BREATHING AND SLOW MOVEMENTS

Sexual excitation speeds up the rate of breathing. This results in pre-mature ejaculation in men. Two thirds of the men suffer from Pre-Mature Ejaculation at one time or the other in their lives.

"How to prolong the duration of the sexual-intercourse?"

is a Million Dollar Question.

A. Tantra Answer

The Ancient Indian Science-Tantra has an effective answer for this question.

Slowing down the rate of breathing can prolong the period of erection as long as one desires.

B. Mental Diversions

By mental diversions the sexual excitation and arousal in the human male can be controlled and orchestrated. This helps in the man's wife in reaching multiple orgasms several times during every time in sexual intercourse. In some African tribes men are able to engage in sexual intercourse with their wives for over ninety minutes.

The mental diversion is achieved during coitus by engaging in varying numbers of shallow and deep thrusts.

For example

2 shallow/1 deep

4 shallow/2 deep

6 shallow/3 deep

Later these thrusts may also vary at random as well, like:

2 shallow/3 deep

5 shallow/2 deep

1 shallow/4 deep, etc.

Moving from proportioned or systematic number of shallow vs. deep thrusts to purely "On-the-Spot Programmed" number of shallow and deep thrusts take the emotional excitement and arousal off the minds of the copulating male and put him on an Integrated Right Left Hemisphere Mode. This psycho-physiological dynamics helps the man to regulate his ejaculatory function. In fact these men perform sexual intercourse for over ninety minutes with two or three intermissions as desired by their wives. The African name for this technique is known as "Khareeza".

Elaborate and systematic, similar procedures have been indicted and recommended by Tạntra.

8. FEMALE PARTICIPATION

A. An Eye-Opener

Many a women feel that they are expected to play a passive partner during sexual intercourse. Some of them in fact keep their eyes closed by closing their eyelids or by the use of their hands. Keeping the eyes open by the wife is very important for her psychological participation in sex. Because of their strict upbringing by their parents some girls detest sex and try to avoid sex. This results in the closure of their eyes during sexual intercourse.

In the following cases also eye closure is likely to occur:

1. When the girls are not able to marry the man of their choice, or
2. When choice is forced on them, or
3. When they don't like the man

Some of the girls who have been sexually abused develop an aversion for sex, and due to their over-generalization, consider the sexual intercourse with their husband as equivalent to raping. All the above girls feel that sexual intercourse with their husband is obligatory, and is one among the household duties. They feel that it is a necessary evil which has to be tolerated however disagreeable and painful it may be to them. This attitude takes the pleasure away from sex not only for the wife but also for the husband. A non-participative, passive, non-responding, dummy- like wife can sexually frustrate the husband and force him to go after another woman. In fact, some of these wives with an aversion for sex persuade their husbands even if the husbands are unwilling to bring another woman into their lives in order escape the stressful sex life.

Keeping the eyes open is the first step in solving all the above problems. This brings such wives to a feeling of "here and now" and experiences their husband fully by seeing them.

B. Touch and Feel

The wife is to touch and feel the body of her husband before, during and after sexual intercourse. Some women keep their hands kept inter-twined beneath their head during sexual intercourse. This is a non-participative, passive position, which is sexually dysfunctional. The wife is to touch, massage, and hug the body and limbs of her husband while having copulation.

C. Kissing Keeps One "Here and Now"

Kissing by the wife whenever possible before, during and after the sexual intercourse enhances the quality of satisfaction for both husband and wife.

D. Hip Titling in Synch

The wife by tilting and moving her hip in synchronization with her husband's hip movements helps in the enjoyment by both.

E. Hip Movement Exercises

To help the women with sexual aversion to come out of it the following exercise will help.

(a) Hip-Tilting: Standing

The woman is to stand with her feet part. With her knees slightly bent, and keeping her palms behind her head, she is to tilt her pelvis forward and up and then backward and up in a rhythmic manner. A set of six such movements can be repeated six times with an intermittent brief rest pause.

(b) Hip-Tilting-Kneeling

Kneeling on the fours, the woman can tilt her pelvis forward and down and backward and up. This is also to be repeated as many times as mentioned earlier.

(c) Hip-Tilting-Lying on Back

Now the hip is to be tilted up and down as many times as referred earlier. These exercises defreeze the stiff muscles, which had frozen and contracted due to an aversive attitude to sex. Once the muscles are relaxed as a result of the above exercises, there is a concomitant positive change in the attitude to sex. Even years of sexual inhibition melt away. A woman with a quarter century of sexual aversion and sexual inhibition blossomed with sexual enthusiasm.

9. FEMALE ORGASM

The wife is to "let go" of herself when she reaches orgasm. Many a women have not experienced orgasm due to various reasons.

A. Faking an Orgasm

One of the best ways a woman can reach an orgasm is to "Fake an Orgasm".

To help a women feel how it would feel when she experiences an orgasm is to ask her to do the following exercise.

B. Holding Ice Cubes in Both the Palms

The woman is asked sit with her eyes closed. She is asked to keep the fingers of both her hands to be closed. She is to imagine that he is holding an ice cube in each of her palms. She is to feel and act as to how it feels to hold the ice cubes in her hand. She is not supposed to throw the ice cubes away. Gradually she will act as if her arms are shivering, her body stiffening with the chillness experienced from the ice cubes. She will shake her head and let out hissing noises. In case she does not produce any of these responses, she can be asked to produce such responses. Then she is asked to open her eyes, and told that a similar set of responses will occur during the experiencing of orgasm. She is asked to imitate similar responses during her sexual intercourse with her husband. After half-a-dozen repetition, she catches up with the experiencing of the spontaneous orgasmic experience. This method is useful in treating women who suffer from frigidity and unorgasmia.

10. POST-COITAL INTIMACY

Most men after experiencing their orgasm immediately go to sleep. This frustrates their wives. They feel that they are being just used as a sex object. The psychological bondage between husband and wife requires Post-Coital Intimacy.

After the sexual intercourse the husband must keep awake and keep interacting with his wife for fifteen minutes. Disengaging activities like going to the toilet, getting dressed or going to sleep are to be necessarily avoided.

Before going to bed one can clear the bladder. After the coitus one can continue to remain nude, touch, hug, kiss, and chat for a period of fifteen minutes. Getting into arguments, planning for the future, sharing one's worries and anxieties, and hurting and insulting are to be voided. Positive feelings are to be created, shared and maintained during this period. A sense of humour will help a great deal during this period. Mutual appreciation will also be of much use. This Post-Coital-Intimacy strengthens the marital bondage.

The practice of the above mentioned behavioural techniques would qualitatively improve the sexual satisfaction of the couple, and in turn contribute significantly to Marital Adjustment, Family Mental Health and Community Mental Health. Psychologists can play a significant role in this direction.

SEX: REPRODUCTION VS. RECREATION

The Western Culture had discovered female Orgasm only some years ago. Females had played a passive-role in the sexual intercourse. Or in other words, the 'Male-Dominant-Societies' through out the World had been concerned only about the 'Male-Orgasm' and had never bothered about the 'Female-Orgasm'.

The predominance of Pre-Mature-Ejaculation, and Secondary Impotence among two thirds of the modern men has resulted in the majority of the women suffering from unorgasmia and frigidity.

The development of erectile competency among men depends more on behavioural procedures than on pharmacological preparations like, Viagra and other sex stimulant pills.

The Erectile Incompetence among men has resulted in several psychosocial anomalies.

An Innovative Behaviour Technology for Maximization of Erectile Duration is described in detail in this paper, which will help in overcoming Erectile Incompetency.

ANCIENT INDIAN TECHNOLOGY FOR ACHIEVING SUPER-SEX

The inspiration for this paper has been drawn from Ancient Indian literature of Maha-Bharatham.

Aswathaman wants to revenge the Pancha Pandavas for causing the death of his father Dhronachari. He gets a sword from Siva and goes after the Pancha Pandavas in order to slay them. But Sri Krishnan saves them, and he could kill all their five sons. Frustrated by his failure to kill them, Aswathaman wants to at least destroy the last child that is in the womb of Dhroupathi. He shoots an arrow, the radioactivity of which causes abortion of the child in the womb of Droupathi.

The Royal Medical Experts suggest that the aborted material be collected and kept in a vase, and when touched by a Nishtika Brahmachari would regain life and grow to be a child. Pancha Pandavas seek the help of their grandfather, Bhishmachari, who is considered to be a Nyshtika Brahmachari for touching the vase. But he says that though he was not married, he had psychologically wavered by being sympathetic to a girl called Ambalika. He suggests them to approach Sri Krishnan, as he is a true Mystical Brahmachari. Pandavas are surprised and curious about how Sri Krisahnan would qualify as Mystical Brahmachari, as he had been known to have had sex with innumerable number of women.

However, they approached Sri Krishnan, who readily obliged their request, and the fetus regained life. To the curious Pandavas, Sri Krishna himself came forward to clear their doubt about his qualification to be considered as a Nyshtka Brahmachari.

Sri Krishnan's explanation leads to the following points:

1. When there is no desire for enjoying pleasure, then one does not enjoy any pleasure.
2. Thus engaging in behaviour without expecting any reward, pleasure, or pay-off, distances the person from the behaviour.
3. A behaviour enacted without emotions does not affect the person emotionally.

   He said that when women had desired him to have sex with them, he had no desire to have sex with them. He only fulfilled their desire and thereby he was emotionally distanced from his behaviour of having had sex with them.

Since he had sought no pleasure, he had never ejaculated, though he had sex. Even with his two wives he had not ejaculated and he did not beget any children.

Where as in the case of Bhishmachari, he was not physically involved even with that single woman, Ambalika, but he had emotionally related to her by his feeling of sympathy.

This intricate and subtle interpretation of the linkage between Emotion and Behaviour can benefit the Modern Psychologists in devising Innovative Techniques in the area of Behaviour Technology to solve several Mental Health related problems.

From the above, it can be understood that it is possible to engage in sex without ejaculation, provided the man does not desire to end up with an ejaculation, which is an emotional pay-off for him.

The possibility of Ejaculatory Control, if not Ejaculatory Denial or Non-Ejaculatory-Sexual-Intercourse becomes evident from the existence of certain present practices in India and Africa.

In India, in Kerala, a community, which stands at the top of social hierarchy, known as Namboodhris have been practicing the Single-Child-Norm. The first and only child is considered as the socially recognized child.

If any one gets more than one child, they are not recognized as the children of that family. This shows that this group of people has known, and has been practicing Ejaculatory Control.

In Africa, a certain tribe engages in sexual intercourse for ninety minutes, with two intermissions in between the period. The method they use is called as Khareeza.

NON–EJACULATORY SEXUAL INTERCOURSE

While the Modern Men have the ejaculation as the ultimate goal of enjoyment every time they engage in sexual intercourse, the Ancient Men of India had their ultimate goal-not to ejaculate during sexual intercourse. This was meant to ensure good physical and mental health for men and women. The Non-Ejaculatory Copulation ensured Health and Longevity for men, and multiple orgasms for females.

Misinformed, or incompletely informed of the Ancient Sex Technology, some of the Modern Men, feel that they will grow weak if they have sex and ejaculate. Hence, some of them due to this superstitious belief avoid sexual intercourse with their wives. This leaves their wives high and dry and sexually frustrated after every sexual intercourse.

To help the Modern Men to shift their focus from the present "Self-Centred", "Ejaculatory-Self-Enjoyment" to "Spouse-Centred", "Non-Ejaculatory-Spouse's-Multiple-Orgasm-Enjoyment", and to help them move from the present "Heightened Sexual Arousal" to "Relaxed Sexual Enjoyment Hosting to the Spouse" the following techniques will help.

As preparatory to reducing the sexual arousal and for prolonging the duration of the period of erection, the final pay-off of ejaculation can be de-emphasized for the males.

Men can develop voluntary control over their sexual arousal by doing the following:

1. Set the Goal of Non-Ejaculation.
2. Relax their fingers and toes.
3. Relax the inner thighs.
4. Relax the abdominal muscles.
5. Relax the lower back muscles.
6. Take "Long-Inhalations" and "Long-Exhalations".

The details of the Behaviour Technology for achieving effective Ejaculatory Regulation in a gradual step-by-step manner is presented in the following Table 1.

The above lovemaking is to be practiced without emission of semen.

The measured strokes will have direct impact on the body, mind and breathing of both the man and the woman. The love-strokes are not to be counted in the mind, because it will block out the experiencing of the sensuality of sex, and also the Awareness "Here and Now".

The strokes can be counted with the help of:

1. A rhythm - such as background music
2. A rosary by the female or male
3. Mnemonic devices
4. Electronic Metronome ringing at termination of a specific pre-set count

The counting of strokes serve the role of Diversion of Attention, and thus as an Arousal Reduction Technique.

The progression in the frequency of strokes per intercourse, intercourse per day and the number of days in succession gradually and systematically desensitizes the sexual arousal of both men and women.

The details of this technique can be provided to married people, as well as the adolescent males and females so as to enable them to take maximum advantage of this.

Table 1

Maximization of Ejaculatory Duration

Method	*Position*	*No. of strokes after whichman withdraws without ejaculation*	*No. of times per day*	*No. of days of practice in succession*
1.	Man on Top: Woman lies on her back (with a cushion beneath her). Man lies over-woman	9	1	1
2.	Same as above.	18	2	2
3.	Woman-on-Top: Woman kneels/squats on man and moves up and down. Man lies on his back	27	3	3
4.	Same as above	36	4	4
5.	Rear-Entry (Kneeling): Woman kneels and keeps her head on the bed. Man kneels perpendicularly and enters her from behind	45	5	5
6.	Same as above	54	6	6
7.	Rear-Entry (Standing): Woman stands and bends forward. Man stands and enters her from behind	63	7	7
8.	Same as above	72	8	8

This technique will be very useful in:

1. Reduction of excessive sexual arousal among men
2. Reduction of lack of sexual arousal among men
3. Prolongation of the duration of erection
4. Prolongation of the duration of sexual intercourse
5. Reduction of Sexual Anxiety among women
6. Reduction of Unorgasmia among women
7. Reduction of Frigidity among women
8. Ensuring Multiple Orgasm for women
9. Reduction of Multi-Partner Sex
10. Ensuring Prevention of STD
11. Ensuring prevention of HIV infection
12. Ensuring Low Fertility Rate
13. Ensuring Population Control
14. Reduction Sex Crimes
15. Reduction in masturbation among men and women
16. Reduction in abnormal sexual behaviour of males and females
17. Reduction in male and female Sexual Dysfunctions
18. Emancipation of males from "Performance Anxiety"
19. Emancipation of males from "Sexual Obsession"
20. Reduction of Pre-Mature Ejaculation
21. Reduction of Secondary Impotence
22. Reduction of Vaginimus and Frigidity among women
23. Reduction of Homosexuality and Lesbianism
24. Reduction in abnormal sexual behaviour of males and females
25. Reduction in male and female sexual dysfunctions

REFERENCES

1. Benson, H. Benson Relaxation Response 1979.
2. Ganesan, V. X-10: Ten Pre-Requisites for Sexual Satisfaction. Unpublished paper, Dept. of Psychology, Bharathiar University, Coimbatore, 1980.

3. Ganesan, V. Management of Aversion to Sex among Females with Self-Defense Technique. Unpublished paper, Dept. of Psychology, Bharathiar University, Coimbatore, 1985.

4. Ganesan, V. Management of Aversion to Sex among Females with Touch Therapy. Un published paper, Dept. of Psychology, Bharathiar University, Coimbatore, 1995.

5. Iyengar, B.K.S.

6. Jacobson, Jacobson's Progressive Relaxation Technique.

23

Adolescent Sleep

Implications for Student Life

V.S. Pramila*

When we think of health psychology we are most likely to think of adults as being in the greatest need and therefore importance is given to improve the health and well-being of adult men and women. In doing so the emphasis is on activities and behaviours that are done while one is awake – like the food we eat, the attitudes we should develop, our habits, the exercises that we need to do, the daily schedule that we should follow, and so on. Hardly any thought is given to the role of sleep in health and well-being. Also, even less importance is given to a significant section of the society – the adolescent. That sleep is essential and necessary for health is something that no one would deny but concern does not go much beyond that. Perhaps, the belief that young people can and should adjust to difficulties (such as a little, or rather, a lot less sleep) and not be the worse for it may underlie apathy toward an important issue!

The quality of life of today's youth, especially the school-going and college-going adolescent leaves much to be desired, especially if after class 10 he decides to go into the engineering stream or the medical stream. As we are already aware, the preference for these two courses is so great that students strive to get into corporate coaching centres to prepare for the common entrance examinations

* Professor, Department of Psychology, Andhra University, Visakhapatnam, Andhra Pradesh.

that are conducted by the state. In Andhra Pradesh alone, in May 2007, more than 2, 00,000 students competed for entrance into the engineering and medical courses. The grind in preparation for entrance to these corporate coaching centres starts as early as Class 9 when they are 13 or 14 years old, (early adolescence stage) and will continue until they are 16 or 17 years old. The typical schedule of a student in the coaching centres is as follows:

Table 1

Daily Schedule of Students in Coaching Centres

Timings	*Activities*
4:00 AM to 4:15 AM	Personal hygiene
4:15 AM to 6:15 AM	Study hour
6:15 AM to 7:00 AM	Bathing and breakfast
7:00 AM to 7:30 AM	Commuting to class
7:30 AM to 8:30 AM	Study hour
8:30 AM to 12:30 PM	Attend classes
12:30 PM to 1:00 PM	Lunch
1:00 PM to 3:00 PM	Self-study and Problem solving
3:00 PM to 5:00 PM	Maths
5:00 PM to 5:30 PM	Break and snacks
5:30 PM to 7:00 PM	Counselling (Clarification of doubts)
7:00 PM to 7:30 PM	Commuting to the hostel
7:30 PM to 8:30 PM	Homework
8:30 PM to 9:30 PM	Dinner
9:30 PM to 11:00 PM	Study
11:00 PM	Bed and lights out

As can be seen from this schedule, of the 19 hours they are awake, 15 hours goes for study, 1 hour for commuting, and the remaining 3 hours are for having their meals or attending to their personal needs. For rest and sleep they have only 5 hours at their disposal. This rigorous programme may start as early as class 9. What is the impact of this kind of schedule that starts in June every year and goes on till the July of two years later with no weekends, no vacations and no holidays on the adolescent? What impact and consequences would such a schedule have on the well-being of a student? I would like to focus on this aspect in the light of research that has been done in the West on adolescent sleep.

Those who are not studying in coaching centres but are taking private tuitions are working almost in the same schedule except that they may wake up at 5:30 in the morning than at 4:00.

Studies in other parts of the world such as Europe (Tynjnln, Kannas and Vnlimaa, 1993), Brazil (Andrade & Barreto, 1997) and America (Manber, Pardee, Bootzin, et al., 1995) show that students sleep at more or less the same time – that is, at 22:04 hrs ±0100 hrs. A sleep habits survey administered to more than 3,000 Rhode Island 9th to 12th graders revealed that the median amount of reported sleep in this group was 7.5 hours (Wolfson and Carskadon, 1998).

The average hours of sleep required by an adult ranges from 7 to 8 hours. The adolescent is still in the development stage when there are a lot of changes taking place in his body. These changes affect every aspect of his life, his functioning and his behaviour.

The Biological Clock – The internal biological clock seems to act against the sleep-wake cycle. The sleep-wake cycle predicts that the longer one is awake the greater will be the need to sleep. However, in the case of teenagers there seems to be an inability to go to sleep at night until 11 or 12 o'clock followed by great drowsiness on waking up at 6 or 7 in the morning. In fact, they like to continue sleeping in bed till late in the morning. This has been called "phase delay." Carskadon et al., (1980), who has done research on adolescent sleep finds that adolescents sleep approximately 9.2 hours, if given the opportunity. This means that instead of a decreasing need for sleep there is an increased need for sleep, more than they had as children. The students who have been referred to above get only 5 hours of sleep which is a little more than 50% of the sleep requirement. The result is what is called a "sleep debt" that accumulates over the week. In the West the adolescent works out the sleep debt over weekends when they sleep in late but in India it is a six-day week and Sunday is the day when the weekly test is conducted. The student has to perform or else lose out in the race to get into the best colleges.

In an interesting study, Carskadon and Dement (1981) described research on college students restricting their sleep to 5 hours a night for several nights. They found that daytime sleepiness increased with each night of restricted sleep, indicating the cumulative effect of sleep loss. The research also showed that even with restricted sleep students felt more alert in the evening, encouraging the tendency to stay up late again. If additional tests of sleep latency are carried out at 8 and 10 p.m., a student who struggled and dozed through the early afternoon becomes energetic and internally stimulated in the evening, often past midnight. The implication of this is that despite sleep loss, the adolescent student may seem to be quite active in the evenings giving the impression that the cumulative sleep debt, if any, has no effect on them.

While sleepiness is the most obvious consequence of sleep loss, the effect of insufficient sleep goes much beyond a drive to go to sleep. Involuntary napping—called microsleeps—takes place and other effects such as gaps in processing information and in behaving reliably also take place. Another consequence is tiredness - a symptom that includes not just fatigue but also a difficulty in initiating certain behaviors. Students who are tired do not have trouble doing something that is compelling or exciting. Tasks that are tedious, such as studying for an exam are much harder to do when sleep deprived. (Graham, 2000).

Learning and Memory – Another area where sleep research is relevant to the student is the effect of sleep on learning and memory. There is plenty of evidence that the brain consolidates and practices what is learned during the day *after* the student goes to sleep. Learning actually continues to take place while a person is asleep. Dr. Stickgold has stated that the brain consolidates the learning during two phases of sleep— slow-wave sleep and REM sleep. Chronic partial sleep deprivation also affects higher level cognitive functions or "executive" functions. These include working memory and verbal creativity. Wolfson and Carskadon (1996) have shown that poorer grades have been associated with short nocturnal sleep lengths. In another study she found that sleep restriction among 9th through 12th graders resulted in depressive mood (Carskadon et al., 1989). In college students she found that anxiety and depression scores correlated with insufficient sleep. These results indicated mood changes are associated with insufficient sleep (Carskadon et al., 1991). People who are sleep deprived are irritable, showing increased anger and lowered tolerance to frustration. The effects relate to both thinking and emotional control.

Neurobehavioural Consequences – Sleep restriction in adolescents leads to a decline in alertness. They also show a decline in vigilance, reaction time, attention, memory, behavioural control, motivation and mood. The effect of this is that it will reflect in the school work and increases his propensity to use alcohol, drugs, coffee and nicotine (Dahl, 1999, Dinges, et al., 1997)

Health Outcomes- Research has also shown that sleep-deprived persons become susceptible to infections, experience metabolic effects, have lowered immune function and tend to use alertness-promoting agents such as caffeine and other stimulant medications.

Having reviewed some of the effects of sleep loss in adolescent students, it would be interesting to study the scenario in the Indian situation. Efforts to conduct a survey in corporate tuition centres were unfruitful. However, a study was conducted on 425 adolescent students in both rural and urban areas in Coastal Andhra region (Ravi Kumar & Pramila, 2006). They were in Classes 10, 11 & 12 and the degree level. These were not students of corporate tuition centres but were staying with their parents while studying. The detailed break-up of students participating in this study is given in Table 2.

Table 2

Sample of Students

Educational Level	*Urban Students*		*Rural Students*		*Total*
	Male	*Female*	*Male*	*Female*	
10th Class	30	30	31	30	**121**
Intermediate	67	33	41	31	**172**
Degree	30	32	34	36	**132**
Total	**127**	**95**	**106**	**97**	
	222		**203**		**425**

A questionnaire survey was conducted on these students on their sleep habits and practices. They were asked to rate their behaviour or practice on a 5-point scale of ranging from "every day/night", "once in two days", "1-2 times a week", "never", and "don't know".

Table 3

Sleep-related Behaviour: Percentage of "Never" Response by Students

Behaviour	*10th Class*		*Intermediate*		*Degree*	
	Rural	*Urban*	*Rural*	*Urban*	*Rural*	*Urban*
Feel satisfied with sleep	19.4 (10.0)	3.3 (13.3)	14.6 (9.7)	17.9 (12.1)	5.9 (5.6)	16.7 (12.5)
Fall asleep in morning class.	64.5 (60.0)	70.0 (86.7)	80.5 (80.6)	71.60 (90.9)	55.9 (77.8)	73.3 (65.6)
Fall asleep in afternoon class	64.5 (73.3)	66.7 (83.3)	75.6 (93.5)	56.7 (78.8)	35.4 (52.8)	73.3 (75.0)
Feeling tired or sleepy during the day	48.4 (33.3)	53.3 (43.3)	63.4 (71.0)	49.3 (29.4)	29.4 (52.8)	36.7 (21.9)
Sleep until afternoon	83.9 (90.0)	66.3 (80.0)	87.8 (77.4)	73.1 (87.9)	82.4 (69.4)	80.0 (71.1)
Stay up all night	54.5 (73.3)	66.3 (93.3)	78.0 (74.2)	56.7 (69.7)	70.6 (63.9)	70.0 (59.4)
Have a hard time falling asleep	48.4 (50.0)	53.3 (50.0)	48.8 (32.3)	61.2 (90.9)	55.9 (63.9)	60.0 (37.5)
Awaken too early in the morning and have difficulty falling asleep	51.6 (50.0)	60.0 (36.7)	48.8 (58.1)	52.2 (81.8)	50.0 (61.1)	46.7 (50.0)

Note: Female percentages are given in brackets.

From Table 3 it is observed:

(A) That a larger percentage of males than females was never satisfied with their sleep (except for the urban 10th class student).

(B) Falling asleep in the morning class was seen to be more prevalent among the rural 10th class and degree students than the intermediate students and looking at the gender factor; the female students seem to be at a disadvantage.

(C) Nearly half the number of students or more feels tired and sleepy during the day.

(D) The practice of sleeping until the afternoon is not very common, but is seen to occur more commonly among the urban students at the 10th class and degree level.

(E) Staying up all night to study occurs more often at the 10th class level both among rural and urban adolescent males, urban male intermediate students, and adolescent females at the degree level in both urban and rural settings.

(F) Significantly large percentages of students at all educational levels, whether male or female, rural or urban, have a hard time falling asleep.

(G) Not being able to go back to sleep after awakening too early is also very widespread among all sections of students.

These results give us new perspectives on behaviour that has been neglected so far as being relevant to health and well-being. First, it clearly shows that sleep problems and "sleep debt" occur among adolescents in our country that could be widely prevalent. Second, it does not seem to be limited to those students who study in corporate tuition centres. The problem must be much more severe among them given the daily schedule that they follow. Third, the perception or impression that among rural students sleep problems may exist at a very minimal level because the lifestyle is more laid back and slow than urban life does not seem to be justified. In fact, in some instances they have more sleep debt than their urban counterparts. Further research is needed to go into the reasons for this phenomenon. Fourth, there is an urgent need for parents and those making policy decisions in educational matters at the government level, at the institutional level to take note of the implications of these findings and take preventive steps to ensure the future generation will be a healthy one.

The rising rate of depression and suicides among adolescent students is an index that things are not as they should be. Sleep, or rather the lack of it, can and does affect mental and physical well-being and unless steps are taken early enough we may soon have a problem that is going out of hand.

REFERENCES

Andrade, M. M. M. and Menna-Barreto (1997). Sleep patterns of high school students living in Sao Paolo, Brazil. Youth Enhancement Services. *International Conference on Contemporary Perspectives on Adolescent Sleep.* Los Angeles: CA.

Carskadon, M.A. and Dement, W.C. (1981).Cumulative effects of sleep restriction on daytime sleepiness. *Psychophysiology* **18:** 107-113.

Carskadon, M.A., Harvey, K., Duke, P., Anders, T.F., Litt, I.F., and Dement, W.C. (1980) Pubertal changes in daytime sleepiness. *Sleep* **2:** 453-460.

Carskadon, M.A. and Mindell, J.A. (1989) Validation of a sleep diary: Effects of transition from daylight savings time to standard time on sleep and mood in college students. *Sleep Research* **18**: 384.

Carskadon, M.A., Seifer, R., Davis, S.S., Acebo, C. (1991). Sleep, sleepiness, and mood in college-bound high school seniors. *Sleep Research* **20**: 175.

Dahl, R.E. (1999). The consequences of insufficient sleep for adolescents: Links between sleep and emotional regulation. *Kappan.* **80** (5):354-359.

Dinges, D., et al. (1997).Cumulative sleepiness, mood disturbance, and psychomotor vigilance performance during a week of sleep restricted to 4-5 hours per night. *Sleep.* **20**(4):267-277.

Manber, R. Pardee, R.E., Bootzin, R.R. et.al., (1995) *Sleep Research.* 24(A) 106.

Mary G. Graham, (Ed.) (2000) National Research Council and Institute of Medicine *Sleep: Needs, Patterns, and Difficulties of Adolescents. Forum on Adolescence.*

Board on Children, Youth, and Families, Commission on Behavioral and Social Sciences and Education. Washington, D.C.: National Academy Press.

Ravi Kumar, M.V. and Pramila, V.S. (2006). Sleep habits of adolescent students in Coastal Andhra . Unpublished master's dissertation. Department of Psychology & Parapsychology, Andhra University, Visakhapatnam.

Tynjnln, J.,Kannas, L., and Vnlimaa, R. (1993). *Health Education Research.* 8 (1): 69-80.

Wolfson, A. and Carskadon, M.A. (1996). Early school start times affect sleep and daytime functioning in adolescents. *Sleep Research* **25**: 117.

Wolfson, A. and Carskadon, M.A. (1998). Sleep schedules and daytime functioning in adolescents. *Child Development.* **69(4):875-887**.

24

Efficacy of Psychotherapeutic Intervention Among Chronic Low Back Pain Patients

An Experimental Study

R.Balakrishnan*, Tarannum Mushtaq, Kumar. P*****

ABSTRACT

The present investigation was carried out to study the efficacy of Psychological intervention on the experience of pain intensity among the chronic low back pain patients. A purposive sample of 200 out-patients of both sexes aged 20-60 years with chronic low back pain of at least 6 months duration was selected from the physiotherapy centre in AYUSH hospital ATLANTA POINT, PORT BLAIR. The patients were requested to self administer the Visual Analogue self-rating scale and their experience of pain before and after the psychological intervention were recorded and mean, SD were computed. The psychological interventions employed in the present study were the active type of psychotherapy which included behavioral counseling, Back care instruction, eye movement desensitization and reprocessing, Jacobson progressive muscular relaxation training and self- instructions. The paired't' test was utilized to analyze the data. The finding shows that there is a statistically significant reduction in the chronic low back pain among

* HOD of Psychology, PSG College of Arts and Science, Coimbatore.

** Research Scholar, Vinayaga Mission Research Foundation, Salem.

*** PG Student of Psychology, IDE, University of Madras, Chennai.

the patients due to the psychological intervention. The present study indicates the efficacy of psychotherapeutic intervention in significantly decreasing the pain experience of the chronic low back pain patients, particularly on a short-time basis. These findings are discussed.

Every one experiences pain at some point in his/her life. The pain can be Acute/short or chronic/longer which does not go away with common pain relieving therapies. Regardless of its duration and experience, it may affect the day to day ability to work, to enjoy with loved ones or to take care of self (Mayilvahanan Natarajan,1996) Back pain is a multifactorial disease. It may be something as straight forward as an arthritic joint or as complex as multiple nerve lesions in a patient with significant psychopathology (Kanner 1997).

The Chronic low back pain is one of the most disabling condition in the modern industrialized society. It has been stated that I million of work population are disabled at any given time due to low back pain: 2.6 million are chronically disabled. The traditional medical and physiotherapeutic approaches for its management have a positive out- come, by reducing the pain intensity and enhancing the ability levels to some extent. By implementing the psychotherapy the result can be maintained by the patient for long duration due to the learned coping skills, which ultimately helps the patients to reduce the dependency on the medicine and medical professionals.

This study stresses the necessity of psychotherapeutic approach as model of treatment, instead of traditional medical model of treatment alone, for the chronic low back pain patients. And also it is necessary for the health care processionals, to know how this psychotherapy approach can reduce the intensity of pain in patients so that chronic low back pain can be managed efficiently by the health care professionals. For, it is observed that psychotherapy helps a person to meet his own needs, to learn more effective ways of behavior, and to develop more adequate desirable defense mechanism.

STATEMENT OF THE PROBLEM

The problem taken up in the present investigation is to study the efficacy of psychotherapy on the experience of pain intensity among the chronic low back pain patients.

OBJECTIVE OF THE STUDY

To examine the efficacy of the psychotherapeutic interventions on the experience of pain intensity among the chronic low back pain patients.

Hypothesis

There will be a significant reduction in the experience of pain intensity among chronic low back pain patients after psychotherapeutic interventions.

Methodology

Research Design

The research design adopted for present study is a one group pretest- post test design, where the effect of the psychological interventions on chronic low back pain was judged by the reduction in the post test (V.A.S) scores.

Sample

A purposive sample of out patients (N=200)aged 20 to 60 years, with chronic low back pain of at least 6 months duration was selected from the physiotherapy department Ayush hospital, Atlanta point, Port Blair. The patients having the low back pain below 6 months of duration or the patients with severe back pain who are unable to concentrate and cooperate for the interventions were not chosen for the study.

Tools Used

1. To measure the level of pain intensity the visual analogue scale (V.A.S) was used.
2. Self made assessment chart was used to obtain the personal data as a part of case history taking.

Description and Administration of Research Tools

1. Self made Chart was used to collect the data regarding Name, age, sex, occupation, duration of pain.
2. The Visual Analogue scale (V.A.S)

This is the simplest pain assessment tool where scalar diagrams on which patients indicate their level of pain where a level on 0-1 indicates no pain an 9-10 indicates worst possible pain. This scale is widely utilized by clinical psychologists, and other health care professionals, who deal the patient with pain; its validity and reliability of the (V.A.S), are well established. There are many other ways in which V.A.S have been presented (Wewers & Lowe, 1990) in the literature

SCORING

The number chosen by the patient from the 0 to10 continuum of the (V.A.S) was considered to be his/her score. The higher the (V.A.S) Score, the higher the experience of pain.

The patients who had been diagnosed as Chronic low back pain, were given the medications and referred for out- patient physiotherapy programme were interviewed and personal data obtained by the help of assessment chart, and also pretest was conducted through the administration of self rating (V.A.S), personally by the investigator, on patients 1st Visit. At the end of the treatment (14 or 15 session) the post test (V.A.S) was conducted and the data was statistically analyzed.

PROCEDURE

After obtaining the necessary permission from the concerned hospital authorities, one of the investigators, a physiotherapist interviewed individually, low back pain patients, obtained their personal data and asked the patients to self administer the self rating V.A.S on patients first visit. The psychotherapeutic intervention was administered to each patient thereafter for 15 sessions. One session per day and each session lasting for one hour. Each patient was directed to practice the techniques as home work. The entire treatment programme went up to 15 days for each patient. At the end of the treatment programme the V.A.S was readministered for each patient.

The techniques employed and the detail instructions utilized in the psychotherapeutic interventions are given here under:

Psychotherapeutic Interventions

The out-patients with chronic low back pain were treated in one hour session with psychotherapeutic techniques, progressively and sequentially for 15 days according to their learning capacity;

throughout the programme the patients were advised to do homework employing the psychotherapeutic techniques as taught by the investigators. The treatment programmes employed in this study were Behavioral counseling, Self instructions, Back care instructions, Eye movement desensitization and reprocessing (EMDR), and Jacobson (1938) progressive Deep muscle relaxation.

Behavioral Counseling

Step-I: The investigator patiently listened to the patient's problem, and gathered information to know how the patient expressed his/her pain behavior, and also to note the myths regarding their pain and treatment etc.

Step-II: Patient was educated regarding the medical diagnosis, anatomy, body mechanics (structure & function of the low back region), various cause of pain, first aid and preventive behavior for back pain, emotional, psychological issues of chronic low back pain, posture and its role in the back pain and self management techniques and finally about necessity of and cognitive behavioral intervention for its management. The investigator exchanged ideas with the patient regarding their back pain and motivated them to participate in the treatment programme. By this process any myths and confusions of the patients regarding pain were clarified to them.

SELF INSTRUCTIONS

This instruction technique for creating cognitive awareness of the posture, by changing the habits and style of work, which can help the patient to reduce the mechanical stress and prevent the recurrence of chronic lowback pain, which involved the following steps:-

Step–I: The investigators loudly and clearly instructed the following "back care instruction "/"postural training instruction" according to the patients, necessity, work style/occupation.

Step–II: The above mentioned instruction are repeated by the patient to the investigator.

Step–III: Patient was instructed to self talk/whisper these instructions and correct his/her posture, when they are assuming that particular posture.

Step–IV: Advised to practice these newly learned instructions.

By following these self instructions, the patients assumed good posture by changing their habits and style of work, which ultimately prevented the recurrence of back pain.

Further the patient was instructed to do home work on this technique and to practice once per day.

Back Care Instruction

The patient was instructed explicitly to adapt and use instructions given below for each posture. The investigators demonstrated the postures appropriately to the patients.

A – Standing

"Stand straight/erect.

Both legs should equally bear the Weight.

Hold the weight near to he body.

If, standing for longer duration, advised to keep the foot on a small stool".

B – Sitting

"Sit straight in the chair, advised not to lean on the chair.

Advised not to lean on the table.

Take the weight of the upper body through the arms to the arm rest of the chair once for very hour.

Advised to keep the foot on the foot rest of the table".

C – Bending

"While lifting the weight, instructed to bend the hips, knees and sit down without bending the back, weight should be adjusted conveniently between the two feet and advised to lift the weight.

Twisting the back should be avoided when lifting the weights".

D – Exercises

"Stretch the back for every two hours, while doing the desk job.

Stretch the back five or six times before lifting the weights.

Advised to perform the exercises according to advice".

Eye Movement Desensitization and Reprocessing (EMDR : Mark Grant)

Step – I: The patient is advised to select a calm environment and switch on the favorite music tape which last for 30 minutes, and lye down in supine position.

Step – II: The patients were instructed to focus their attention on pain or some aspect of how the pain has affected the sufferer's life, at the same time, advised to listen to the music tape for 30 minutes.

Many people find this aspect most difficult, but literally they don't have to do anything other than pay attention to their experience. Each person will process information uniquely, based on personal experience and values.

Before starting the procedure the patient was cautioned about increase in pain experience and about different sensations felt during the EMDR session and assurance was given about the reduction in the level of the disturbance at the end of the EMDR session.

Patient was instructed to do home work on this technique, to practice once per day.

Jacobson Progressive (Deep) Muscle Relaxation(JPMR)

General instructions were given to the patient regarding the internal environment (empty bladder, and not with the hunger or thirst) and external environment (the room which is free from distractions and with well ventilation) before starting the procedure.

The patient is advised to follow the following sequence of JPMR practices, while lying supine on the floor.

Step – I: The investigators instructed the patient to squeeze his/her own right hand make a fist and asked to experience the tightness for 10 seconds and suggested him to relax by opening the fingers and experience the relaxation in his/her right forearm muscles & hand for 20 seconds advised to perform another time.

Step – II:" Repeat the step –I on the left hand for 2 times".

Step – III : Instructed to, bend both the elbow's inside, suggested to feel the tightness for 10 seconds in the biceps muscle on both the arms and asked to stretch out both the elbows and advised to experience the relaxation in the arms for 20 seconds; advised to perform another time.

Step – IV: Instructed to press both the arms against the floor & feel the tightness in both the triceps for 10 seconds and advised to relax for 20 seconds and experience the relaxation n both his arms– instructed to repeat the same process for another time.

Step – V: Instructed to relax the hands and arms maximally and also to relax the rest of the body and to concentrate on the feeling of relaxation.

Step – VI: Instructed to wrinkle the forehead by raising the eyebrows, maintain it for 10 seconds and advised to feel the tightness and then relax by smoothing it out for 20 seconds; to repeat the sample process another time.

Step – VII: Instructed to frown and crease the brows and feel the tightness for 10 seconds, then relax for 20 seconds by smoothing the forehead; repeated the same process another time.

Step – VIII: Instructed to close both the eyes tightly for 10 seconds and then relaxed by keeping them gently and comfortably closed for 20 seconds; repeated the same process another time.

Step – IX: Instructed to clench the patients teeth together and feel the tightness in the jaw muscles for 10 seconds and suggested to release the tension and feel the relaxation for 20 seconds; advised to repeat it for another time.

Step – X: Instructed to press the tongue tightly against the roof of the mouth for 10 seconds and then release the tension and advised to experience the relaxation for 20 seconds; repeated the same process another time.

Step – XI: Instructed to press the lips tightly together for seconds and relax for 20 seconds; same was repeated for another time.

Step – XII : Instructed to relax all the facial muscles and also the rest of the body and concentrate on the feeling of relaxation.

Step – XIII: Instructed to press the head against the floor as far as possible for five seconds and advised to feel the tightness, then relax the neck muscles for 20 seconds; and repeat the same for another time.

Step – XIV: Instructed to raise both the shoulders; advised to hold them and feel the tightness for 10 seconds, then drop them for relaxing them to 20 seconds; repeated the same process for another time.

Step – XV: Instructed to move both the shoulders in a rotatory movement - upwards, forwards, downwards and back wards for 10 seconds; then relax for 20 seconds in a comfortable position – repeated the procedure for another time.

Step – XVI: Instructed to relax all neck, shoulder and back muscles and the rest of the body and to enjoy the sensation of relaxation.

Step – XVII: Instructed to concentrate on breathing pattern, inhale and hold the breath for 10 seconds and exhale and relax for 20 seconds; repeated the procedure for another time.

Step – XVIII: Instructed to tighten the stomach muscles by pushing them outward for 10 seconds, then relax for 20 seconds; repeated the procedure for another time.

Step – XIX: Instructed to tighten the stomach muscle by drawing them in tightly for 10 seconds and then relax for 20 seconds; repeated the procedure for anther time.

Step – XX: Instruction was given to feel the smooth movements of the fingers on the chest and stomach and relax as much as possible.

Step – XXI: Instructed to arch the lower back by lifting it up, and feel the tightness in the lower back for 10 seconds then rest it comfortably and experience the relaxation fro 20 seconds; repeated the same for another time.

Step – XXII: Instructed to relax chest, stomach and lower back and also the rest of the body and to concentrate on the deeper state of relaxation; advised to enjoy the relaxation.

Step – XXIII: Instructed to press right heel into the floor and feel the tightness in the right thigh muscles for 10 seconds then suggested to relax for 20 seconds; repeat the process for another time.

Step – XXIV: Repeated the step XXIV on the left leg – two times.

Step – XXV: Instructed to press feet and toes towards the face, feel the stretch in the calf muscles for 10 seconds then relax for 20 seconds; repeated the same process for another time.

Step – XXVI: Instructed to bend the both feet and toes away from the face and feel the stretch in the shin muscles for 10 seconds and relax for 20 seconds ; repeated the same for another time.

Step – XXVII: Instructed to focus the patient's mind sequentially from toes, legs, tights, buttocks, lower back, stomach, chest, face, neck, and both the upper limbs and advised to enjoy the relaxation for 25 seconds.

Step -XXVII: Instructed to close the eyes take the breath in, hold the tightness for 10 seconds and relax by exhaling the breath out for 20 seconds –repeated the same process for two more times.

Step – XXIX: Instructed to relax completely; advised to think of the effort that is required to raise the shoulder and arm, advised to think, notice the tension in the shoulder and arms.

Step – XXX: Patient was instructed not to lift the hand, advised to relax and observe the relief and disappearance of tension.

Step – XXXI: Instructed to relax completely, if patient want to get up, advised to count backward from 5-1, if he wants to sleep, he can just relax and sleep.

- Patient was instructed to do home work employing this technique once per day.

RESULTS AND DISCUSSION

The present investigation was undertaken to examine the efficacy of psychotherapeutic effects on experiencing pain intensity among chronic low back pain patients; the data included pre and post test results on V.A.S from 200 subjects was analyzed with the paired t- test and it is presented below.

Table 1

Showing Mean, SDd, t ratio on (V.A.S) scores of the out-patients in the pretest and posttest sessions

Sessions	*N*	*Mean*	*Mean Diff*	*SDd*	*t-ratio*	*Level of significance*
Pretest	200	8.000	7.000	7.035	14.080	<.005
Posttest	200	1.000				

The table 1 shows that the't' value observed is 14.080 and it is significant at <.005 level. The mean for pretest is 8.000 and post test is 1.000. There is a significant difference in the mean V.A.S score, which indicates that there is a decrease in the experience of pain intensity among chronic low back pain patients as hypothesized in the present study.

The findings may be interpreted to mean that the psychotherapeutic interventions employed in the present study as enhanced the patients body awareness, the assumption of the new body posture, inner muscular and mental control.

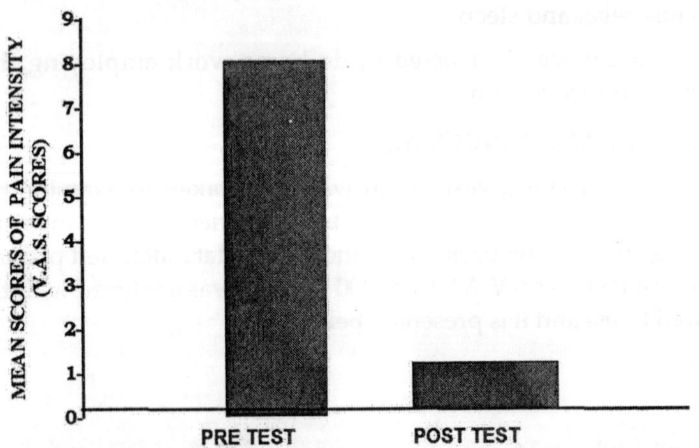

Graph Representing pre and post interventions difference inrelation to the experience of Pain Intensity among Chronic low back pain patients (V.A.S. SOCRES)

CONCLUSION

There is a significant reduction in the experience of pain intensity among chronic low back pain patients due to the application of psychological interventions to them.

REFERENCES

Chronic pain – Physical Medicine & Rehabilitation as – Methodist Health Care System H. page 1-6.

Daniel Bruns, Kevin J. Gaffney 1998- National Guidelines for the psychological Assessment and treatment of the influided patient – www.healthpsych.com, page 1-3.

Jacobson,E.(1938) *Progressive relaxation:* University of Chicago press.

Kanner,R. (1997) *Pain management secrets*. Philadelphia: Hanley & Belfus, Inc.

Mark Grant, MA.(1999), overcoming pain and stress, based on eye movement desensitization and reprocessing (EMDR).- http://www.emdr.com/refs.htm.

Mayilvahana Natarajan (1996). *The Text Book of orthopedics and Traumatology, Backache*. Page - 147-149.

Sunder,S. (1998) *Lecturer Note on rehabilitation Medicine, pain,* Page -61-75.

Wewers,M.E., & Lowe,N.K(1990). A Critical review of visual analogue scales in the measurement of clinical phenomena. Research in Nursing and Health, 13,227-236.

25

Healthy Living
A Preventive Life Style

Nibedita Jena*

ABSTRACT

The concept of health that struck the biopsychosocial perspective has brought into focus on emotional, physical, spiritual and psychological well-being. Healthy living according to Upanishad – "he who desires to live on this earth for more than hundred years should follow a path to action and accordingly a man should act". Wellness by definition involves experience of somatic comfort (emotions, mood, calmness, pleasure, joy, relief, happiness) and a functional ability level at or near the person. From time immemorial mankind has remained puzzled on the subject of wellness. It has been one of the most difficult metaphysical riddles to solve because it is a multidimensional holistic approach to living. The present study aimed to focus on the relationship between life style and holistic health, to explore the characteristics and components of a healthy life style, and to examine the predominant personality type. A total of 60 subjects consisting of male and female younger (20-30 years) and older (60-70 years) age groups were administered the standardized inventory developed by David and Frawly (1979) and another one was specially designed to record health habit index with a survey method. Analysis of results based on factorial design showed that out of 60 subjects irrespective of age and sex, 4 persons maintained a balanced lifestyle and were

* **Reader in Psychology, Reveshaw University, Cuttack, Orissa.**

healthier both in mind and body. Results also revealed that people who followed a regular life style were having healthier personality type than others. Thus achieving wellness is a process involving voluntary choice of thought, attitude, feeling and life styles.

Attainment of happiness is the innate desire of every human being, but our life style, attitude and values have undergone a radical change with rapid modernization and move more and more towards consumerist culture. Everything has to be done in a hurry- fast food, fast track, fast buck and first life to find quick-fix solutions for everything under the sky, but in the process we lose the perspective and balance in life. In this midline an alternative way of thinking comes to mind. Can life style modification help some one? But the question is how do we define the term life style? In a general way, life style means the way of life, the pattern of living of a person-how he spends his time from moment to moment. It also means the food we take, drinking habit, exercise, diet-particularly overeating and consuming too many high fat, low fiber food- constantly facing high stress situations and likes and dislikes of a person. These result from a lifestyle of experience, beginning in early childhood, evolving through adolescence and adulthood. Besides the genetic makeup and personal habits, other factors like family, school, society, culture and education have significant roles in determining the life style of an individual. A healthy life style holds the key to the prevention of many diseases. So we should try to do every thing possible to incorporate healthy habits in the formative years of life. There is a life style circle consisting of AHAAR, VIHAAR, DIET, ACTIVITY, HABITS, THOUGHTS, ACHAAR, and VICHAAR. In a healthy life style all these are perfectly balanced to bring equilibrium in our living, in our mind and body and that we can do only by adapting a holistic approach. Healthy living according to Upanishad – "he who desires to live on this earth for more than hundred years he should follow a path to action and accordingly a man should act".

A well year is a year of life free of diseases. A person might not have identifiable pathology and yet not be healthy. So health is not just the absence of illness. But it is a condition of how well all the body's components are working. Wellness is a multidimensional holistic approach. It is a dynamic process of developing awareness that health and wellness are interdependent. Holistic health means spiritual, physical and social wellbeing. Personality and individual's behavior style plays a crucial role in health habits. The role of behavior in health has received increasing attention since the turn of the century. If people would practice a few health related behavior such as reducing smoking and alcohol consumption, eating more healthy diets and getting sufficient exercises, there is no doubt, we will have a healthy society. We are killing ourselves by our own careless habits and we are killing ourselves by carelessly polluting the environment and by permitting harmful social conditions.

Physical and mental health: There is intimate connection between the mind and body. Any ill feelings or bitterness towards another person will at once affect the body and produced some kind of diseases in the body. Intense passion, hatred, long standing jealousy actually destroys the cells of the body and induces diseases of the heart, liver, kidneys, spleen and stomach.

Removal of hatred through cosmic love, service, friendship, mercy, sympathy and compassion, removal of greediness through generous acts and charity, removal of pride through humanity will help a person in achieving good mental health. Laughter and cheerfulness increase the circulation of blood. A person when wants to have a wonderful physical and mental health, he should be cheerful, tolerant and meditate. He should do pranayams, Asanas.

Ill health is a myth: During illness detach yourself from the body. Connect the mind with the soul. Feel always "I am healthy in body and mind".

Vedanta for health: Auto suggestion is only an offshoot of vedantic assertion and affirmation.

Health and the elements: This body is composed of five elements such as earth, water, fire, air, and ether. It has a natural power to heal itself. If we help this power by means of above five elements, the work of healing will be accelerated.

How to utilize air:

(i) By wearing few clothes

(ii) By exploring the body to fresh air

(iii) By taking morning and evening walk

(iv) By keeping the windows fully open in working place and while in sleep as well.

(v) By deep breathing exercise.

Use of water:

(i) In the form of hot bath, cold bath, vapor bath, herbal bath.

(ii) By taking a glass of water on getting up from bed and while retiring to bed and before and after meals. The body requires a minimum of 10 liters of water a day.

How to utilize light:

One should expose their body to the morning sun and get vitamins from it. Chromopathy can cure many diseases.

Use of earth:

Earth contains magnetic current and many properties of curing disease. It is used as cold or hot packs.

Ideal physical health: Eating in a healthy way though is not easy but it can be done. It is not uncommon for people to be confused, about the best way to eat. Breakfast has been shown to be the most important meal of the day because the body has been in a fast since a man went to sleep at night. Our body's primary energy is glucose, which is stored in our liver and muscles. By morning all our body glucose has been used up, so it is important to fill up our stores before we starts the day.

Fruits and vegetables are loaded with physiochemical, antioxidant, vitamins, minerals and fiber. More colorful fruits and vegetables are more nutrious.

More planning is often difficult for many people, but it is needed urgently for maintaining healthy life.

A balanced diet is simply one in which foods of various types are present in sufficient quantity to give all the nutrients which are needed in the right amount.

There are several questions that had long been asked about the benefits and danger of vigorous exercise. Does exercise enhance health? Does it contribute to longevity? How much is necessary to maintain good health? There are no simple answers to this questions, but it is essentially needed for healthy life. There are five types of exercise like isometric- It is performed by contracting muscles against an immovable object and thus gain strength. Pushing hard against a solid wall is an example of isometric exercise. Isotonic exercise- It requires the contraction of muscles and the movement of joints. Isokinetic exercise is superior to either isotonic or isometrics in promoting muscles. The main disadvantage to isokinetic exercise is the inconvenience and expense of its elaborate equipment.

An aerobic exercise is an exercise that does not require an increased amount of oxygen. It includes short distance running, jogging, dancing, rope skipping, swimming and cycling. The most important characteristics of aerobic exercises are intensity and duration. Exercise influences physical fitness, muscle strength, muscle endurance, flexibility, weight control, decreased depression, reduced anxiety, increased self-esteem, protection against colon cancer, and prevention of osteoporosis.

The word yoga means union, harmonious integration and equilibrium. Yoga psychology has been claimed as the Indian practical psychology, as it not only enunciates the laws and principles of controlling the divergent modification of the mind, but also teaches how to translate them into action. The Bhagavad-Gita presents an integrative synthesis of different categories of yoga, such as Jnan Yoga (the philosophical technique of the rational and the scientific intellect in unraveling the secrets of nature and living a life of harmony, wisdom, truth and justice), Karma Yoga (the principles of unattached action), Bhakti Yoga (the techniques of selfless affection and devotion), and Patanjali. Ideal spiritual health includes Yoga, Meditation, and Self-realization. Self-realization has 3 stages such as self observation, self evaluation, and self reinforcement.

Ideal psychological health: It requires three aspects such as full expression, harmonization, and common end. Besides this Carl Rogers states mentally healthy persons should have (a) acceptance of feelings, self-esteem, openness to new ideas, and creativity. Erickson states that mentally healthy persons are

- Trust others and also themselves
- Capable taking responsibility
- Have a clear, integrated identity

Thus as long as there is life, there is hope for a better life and as long as we care for one another our life will become more colourful.

Three types of preventions such as primary prevention, secondary prevention and tertiary prevention have a predominant role in maintaining healthy living. Primary prevention is a term that gained considerable popularity in the recent years, refers to the activities that are undertaken by apparently diseases free individual with the intent of helping them to achieve maximum wellness). Secondary prevention involves efforts directed toward detecting early signs or symptoms to prevent a more serious condition. Tertiary prevention involves measures designed to cure the diseases or to control the progress of disease.

Bio-feedback is the treatment technique in which people are trained to improve their health by using signals from their own bodies, it also aims at achieving various control over such visceral activities as heart rate, blood pressure etc.; it prevents migraine, disorder of the digestive system. It is a tool and reminds physicians that behavior, thought and feelings profoundly influence physical health. In order to prevent ourselves from disease we should aware and manage ourselves. Lack of management leads to heart disease and sexually transmitted diseases.

OBJECTIVE

The main objective of this study is to investigate the relationship between life style and holistic health, to explore the characteristics and components of a healthy life style, and to examine the predominant personality type.

METHODOLOGY

An exploratory study was conducted by taking older and younger age group individuals in the areas of holistic health, life style and predominant personality type. The total sample consists of 60 male and female with younger and older age group. The mean age groups of younger males were 24.7 years, younger females were 23.5 years, older males were 59.4 years and older females were 59.2 years.

INSTRUMENT

Three questionnaires were used in the present study to collect data with survey method. The first two questionnaires were based on the psychological and physical symptoms (David Frawly, 1979). The third questionnaire was designed to measure health habit index. Questionnaire-1 described (according to vata, pitta and kapha), physical frame, weight, chest, appetite, voice, speech, memory, emotional tendencies, sleep, faith, dream, activity, strength, exertion, sensitivity, resistance to disease, and sexual nature. It consisted of 20 items, each having 3 alternatives; A=Vata, B=Pitta, C=Kapha.

Questionnaire-2 described (according to vata, pitta and kapha) pain, fever, bodily discharge, mouth, throat, stomach, intestines, feces, urine, onset of disease, time of day when diseases get aggravated. It consist of 15 items, each having 3 alternatives like A=Vata, B=Pitta, C=Kapha. The subjects were asked to select any one alternative for each item.

Questionnaire-3 consisted of 20 items describing positive health, daily habits. Each item has 3 alternatives, always (scored-2), sometimes (scored-1), never (scored-0). Subjects were asked to select any one alternative for each item.

The subjects were also regulated to check one alternative under each item that describes them accurately. They were given two weeks time to complete. Diet and nutrition are very important for healthy living. So a balanced diet chart and daily nutrient requirements chart were also taken to study healthy living.

RESULTS AND DISCUSSION

The quality of diet determines how a person looks and feels. Chemicals, water, carbohydrates, protein, fats, vitamins, and minerals make identifiable contribution to the metabolic process of the body (Greenfield, 1985). So a balanced diet chart and daily nutrient chart are taken in the present study (See table-1 and table-2). Poor diet can lead to cancer, hypertension, arteriosclerosis and many more other diseases.

Table 1

Balance Diet: (Qualities in grams)

	Average man	*Average woman*	*Adolescent*	*Child*
Cereals	450	350	500	200
Pulses	50	45	60	35
Green vegetables	75	100	100	60
Other vegetables	75	50	50	40
Roots	75	50	50	30
Milk	200	200	200	250
Fats & oil	20	20	22	25

Table 2

Our daily Nutrient requirements

	Calories	*Protein*	*Fat*	*Minerals*	
				Calcium	*Iron*
Average man	2875	60	20	400	28
Average woman	2225	55	20	400	30
Adolescent boy	2447	67	22	600	41
Adolescent girl	2056	62	22	600	28

Psychological and physical symptoms representing 3 humor vata, pitta, kapha questionnaire of David Frawly were administered on two age group males and females and response were analyzed on the basis of each personality type. Another questionnaire was administered to measure health habit index of vata; pitta and kapha dominant people in the total sample (see table-3).

Table-3 presents in younger age group that 18 persons are having vata personality, the mean good health scan is 22.5, 6 persons are having pitta personality with the mean good health scan 29.5 and 6 kapha personality with mean good health scan 24.1 where as in older age group 13 are having vata personality with mean good health scan 24.0, 9 pitta personality with mean good health scan 19.0 and 11 kapha personality with mean health scan 22.2.

Table 3
Mean good health score of younger and older adult showing predominant personality types

Age Group	*Personality type*	*N*	*Mean good health scan*
Younger Group 20-30	Vata	18	22.5
	Pitta	06	29.5
	Kapha	06	24.1
Older Group 55-65	Vata	13	24.0
	Pitta	09	19.0
	Kapha	11	22.2

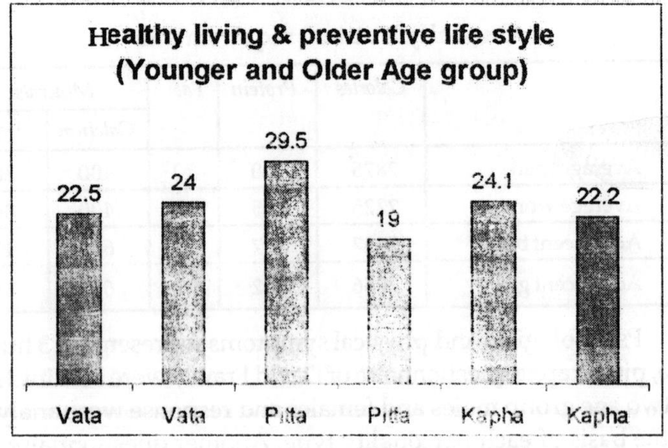

Table 4
Mean health habit index score of vata, pitta and kapha dominant people in the total sample

Predominant Humor	*N*	*Mean Health Habit Scan*
Vata	21	17.52
Pitta	14	23.25
Kapha	21	24.90
Balanced	4	25.50

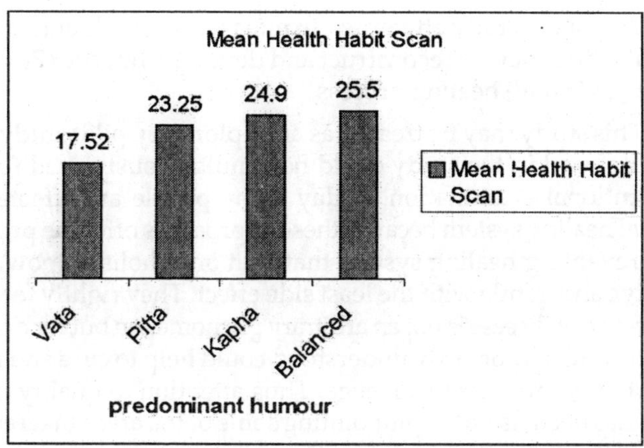

This shows that the mean health good score of younger and older persons showing predominant personality type.

This result shows out of 60, 21 vata predominant humors having 17.52 mean health habit score, 14 pitta predominant humor having 23.25 mean health habit score, 21 kaphá predominant humor having 24.90 mean health habit score and 4 balanced personality having 25.50 mean health habit score. So we can say that 4 persons who maintain a balanced personality in their life style were healthier than any other predominant personality type.

GENERAL DISCUSSION, CONCLUSION AND IMPLICATION

The main objective of this study was to determine the relationship between lifestyle and healthy living. A daily routine of life style check list, disease check list and mental and physical health check list used for this purpose. The hypothesis that people who followed the ideal healthy life style were healthy than other people who does not follow the healthy life routine. Though only 60 subjects were taken, but the findings were very encouraging. The mean score of 15 younger male is 24.7 and the mean score of 15 younger female is 22.6. The mean score of 15 older male is 26 .3 and the mean score of older female is 23.1. It has been found out that people who followed a healthy life style were healthier than other people irrespective of age and sex.

This small study attempted to integrate life style and holistic health, with a view to reconstruct and develop a holistic (Physical, mental, spiritual) healing process.

This study may be treated as an exploratory pilot study. The measure used in the study could he simultaneously used for the constitutional examination. Today many people are affected by oriental healing system because these approaches offer the promise of a preventing healing system that is at once holistic, powerful, effective and gentle with the least side effect. They rightly feel that occurrence of disease is not an arbitrary phenomenon but for definite reason, which if correctly understood could help to cure and more importantly, prevent recurrence. Thus attention to quality of life issues has been useful in pinpointing some of the areas that require particular attention and interventions.

REFERENCES

Abhedananda, Swami (1967). Yoga psychology, Calcutta (India); Rama Krishna Vedanta Matha.

Acharya, S.B. (1995). Personality, Motivational, and Cognitive competences of invulnerable children. Unpublished Doctoral Research Report, Utkal University.

Brodov, V. (1984). Indian Philosophy in modern times. Moscow: Progress publishers.

Campbell, A.; Converse, P.E.; & Rodgers, W.L. (1976). The Quality of American life, Newyork: Russel stage Foundation.

Debroy, B. & Debroy, D. (1990). The Upanishads: Books for All, New Delhi, India.

Frawley, D. (1990). Ayurvedic healing A comprehensive guide; Saltlake city, Vatah, Pallage press.

Mc Reynolds, W.T. (1982) Towards a psychology of obesity: Review of research on the role of personality and level of adjustment, International journal of eating disorders, 2:37-57.

Mc Reynolds, W.T. (1982) towards a psychology of obesity: Review of research on the role of personality and level of adjustment, international Journal of Eating disorders, 2:37-57

Miler, S.M Brody, D.S and summerton, J. (1987) styles of coping with threat : implications for health, Journal of personality and social psychology. 54: 142-8

Moos, R.H. and schaler, J.A (1984) the crisis of physical illnesses. An overview and conceptual approach, in R.H Moos (ed), coping with physical illness: New perspective, Vol-2, pp: 3-25, New York: Plenum.

Moos, R.H and swindle, R.W, Jr (1990) stressful life circumstances : concepts and measures, stress medicine, 6:171-8.

Murray, M. and Mc Millan, C. (1993) Health beliefs, locus of control, emotional control and women's cancer screening behavior, British journal of clinical psychology. 32:87-100.

Norman, P. and Corner, M. (1993) The role theory of planned behavior and exercise: an investigation into the role of prior behavior, behavioral intentions and attitude variability, Europeon journal of social psychology, 25:403-15.

Norman, P. corne, M. and bell, R. (1999) the theory of planned behavior and smoking cessation, Health Psychology, 18:89-94.

Normandue, S, kalinins, I., Jutras, S. and hanigan, d. (1998) a description of 5 to 12 year old children conception of health within the context of their daily life, Psychology and health, 13:883-96.

Ogden, J. (1995b) changing the subject of health psychology, psychology and health, 10:257-65).

Ogden, J., (1995c) psychological theory and creation of the risky self, social science and medicine, 40:409-15.

Ogden J.,(1999) body dissatisfaction, counseling news, January-20-1.

Ogden, J., and wardle, J. (1991) cognitive and emotional responses to food, international journal of eating disorders, 10: 297-311.

Ogden, J. and steward, J., (2000) the role of the mother / daughter relationship in explaining weight concern, international journal of eating disorders, 2:78-83.

Ogden., J., Andrade, J., Eisner, M. et al, (1997) to treat? To be friend? To prevent patent's and Gps views of the doctors role, Scandinavian journal of primary health care, 15: 114-17.

Paxton, S.J., browning, C.J and O' connel, G. (1997) predictors of exercise prpogramme participation on older women, psychology and health, 12-543-52.

Petrie, K.J., Booth, R.J. and pennebaker, J.W (1998) the immunological effects of thought suppression, Journal of personality and social psychology, 75: 1264-72.

Shaw, C., Abrams, K. and marteau, T.M (1999) psychological impact of predicting individuals risk of illness: A systematic review, social science and medicine, 49: 1571-98.

Sheeran, P. and orbell, S. (1998) implementation intentions and repeated behavior : augmenting the predictive validity of the theory of planed behavior : augmenting the predictive validity of the theory of planned behavior, European journal of social psychology, 28: 1-21

Weinman, J., Petrie, K.J., Moss-morris, R. and horne, R. (1996) the illness perception questionnaire: a new method of assessing the cognitive representation of illness. Psychology and health, 11: 431-46.

26

Psychological Well Being Among Tuberculosis Patients

B. Prasad Babu*

ABSTRACT

The present study was conducted to examine the psychological wellbeing among tuberculosis patients. The study was intentionally done on newly diagnosed tuberculosis patients since the follow up of patients to the hospital is not encouraging. The study was conducted on a sample of 182 newly diagnosed tuberculosis patients, among them 130 patients were males and 52 were females. They were administered Wellbeing questionnaire to measure anxiety, depression and energy. The treatment supporters who came along with the patients were administered a schedule to examine the type of support they would provide to the patient. The results indicate that younger patients as compared to their older counterparts experienced more depression and anxiety. There was no significant influence of gender on well-being. With regard to availability of treatment supporter, it is found that patients without treatment supporter had higher levels of anxiety. Significant interaction of the gender of the patient and availability of treatment supporter was obtained. Female patients without treatment supporter reported higher levels of depression, anxiety and low total general well-being.

* **Rehabilitation Counsellor & Head of Office, Rural Rehabilitation Extension Centre for Handicapped, Thiruvallur - 602 001.**

Health Psychology is the branch of psychology that studies the psychological factors and behaviors that relate to physical and mental health. Health psychology studies the effect of behaviour on health and the effect of health issues on behaviour and psychological well-being. Health psychology examines behaviour related to wellness, illness, prevention of illness, and diagnosis.

Psychological well being is a subjective term that means different things to different people. From all of the research I've done for this answer the terms is used throughout the health industry as kind of a catch-all phrase meaning contentment, satisfaction with all elements of life, self-actualization (a feeling of having achieved something with one's life), peace, and happiness.

Tuberculosis (TB) is an infectious disease caused by a Bacterium, Mycobacterium tuberculosis. It is spread through the air by a person suffering from TB. A single patient can infect 10 or more people in a year.

Davis (1967), Davis et al (1967) reported that patient compliance depends on many psychological and sociological factors, including the age and educational level of the patient, the inter-action between the patient and doctor, and patient's own attitudes and ideas about his disease. Pratt et al (1957), Wilmer (1949) and Barnes (1957) have reported the utility of psychological support, counselling and personality make-up of the patients as a helping factor in the therapeutic plan.

Tuberculosis was initially considered as a fatal disease and patients suffering from this illness were often segregated to protect the other members of the family and society from this disease. Many patients showed associated depression and apprehended death. This depression used to lead to retardation in general behavioural and emotional functioning (Wilmer, 1949). With the discovery of effective chemotherapeutic drugs, the gloomy picture has improved. Now the patients can be adequately treated at home. On the psychological front very few studies have been conducted so far, specially in India, where the nature of the work is limited.

OBJECTIVES

The objectives of the present study are the following:

1. To examine the sense of well being among tuberculosis patients
2. To study the influence of age and gender of the patients on their well-being
3. To examine the influence of the role of the treatment supporter on the patients' and their well-being.

METHODOLOGY

Sample

The study was conducted on a sample of 182 patients with Tuberculosis disease (Sputum positive) at the District Tuberculosis (TB) Centre, Visakhapatnam. The sample included those who had undergone sputum examination and were confirmed sputum positive. The total sample of the study consisted of 182 tuberculosis patients among them 130 patients were males and 52 were females. The mean age of the total patients is 38.61 years, while the mean age of male patients is 40.57, and the mean age of female patients is 33.71 years. When total patients' mean age is compared, the male mean age is high and female mean age is low.

TOOLS

Keeping in view the objectives of the study and the nature of the research, questionnaire seems to be an ideal choice. Wellbeing questionnaire is adapted to suit the specific needs of the study as well as the sample to be investigated. The general information regarding the patients, namely, their name and address, age, gender and occupation was obtained.

WELL BEING QUESTIONNAIRE

The Well-being questionnaire was developed by Bradley (1990), to provide a measure of depressed mood, anxiety and various aspects of positive well-being. The scale consists of the 22 items with four subscales i.e. depression, anxiety, energy and positive well being.

TREATMENT SUPPORTER SCHEDULE

This schedule was developed by the investigator and was administered to all the treatment supporters who had come along with the patients to the hospital. The information regarding the gender of the treatment supporters and their relationship to the patient was obtained. The schedule included questions regarding the following aspects: Knowledge about tuberculosis, Type of support to the patient, Responses to disease.

PROCEDURE

The present study was conducted to examine the wellbeing among tuberculosis patients. The study was intentionally done on newly diagnosed tuberculosis patients since the follow up of patients to the hospital is not encouraging. The study was conducted on a sample of 182 newly diagnosed tuberculosis patients, who presented themselves at the District Tuberculosis Centre, Visakhapatnam. After the diagnosis of the disease, the doctor informs the diagnosis of the disease to the patients. The investigator approached these patients and requested them to participate in this study. The patients were made to feel at ease and an initial rapport was established. The questionnaire was given to patients and they were asked to fill it as per the instructions. The treatment supporters who came along with the patients were administered a schedule to examine the type of support they would provide to the patients.

DATA ANALYSIS

The data obtained from the sample of 182 patients was scored and analyzed and the analysis involved the application of t-tests, ANOVA, MANOVA and Chi-square tests.

RESULTS AND DISCUSSION

Psychological wellbeing among tuberculosis was examined by studying the influence of the patients' age, gender and availability of treatment supporters on wellbeing. Tables 1, 2 and 3 provide the results regarding the influence of patients' age, gender and availability of treatment supporters on Well-being.

Table 1
Influence of Age on Well-being

Variable		*Group 1 (n=48)*	*Group 2 (n=62)*	*Group 3 (n=45)*	*Group 4 (n=27)*	*F-Value*
Depression	Mean	9.56	8.50	8.22	7.07	3.664**
	S.D.	4.16	2.73	3.10	2.46	
Anxiety	Mean	11.75	10.81	10.20	9.04	3.605**
	S.D.	4.46	3.16	3.60	2.58	
Energy	Mean	5.50	6.15	6.00	6.44	0.934
	S.D.	3.10	2.41	2.20	2.49	
Positive Well being	Mean	9.13	10.11	9.51	10.52	0.990
	S.D.	4.43	3.81	3.99	2.87	
Total General Well being	Mean	29.31	33.08	33.09	36.85	2.666*
	S.D.	14.55	10.31	10.95	6.93	

Note: Group 1 = Age below 30 yrs.

Group 2 = Age 31 to 40 yrs.

Group 3 = Age 41 to 50 yrs.

Group 4 = Age above 50 yrs.

* = p<.05

** = p<.01

AGE

The sample of patients was divided into four groups on the basis of their age. Group 1 consists of patients aged below 30 years; Group 2 consists of patients between 31-40 years, Group 3 consists of patients between 41-50 years and Group 4 consists of patients above 50 years. The table indicates significant influence of the age of the patient on depression, anxiety and total general well being of the patient (significant F value).

A comparison of the individual groups (Scheffe's test) indicated that Group 1 patients (those aged less than 30 years) had significantly higher scores than Group 4 patients (those aged more than 50 years) on depression and anxiety ($p<.05$). On the other hand, the older patients (Group 4) had a significantly higher mean score on the total general well-being score ($p<.05$) than the younger patients (Group 1).

These two findings suggest that younger patients as compared to their older counterparts experience greater depression and anxiety but lesser general well-being. This is possible because the younger patients might react more to the diagnosis by virtue of their age. They are likely to experience higher levels of stigma attached to this disease and hence feel depressed and anxious. On the other hand, the older patients, in view of their present health and attitude towards work and life may not experience the effects of the diagnosis as much as their younger counterparts.

The findings indicate that the age of the tuberculosis patients significantly influence their levels of depression and anxiety, with the younger patients experiencing more of the same.

Table 2

Patients' Gender and Well-being

Variable		*Male* (*n=130*)	*Female* (*n=52*)	*t-value*
Depression	Mean	8.34	8.90	1.054
	S.D.	3.17	3.50	
Anxiety	Mean	10.75	10.38	0.601
	S.D.	3.37	4.33	
Energy	Mean	6.01	5.92	0.200
	S.D.	2.67	2.35	
Positive Well being	Mean	9.85	9.54	0.491
	S.D.	3.89	4.00	
Total General Well being	Mean	32.84	32.17	0.351
	S.D.	11.14	12.50	

GENDER

A gender wise comparison showed that males have higher anxiety, energy, positive well-being and total general wellbeing and females were found to have higher depression only, but no significant difference was found (see table 2). The gender of the patients does not significantly influence their wellbeing to the disease.

Table 3

Availability of Treatment supporter and Well-being

Variable		*Unavailable (n=74)*	*Available (n=108)*	*t-value*
Depression	Mean	9.01	8.15	1.764
	S.D.	3.56	3.02	
Anxiety	Mean	11.38	10.14	2.269**
	S.D.	3.56	3.66	
Energy	Mean	5.93	6.02	0.221
	S.D.	2.70	2.50	
Positive Well being	Mean	9.30	10.08	1.335
	S.D.	3.98	3.85	
Total General Well being	Mean	30.84	33.89	1.766
	S.D.	11.82	11.18	

Note: * = p<.05

** = p<.01

TREATMENT SUPPORTER

The influence of the availability of a treatment supporter on the patients' wellbeing to the disease was examined and the result is provided in table 3. It can be observed that patients who are accompanied by somebody showed significantly lower anxiety than the patients who came alone and unavailability of treatment supporter gives higher depression and anxiety. It shows treatment supporter plays a major role in their well being. The table also shows that availability of treatment supporter help the patients to enhance their energy, positive well being and total general well being. It indicates that unavailability of treatment supporter leads to some problems in the patients and availability of treatment supporter leads to more positive wellbeing. But, no significant differences were found only mean differences were observed.

Table 4

Interaction of Age and Treatment supporter on well-being

		Unavailable (n=74)		*Available (n=108)*		
Variable	*Group*	*Mean*	*S.D.*	*Mean*	*S.D.*	*F-value*
Depression	Group 1	10.29	4.22	8.55	3.95	0.872
	Group 2	8.39	3.10	8.59	2.44	
	Group 3	8.30	2.45	8.20	3.18	
	Group 4	7.63	2.88	6.84	2.32	
Anxiety	Group 1	12.61	4.09	10.55	4.78	1.322
	Group 2	10.96	3.11	10.68	3.25	
	Group 3	9.70	3.68	10.34	3.61	
	Group 4	10.63	1.30	8.37	2.71	
Energy	Group 1	5.54	3.31	5.45	2.87	0.316
	Group 2	5.96	2.28	6.29	2.54	
	Group 3	6.60	2.22	5.83	2.19	
	Group 4	6.38	2.39	6.47	2.59	
Positive Wellbeing	Group 1	8.54	4.32	9.95	4.55	1.114
	Group 2	10.04	3.83	10.18	3.85	
	Group 3	10.00	4.00	9.37	4.03	
	Group 4	8.50	3.16	11.37	2.34	
Total General Well being	Group 1	27.18	14.37	32.30	14.65	0.892
	Group 2	32.64	10.15	33.44	10.57	
	Group 3	34.60	10.20	32.66	11.26	
	Group 4	32.63	6.35	38.63	6.51	

Unavailable: Group 1 (n=28)
Group 2 (n=28)
Group 3 (n=10)
Group 4 (n=08)

Available: Group 1 (n=20)
Group 2 (n=34)
Group 3 (n=35)
Group 4 (n=19)

The interactive influence of age, gender and availability of treatment supporter on well-being of patients was examined. Two multiple analysis of variances were performed to examine the interactive influence. They are the influence of age and treatment supporter (table 4), gender and treatment supporter (table 5). However, significant findings were observed as far as the interaction of gender and availability of treatment supporter was observed.

Table 5

Interaction of Gender and Treatment supporter on Well-being

		Unavailable (n=74)		*Available (n=108)*		
Variable		*Male (n=61)*	*Female (n=13)*	*Male (n=69)*	*Female (n=39)*	*F-value*
Depression	Mean	8.44	11.69	8.25	7.97	9.254**
	S.D.	3.13	4.35	3.23	2.64	
Anxiety	Mean	11.08	12.77	10.45	9.59	3.746*
	S.D.	3.27	4.57	3.45	3.99	
Energy	Mean	6.03	5.46	5.99	6.08	0.490
	S.D	2.71	2.70	2.65	2.24	
Positive Wellbeing	Mean	9.67	7.54	10.01	10.21	2.679
	S.D	3.77	4.61	4.01	3.51	
Total General Well being	Mean	32.18	24.54	33.42	34.72	4.652*
	S.D.	10.72	14.95	11.54	10.65	

Note: * = p<.05

** = p<.01

Table 5 shows that gender and availability of treatment supporter together influence the depression, anxiety and total general well-being of patients. The mean values indicate that depression and anxiety are highest for females for whom treatment supporter was unavailable. The least amounts of depression and anxiety are observed for female patients who had treatment support. The findings with regard to Total general well-being are in line with the above findings. The mean values regarding this variable indicate that general well-being is highest for female patients with treatment supporter and least for those without treatment supporter.

The results of the multivariate analysis suggest that the gender of the patient and availability of treatment supporter are critical for their mental state and well-being, and this is all the more critical in the case of female patients.

CONCLUSIONS

The younger patients as compared to their older counterparts experienced more depression and anxiety. There was no significant influence of gender on well-being. With regard to availability of treatment supporter, it is found that patients without treatment supporter had higher levels of anxiety. There was significant interaction among gender of the patient and availability of treatment supporter. Female patients without treatment supporter reported higher levels of depression, anxiety and low total general well-being. It is possible that over time, the patients would be able to adjust to the disease and its restrictions on their life style and make the necessary changes.

REFERENCES

Avinash, C.M., and Pershad, D. (1972). Psychosocial survey of tuberculosis. *Indian Journal of Tuberculosis*, 19, 34-38.

Barnes, G. (1957). A study on psychological support to the tuberculosis patients. *Bulletin of National Tuberculosis Association*, 43, (p, 61).

Bergstrom. K. (2002). *Training for Better TB control*. World Health Organization, Geneva.

Bradley, C. (1990). *Hand Book of Psychology and Diabetes*. Harvard Academic Publishers. Switzerland.

Davis, M.D. (1967). Attitudes and ideas about the tuberculosis disease. *Journal of Health and Social Behavior*, 8, (p. 265).

Dubey, B.L. (1975). Psychsocial survey of tuberculosis patients. *Indian Journal of Tuberculosis*, 22, 83-85.

Lomachenkov, V.D., and Kosheleva, G.I. (1997). Psychological features of new male and female cases of pulmonary tuberculosis and their social adaptation. *Problems of Tuberculosis*, 3, 9-11.

Moudgil, A.C. and Pershad, D. (1972). Psychosocial survey of tuberculosis patients of a sanatorium. *Indian Journal of Tuberculosis*, 19, 34-38.

Narayan, R., and Srikantaramu, N. (1987). Significance of some social factors in the treatment behaviour of tuberculosis patients. *NTI Newsletter*, 23, 76-90.

Prasad Babu, B., Madhu,K., and Bhaskara Rao, D. (2007). *Psychological Adjustment and Wellbeing*. Discovery Publishing House, Delhi.

Prasad Babu, B., Raju, MVR., and Bhaskara Rao, D. (2007). *Behavioural Problems among School Children*. Discovery Publishing House, Delhi.

Prasad Babu, B., Santhanam, T., and Bhaskara Rao, D. (2007). *Children with Learning Disabilities*. Discovery Publishing House, Delhi.

Prasad Babu, B., Vimala, T.D., and Bhaskara Rao, D. (2007). *Stress, Coping and Management*. Discovery Publishing House, Delhi.

Prasad Babu, B., Santhanam, T., and Bhaskara Rao, D. (2007). *Learning Disabilities and Remedial Programme*. Discovery Publishing House, Delhi.

Tondon, A.K., Jain, S.K., Tondon, R.K., Asare, R., and Asare, R. (1980). Psychosocial study of tuberculosis patients. *Indian Journal of Tuberculosis,* 27(4), 172-174.

Veena, S, Sridhar G.R. and Madhu, K. (2001). Gender differences in Living with Type 2 Diabetes. *International Journal of Diabetes in Developing Countries*, 21, 97-102.

Wilmer, H.A. (1949). As a patient sees it: A study in introspection in emotional problems in tuberculosis. National Tuberculosis Association, (pp. 279-284).

SECTION—3
ORGANIZATIONAL AND EDUCATIONAL

27

Home Environment Status and Developmental Trend in Children

A Study on Orphanage

Namita Mohanty* Arpita Sahu**

ABSTRACT

Orphanage provides shelter and care to children who have lost their parents or are abused, abandoned and neglected. Children of unwed mothers, illegitimate children, children born with disabilities and girl children in patriarchal societies are left in the orphanage. Although inferior in quality compared to foster care and adoption centers, it plays a significant role in providing home and hopes to millions of children all over the world. Orphanages are either funded by the government agencies or non- government organizations. Some are even supported by religious organizations. There is an increasing trend among the parents and couples to adopt children from the orphanages of the third world countries.

The home environment of these orphanages has a tremendous impact on the all round development of the children living in it. The home is not just a resting place but it is a place characterized by unconditional positive regard, care and affection shown by the parents and other members towards the children. The environment is the surrounding in which the individuals live. This in turn stimulates the growth and development of the children. A study

* Reader Ravenshaw University, Cuttack, India.

** Reader, Ravenshaw University, Cuttack, India.

was undertaken by Katherine et al., (2003) in Alberta , Canada on children adopted from Haiti as infants or toddlers. Prior to adoption they lived in orphanages. This study was designed to examine the English speech and language skills in young children in age group of two and half to eight years. According to the standardized test results, only 18% children scored below average and 29% scored above average on two or more tests. Gender, age at the time of adoption and length of time in the permanent home (1 to 5 years) were not significantly correlated with English language over all test scores. The low scoring children appeared to have more difficulty with grammatical skills than with vocabulary skills. On the whole their articulation (speech sound production) skills were strong.

In another study called as "Not by bread alone" project (Taneja, Beri and Puliyel, 2004), it was revealed that a simple program of structured play accelerated the motor and mental development of children in an orphanage. However, it requires a highly motivated and dedicated play therapist to rejuvenate the play program over long periods. Research reviews indicate that institutional care negatively affects child development and adult productivity (Frank, Klass, Earls and Eisenberg , 1996). Sroufe (1991) found out that institutionalized children deprived of a consistent relationship with a caregiver had a risk for developmental problems and long-term personality disorder.

Institutionalized children were ill prepared for the outside world and it cost over three times more than a permanent loving, adoptive family (Ford & Kroll,1995). On an average institutionalized children were cared for by more than 10 different caregivers per year (Hodges & Tizard, 1978). It has also been observed that there were high staff turnover, poor staff training and few opportunities for professional advancement among caregivers (Cohen, 1986). Against this backdrop, the present investigation sought to find out the status of existing home environment in the orphanage and trend of developments among the children living in it. Developments were measured in four major domains namely gross motor, fine motor, language and personal-social.

METHOD

Sample

The present study was conducted on a group of 30 children in an orphanage named "Vasundhara" situated at Cuttack, Orissa. The sample consisted of both boys and girls and their age ranged from 4 to 5 years. Their mean age was 4.5 years (54 months) . All the subjects were orphans and were taken care of by the orphanage. They were imparted education at the orphanage and were exposed to the learning of languages like Oriya, English, Sanskrit and numerical.

MEASURES

Home Observation for Measurement of the Environment (HOME) developed by Bradley and Caldwell (1994) was used for gathering information about the quality of the children's lives. It has 3 sections. Section 'A' relates to personal information, Section 'B' to family information and Section 'C' consists of 8 subscales measuring information about physical stimulation, language stimulation, general day-to-day stimulation, modeling, encouragement of social maturity, stimulation of academic behavior, pride, knowledge about degree of affection and warmth the child receives, physical environment (safe, clean and conducive to development) and avoidance of physical punishment. Information was collected on the basis of observation and responses of the caretakers. Each 'Yes' answer earned a score of 1 and 'No' a zero. The maximum possible score was 60. The higher the score on the scale, the better was the quality of child's home environment.

Denver's Developmental Screening Test (DDST) developed by Frankenburg and Dodds (1969) provides a quick developmental screening for early detection for normal, delayed or abnormal developments of infants and children from one month to six years of age. The test measures developmental status of children in four major areas namely a) gross motor development, b) fine motor development, c) language development and d) personal and social development. Age appropriate behavior in each of these areas was given in the scale and children were assessed against these dimensions of the scale. Thus the development milestones of children were assessed and compared with standard behavior of children with normal development appropriate for their age. This helped in finding out if the development of the children in orphanage were normal, superior or lagging behind normal children of their age.

PROCEDURE

Initial rapport was established with the children at the orphanage and gradually they were helped to play, talk and enjoy with the researchers. This helped in collecting the data comfortably and easily. Children accepted the researchers with their innocence and a sense of confidence and a bond of attachment were formed. The children were observed one at a time. Nearly two hours were spent each day to collect data. Besides collecting personal data, each child required at least half an hour to 45 minutes to take the tests. For 30 children nearly 15 days were spent for the completion of tests. Data were collected through observation and questioning to the house mothers using the home environment checklist. By asking children to do certain activities and also by observing their development in different areas, assessment was done. Results of assessment were separately recorded for each child.

RESULTS

Data of the present study are analyzed using different statistical measures like mean, percentage and 't' test .Home environment status is assessed by using the scoring key. The scores are given in Table 1.

Results in Table-1 reveals that children receive very poor stimulation in academics (16.66%), language (25%) and variety in daily stimulation (30%).Other living conditions vary from 50% to 75%.The overall home environment condition is 46.66% which is not conducive for developments in children.

Table 1

Total Scores and Percentage of Each Subscale and Grand Total of HOME Checklist

Home environment subscale	*Total score of each subscale*	*Maximum score*	*Percentage*	*Grand total obtained*	*Percentage*	*Interpretation*
1. Stimulation through toys, games and reading materials	6	10	60%	28	46.66%	The home environment is neither stimulating nor conducive for all round development of children
2. Language stimulation	2	8	25%			
3. Variety in daily stimulation	3	10	30%			
4. Modeling and encouragement of social maturity	3	6	50%			
5. Stimulation of academic behavior	1	6	16.66%			
6. Pride, affection and warmth	4	8	50%			
7. Physical environment: safe, clean & conducive to development	6	8	75%			
8. Avoidance of physical punishment	3	4	75%			

Table 2

Developmental Data Measured Through Denver's Developmental Screening Test

Total no. of subjects	*Mean age in Months*	*Domains of development*	*Mean scores of development in months*	*Percentage of development with respect to age*
30	54	1. Gross motor	40.8	75.5%
		2. Fine motor	33.2	61.5%
		3. Language	30.2	56%
		4. Personal-social	43.3	80%

Table 2 indicates that language development is badly affected (56%) and it is followed by fine motor area (61.5%).Personal-social development was least affected (80%) and the next in the development is gross motor domain.

Figure

Developmental Status of Children in Orphanage

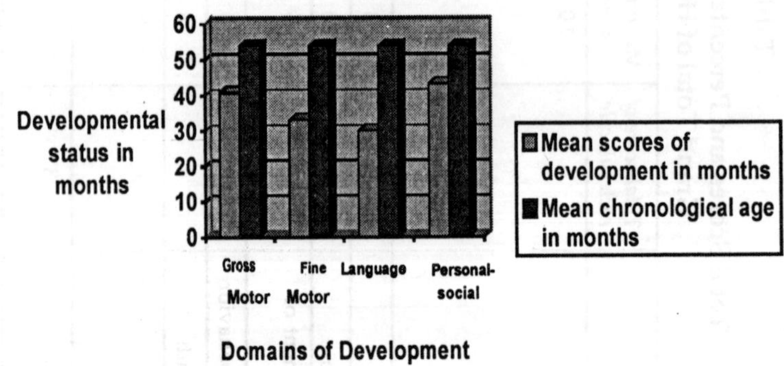

Table 3

Deviations of Development From Mean Age and 't' Values for Different Developmental Domains

Developmental domains	*Mean age in months*	*Mean of Developments in months*	*Mean difference of developments in months*	*SDs*	*'t' values*
1. Gross motor	54	40.8	13.2	21.1	2.4*
2. Fine motor	54	33.2	20.8	34	2.5*
3. Language	54	30.2	23.8	41.2	2.6*
4. Personal-social	54	43.3	10.8	17	1.9 NS

df = 29, *p<. .05 , NS = Not significant

Table-4 provides information about mean scores of development in four different areas, mean of deviations from the mean age of the children and 't' values along with the degrees of freedom and significance level. As indicated by larger Standard Deviations, the data exhibit characteristics of non normal distribution However, Pitman (1937) has shown that for N1 and N2 , if the large sample is not more than five times larger than the smaller sample, then the randomization distribution of (N1 + N2)/ 2 possible outcomes is closely approximated by the t-distribution. Accordingly, Student t distribution statistics have been used in the place of nonparametric test of the Randomization test for two samples. In case of gross motor development ('t' = 2.4,df = 29, p < .05), fine motor development ('t' =2.5, df =29, p < .05) and language development ('t' =2.6 , df = 29, p , .05) children of orphanage lag behind compared to their age. However there is an exception. In personal-social development the children are least affected and they do not significantly lagged behind in development compared to their age ('t' =1.9 ,df =29 , p > .05).

DISCUSSION

The results of the study present a grim picture about the existing environment in the orphanage and the delay in the onset of developmental milestones .There is lack of adequate stimulation for facilitating the process of development among the inmates.

Though there are no potentially dangerous health hazards like rat holes, slippery floor, and dark rooms and unsafe play materials, the living place is less than 100 square feet per child. The neighborhood is clear with trees, grass and garden. There are not enough of affection, warmth, story telling, good conversation and interaction between the caretakers and children. There is also the paucity of spontaneous rewards .The home does not have enough books, newspapers and magazines to encourage them to get exposed to the world of knowledge.

Children are not encouraged for academic growth, social maturity and language development. They are not stimulated enough to learn colors numbers, rhymes ,draw or recognize shapes and spatial relationships such as up , down, under , big or small. Children are not using simple words like ' 'hello', 'ta-ta ' or 'bye-bye'. Grammatical errors and pronunciation are not rectified .Children's enquiries are not attended to and were scolded for expressing their needs to explore. There is the total absence of social interactions like going on a picnic, shopping, trip to art museum, science park and places of historical importance.

Orphanage is not an appropriate place for children to live and grow .It is an inferior alternative to foster care centers. Therefore, we could not expect such an institution to provide and fulfill each and every need and requirement of each child compared to the real family environment of the child. It could not provide ample scope for development and this in turn definitely affected the child physically and psychologically.

In the present study showed that the worst affected domain of development compared to normal age dimension was language (23.8 months behind) , followed by fine motor (20.8 months behind),gross motor (13.2 months behind) and personal-social (10.8 months behind) .The poor language development could be attributed to the poor language structure spoken at the orphanage. Their vocabulary was restricted, most of their questions were left unanswered, linguistic input from the caregivers was of very poor quality as they themselves were from low socio-economic status. Caregivers used restricted language code. Their conversations were brief and minimum without description or elaboration (Bernstein, 1960). Children lagged behind in fine and gross motor development because they did not have much play equipment to play with and manipulate them. They did not have many opportunities for free play like out door and indoor games. They were also not taught minor activities like holding a spoon, tying shoe lace and buttoning their clothes etc. that were usually taught by the mother in daily life.

In the present scenario all children from orphanages should be considered as children with special needs .They should be provided with extra parental time and energy for fostering development. Each month a child spends in an orphanage contributes to lower intellectual problem and more of behavioral problems. Therefore the early interventions will prevent future damage.

Children adopted from orphanage should enter special infant development programs or special preschool programs for older children which include parent participation. A program should include parent-child attachment, teaching social behavior, distractibility, hyperactivity and friendliness with strangers which may lead to child abuse. Community resources, counselors, parenting courses, speech therapy and special education should be the important components of support groups working for the betterment of the orphanages.

REFERENCES

Bernstein, B. (1960). Language and social class. *British Journal of Psychology, 11.*

Bradley, R. & Caldwell, B. (1994) . *Home Observation: The Measurement of the Environment (Revised),* Little Rock, Arkansas : University of Arkansas.

Cohen, N. (1986). Quality of care for youths in group homes. *Child Welfare,* 65 (5), 481 - 494 .(North American counsel on adoptable children.www.nacac.org/policy/orphanages.html .)

Ford, M. &Kroll, J. (1995). "There is a better way : Family based alternatives to institutional care" *.(North American Counsel On Adoptable Children, Research Brief # 3 (March).*

Frank , D.,Klass, P.,Earls, F., & Eisenberg, L. (1986). Infants and young children in orphanages : One view from Pediatrics and Child Psychiatry. (www.nacac.org/policy/orphanages.html.)

Frankenburg, W.K. & Dodds, J. B. (1964). *Denver's Developmental Screening Test,* Medical Centre, Colorado University, Denver , Colorado, U.S.A.

Hodges, B. & Tizard , J. (1978).www.nacac.org/policy/orphanages.html

Katherine, G.C., Caroline, Z., Pollock, K.S., Fast, S. & Reay , M. (2003). Speech-language development in children adopted from Haiti. Department of Speech Pathology and Audiology, University of Alberta,Canada. (http://www.rehabmed.ualberta.ca/spa/phonology/Haiti.htm.2006.)

Pitman, E.J.G. (1937). Significance tests which may be applied to samples from many populations. Supplement to *Journal Report of Statistical Society, 4* , 119-130.

Sroufe, (1991).www.nacac.org/policy/orphanage.html.

Taneja, V.,Beri, R.S., & Puliyel, J.M. (2004).Not by bread alone. *The Indian Journal of Paediatrics,71,4,297-299.*

Triseliotis, J. and Russel, J. (1984). North American Counsel On Adoptable Children.www.nacac.org/policy/orphanages.html.

28

Effect of Sociability on Psychological Well Being in the Present Socio-Cultural Scenario

Geetika Patnaik*

ABSTRACT

Living is an art, a skill, a technique. The search for wellbeing is our human right. In one way or another, everyone is looking forward for a sense of satisfaction and contentment in life; the sense of feeling at peace with ourselves. Persons enjoying sense of ***wellbeing*** tend to minimize their worries and complaints, and are relatively free from self-doubt and disillusionment. ***Sociability*** refers to compatibility, activeness, conformity, mixing nature, flexibility, cordiality, and heartiness. Sociable persons are outgoing, courteous, liberal in their thoughts, receptive to new ideas, and generally keen to develop inter-personal relationships (Gough, 1957). Research in the Journal of Epidemiology and Community Health reveals that socializing with friends is beneficial. It has been found that having friends around in old age can do more for life expectancy than having family members around, and that friends may encourage people to look after their health, and help in reducing feelings of depression and anxiety (Times News Net Work). Sociability enhances ***networking***. Networking is defined as the, "Co-ordination of knowledge and effort between two or more people for the attainment of a definite purpose". In other words, it is the art of

* **Senior Reader in Psychology, B.J.B. (Autonomous) College, Bhubaneswar, Orissa.**

talking to one another, sharing ideas, information, and resource for the purpose of individual and collective success. Networking is the process of "getting together to get ahead". It is the building of mutually beneficial relationships (Etuk, 2006).

Look at the "Ocean" and not at the "wave". Although we appear as little waves, the whole ocean is at our back and we are one with it. No wave can exist of itself. This whole universe is my body; all health, all happiness is mine, because all is in the universe, say, "I am the Universe".

—Swami Vivekananda

Living is an art, a skill, a technique. The search for wellbeing is our human right. In one way or another, everyone is looking forward for a sense of satisfaction and contentment in life; the sense of feeling at peace with ourselves. Persons enjoying sense of wellbeing tend to minimize their worries and complaints, and are relatively free from self doubt and disillusionment. According to Ryff (1995), psychologically healthy people have positive attitudes toward themselves and others. Psychological well being is defined as people's affective (moods and emotions) and cognitive evaluations of their lives. Under this psychological meaning, it is not necessarily what in reality happens to people that determines their happiness or subjective wellbeing, but instead how they emotionally interpret and cognitively process what happens to them (Luthans, 1981). This subjective sense of wellbeing, or happiness, is a person's evaluation of his or her own life (Diener, 2000). Except among the very poor, wealth seems to make little difference in happiness, but social support, friends and spouses and religiosity do. So do certain personality traits, such as extraversion, and the quality of a person's work and leisure experiences (Csikszenmihalyi, 1999; Diener, 2000; Myers, 2000). Of late the focus is more on the processes that underlie life satisfaction.

Sociability refers to compatibility, activeness, conformity, mixing nature, flexibility, cordiality, and heartiness. Sociable persons are outgoing, courteous, liberal in their thoughts, receptive to new ideas, and generally keen to develop inter-personal relationships (Gough, 1957). Sociability enhances ***networking***. Networking is defined as the "co-ordination of knowledge and effort between two or more people for the attainment of a definite purpose". In other words, it is the art of talking to one another, sharing ideas,

individual and collective success. Networking is the process of "getting together to get ahead". It is the building of mutually beneficial relationships (Etuk, 2006). Meaningful life or life affiliation questions how individuals derive a positive sense of wellbeing, meaning, and purpose from being part of and contributing back to something larger and more permanent than themselves. (e.g. family, friends, social groups, organizations, movements, traditions, belief systems, etc.

According to ***social convoy theory*** people move through life surrounded by social convoys circles of close friends and family members of varying degrees of closeness, on whom they can rely for assistance, wellbeing and social support, and to whom they in turn also offer care, concern, and support (Antonucci & yama, 1997; kah & Antonucci,1980). All of these factors contribute to health and wellbeing (Antonucci, Akiyama & Merline, 2001). ***Socioemotional selectivity theory*** indicates a life-span perspective on how people choose with whom to spend their time. According to Carstensen social interaction has three main goals. These are as follows: (1) It is a source of information; (2) It helps people develop and maintain a sense of self; and (3) It is a source of pleasure and comfort, or emotional wellbeing. By middle age, although information-seeking remains important, the original emotion-regulating function of social contacts beings to reassert itself (Fung, Carstenses, and Lang, 2001). In other words middle-aged people increasingly seek out others who make them *feel good*. Moreover, middle aged and older adults place greater emphasis on emotional affinity in choosing hypothetical social partners than young adults (Carstensen et al, 1999).

Some findings suggest that people who are optimistic, extraverted, and avoid undue worrying tend to be happier than those who are pessimistic, introverted, and prone to worry excessively (DeNeve and Cooper, 1998). Research in the journal of Epidemiology and community Health reveals that socializing with friends is beneficial. It has been found that having friends around in old age can do more for life expectancy than having family members around, and that friends may encourage people to look after their health, and help in reducing feelings of depression and anxiety. (Times News Net Work).

OBJECTIVE

Basing on the rationale of Social Convoy theory and Socioemotional Selectivity theory, the present study aims at investigating the effect of sociability on psychological well being of middle-aged subjects.

METHOD

Sample: The sample consisted of 50 male and 50 female middle-aged subjects (Range = 40 to 50 years) from professional and non-professional status.

MEASURES

California Psychological Inventory (CPI) of sociability (SY) and psychological wellbeing (ps-wb) were administered to a group of 100 adults. The subjects were comprised of equal number of males and females from middle socio-economic status.

Table 1

Description of the Testing Procedure

N = 100

Testing Session	*California Psychological Inventory (CPI)*	*Testing Condition*
I	Sociability	In groups of 10-15 subjects
II	Psychological well being	In groups of 10-15 subjects

PROCEDURE

The subjects were tested in small groups of 10-15subjects in each. They were informed that they would be administered some psychological tests and that their responses to these testing would be used only for research purposes which would be treated as confidential. However, if they themselves would like to get some general feedback about their performance, they were instructed to contact the investigator after two weeks. Once the general instructions were over, each subject was given a test booklet which contained the Sociability and Psychological well being Inventory. The investigator then read out the specific instructions for these

Inventories and the subjects were asked to clarify any of their doubts about their assigned task. Most of the subjects completed the task in an hour and half, though there was a little variation observed in some subjects.

RESULTS AND DISCUSSION

The extent of relationship between Sociability and Psychological well being was assessed by finding out the coefficient of correlation between the two sets of scores obtained from Sociability and Psychological well being CPIs. This coefficient of correlation was found to be 0.65 in the present investigation.

Table 2

Coefficient of correlation between Sy and Ps-Wb (CPIs)

CPI	*N*	*Correlation Coefficient*
Sy-1	100	0.65
Ps-wb1		

The investigator had adopted the Product-moment method in determining the correlation coefficient. Such high coefficient confirms the expectation that sociability as a personality trait plays a significant role in affecting the Psychological well being of the subject.

Further study may be undertaken to examine the reliability of such finding following the test-retest method. High reliability coefficient will confirm the objectivity, predictive capability, and consistency of the present finding. It also indicates that the individual remains rather uniform, or maintain their typical trait characteristics under repeated measurements. On the other hand, a low re-test reliability coefficient means that the traits measured through the test changes from time to time or the test as an instrument is affected by some other extraneous variables. Since the California Psychological Inventory has been widely accepted as a Standardised Measure of Personality traits, having high validity, the present investigation may be considered as a valid study for the purpose.

Moreover, every person is an unique entity with his own lifestyle and idea of well being. Of late, there has been a change in perceiving psychological wellbeing. The importance of ***"interdependence"*** has been realized along with its increasing influence on coping and on adopting healthy lifestyle. Interdependence is the connectedness of individual with the social environment. It is the "belongingness" and "connectivity" to others that help us in experiencing and nurturing the sense of wellbeing within us.

Man does not like to stagnate; he always likes to develop into something better. There are some ways to achieve this metamorphosis in one's life. Moreover, since any trait in the personality structure is not a fixed entity, it can also be encouraged if conscious effort is made for the same. This type of personality renovation and manipulation will not only help the individual to excel in the work situation but also add to his psychological wellbeing. That people differ from each other is obvious. How and why they differ is the concern of the study of personality. A careful organization, participation, provision for incentive for the subjects to keep up their motivation, encouragement from the investigator, etc. may have a positive effect on the effectiveness of manipulating sociability trait that enhances psychological wellbeing.

REFERENCES

Antonucci, T.C & Akiyama, H. 1997. Concerns with others at midlife: Care, Comfort, or Compromise. In M.E.Lachman & J.B.James (Eds), ***Multiple paths of midlife development.*** Chicago: University of Chicago.

Antonucci, T.C & Akiyama, H. & Merline, A. 2001. M.E. Lachman (Ed.). ***Handbook of midlife development.*** New York: Wiley.

Carstensen, etal. 1999. Taking time seriously: A theory of socioemotional selectivity. ***American Psychologist*, 54,** 165-181

Csikszenmihalayi, M. 1999. Diner, 2000: Meyrs, 2000. If we are so rich, why aren't we happy(***American Psychologist, 54,*** 821-827

Diener, E.2000. Subjective wellbeing. The science of happiness and a proposal for a national index. ***American Psychologist , 55*** , 34-43.

Etuk, E.S. 2006. Recipe for success. The 21 indispensable things that can help you suceed in life. ***Emida_International_Publishers*** . Thomson Press, NewDelhi.

Etuk, E.S. 2006. Recipe for success. The 21 indispensable things that can help you succeed in life. ***Emida International Publishers*** . Thomson Press, NewDelhi.

Fung, H.H., Carstensen, I.I. & Lang, F.R. 2001. Age-related patterns in social networks among European-Americans and African-American: Implications for socioemotional selectivity across the life span. ***International Journal of Aging and Human Development,*** 52, 185-206

Gough, H.G 1957. ***Manual for the California Psychological Inventory.*** Palo Alto, California Consulting Psychologists Press.

Luthans, F. 1981. ***Organizational Behaviour.*** Mc Graw-Hill.

Ryff, C.D. 1995. Psychological wellbeing in adult life, ***Current Directions in Psychological Science, 4*** , 99-104.

Times News Network.

29

HRM Strategies for Organizational Health

Towards Building Synergy

Soumya Mishra*

ABSTRACT

Managing' people at work places along with sustaining an optimum level of organizational health and effectiveness remains a challenge for both management experts and organizational psychologists. OB research in the last decade has shifted the focus from HRD to HRM (Human Resource Management). The objectives of the present study were (i) to understand and explain the dynamics and differences in the HRM practices and their influence on the eleven factors of organizational health in technical institutions. Two hundred faculty members and promoters from twelve technical institutions (engineering, IT and Business administration) served as the respondents. Standardized measures were used to collect information (Udai Pareek, 1997; D. Duttaray, 1991). The results indicated that HRM practices do have highly significant effects on several aspects of organizational health such as trust, coping, environmental awareness, environmental satisfaction, organizational satisfaction, involvement, autonomy and autonomy. Performance appraisal systems, opportunities for training and career planning and organizational climate as part of HRM strategies

* **MDP and Soft Skill Facilitator, Centre for Good Living, B-14, Utkal University, Campus, Vani Vihar, Bhubaneswar - 751004.**

seemed to enhance synergy of the employees. The findings also suggested certain HRM and OD intervention strategies which could improve organizational health and build up a synergistic work culture in place of a soft work culture.

In India, a growing and internationally competitive corporate sector and prosperous and ambitions middle-class including very well placed NRIs co-exist with widespread poverty, ill health, illiteracy in the long-deprived socially and economically exploited bottom 50% of its one billion strong population - especially women and children in rural areas and city slums. At the same time, mega shifts are taking place in management thinking, execution and implementation; from stock holders to take holders; command and control to facilitation and coordination; authority.

To empowerment; centralization to decentralization; local to global perspective; hierarchy to network; and theory X to theory Y.

CHANGE PROCESS

"You cannot manage change; you have to go ahead of it", wrote Peter Drucker (1999) in his famous book 'The' Management Challenges for the 21st Century'. The focus in the change is from labour cost to human resources. The most visible articulated change pertains to the attitude of corporate managers towards employees, now called associates or partners, who are now resources and assets instead of mere factors of production or elements of cost (Sahoo, 2007). This change process has generated very important conceptual diversions in the areas of human resource management (Saini & Khan, 2000). By the beginning of the 21st century, human asset and resource strategies have taken roots in management paradigms. HR-focused management put emphasis on MBO, MBT, Team work, empowerment, corporate social responsibility, BPR, benchmarking and knowledge management.

RATIONALE OF THE PRESENT STUDY

Considering the importance of HRM, there is a need to explore it's links with organizational health and synergy. Indian organizations do believe mostly in a soft work culture (Sinha, 1991). Since globalization ahs generated a global competitiveness in the frame work of a liberalized economy in India, it is apparent that HRM strategies must improve organizational health and synergy in order to survive and grow. The objectives of the present study were to understand and explain the dynamics and differences in the HRM practices and their influence on the eleven factors of organizational health in technical institutions.

SAMPLE

200 faculties and promoters from twelve technical institutions (Engineering, IT and Business Administration) served as respondents.

METHODOLOGY

Standardized measures were used to collect data. For assessing HRM practices and strategies, MAO-A developed by Udai Pareek (1997); and for organizational health, the Q,ganizational htealth Questionnaire, developed by D.Buttaray (1991) were used.

Motivational Analysis of Organizations - Atmosphere (MAO-A) is defined as the perceived effectiveness of organizational climate. Organizational climate is proposed in terms of six motives and ten organizational processes. The six motives are achievement, influence, extension, control, affiliation, and dependency. The ten processes are orientation, interpersonal relation, supervision, managing problem, managing mistake, managing conflicts, communication, decision-making, trust, and rewards. The instrument has 120 items, one for each of the ten organizational processes, for each of the six motives and each of the two orientations (approach and avoidance). Respondents are asked to rate each item on a 5-point scale. Operating Effectiveness Quotient (OEQ) can be calculated for the motivational atmosphere by looking at the totals (means) of the six motivational aspects. Approach and avoidance aspects can be used in calculating OEQ of a motivational aspect by using the formula:

$$\text{OEQ} = \frac{\text{Approach} - 10}{\text{Approach} + \text{Avoidance} - 20} 100.$$

Organizational Health Questionnaire contains 57 items. The eleven factors include trust, organizational awareness, autonomy, creativity, evaluation, involvement, physical health, coping, environmental awareness, environmental satisfaction, and organizational satisfaction. It is rated on a 5-point scale. A higher score indicates greater positive perception of that factor as an index of organizational health.

RESULT AND DISCUSSION

OEQ for faculties and promoters were found out. These are presented in the following two tables.

Table 1

Showing OEQ Profile of Faculties of Technical Institutions

Motivation	*Organizational Processes*										
	1	2	3	4	5	6	7	8	9	10	*Mean*
A	52	63	51	49	58	58	59	53	56	53	55
B	72	62	61	63	67	74	67	56	64	73	66
C	44	61	78	61	56	41	63	67	64	49	59
D	47	69	81	72	51	63	47	70	63	49	61
E	55	69	73	78	65	61	51	62	69	56	64
F	59	48	70	55	69	53	56	51	53	61	58
Mean	55	62	69	63	61	58	57	60	62	I 57	

Achievement seems to be the lowest motivational factor. Both extension and dependency are quite high among the faculties. A comparative micro analysis shows that faculty of engineering colleges have lower achievement motivation than faculties of IT and business administration institutions. IT faculties have the highest degree of positive or approach orientation among the three groups.

Table 2
Shows OEQ Profile of Promoters

Motivation	*Organizational Processes*										
	1	*2*	*3*	*4*	*5*	*6*	*7*	*8*	*9*	*10*	*Mean*
A	61	62	63	67	66	65	62	68	63	64	64
B	73	63	64	67	74	68	69	73	71	70	69
C	47	51	61	62	58	57	58	61	60	57	57
D	49	54	64	67	79	78	62	49	47	52	60
E	56	69	72	77	64	61	52	55	52	58	62
F	57	52	72	55	68	54	56	54	52	60	58
Mean	57	58	66	66	68	64	60	60	57	60	

Both ex-power power or influence and achievement motivation seem to be .dominant with the promoters of technical institutions. Control seems to get the lowest weightage. Here, the promoters of engineering colleges have a higher score than the promoters of IT and business administration. The HRM practices and strategies are positively oriented in IT and business management organizations imparting degrees of MCA, MBA and PGDBM. Synergy in terms of these ten organizational processes seems to be better among the faculties and promoters of IT and business administration institutions compared to engineering colleges.

Compared to faculty members, the promoters institutions perceive organizational health of all three categories of more positively. The IT faculties perceive most of the facets of organizational health more positively than engineering and business administration faculty member. But, in case of promoters, the engineering group scores the highest. This may be due to the fact that the infrastructure of engineering colleges is better than IT and business administration units. The AlMA parameters such as infrastructure, intellectual capital, governance, placement and growth are maintained better by these intuitions (AlMA, 2007).

Table 3

Showing mean values of eleven organizational health factors for the faculties and promoters of technical institutions

Factors	*Faculties*			*Promoters*		
	Engg.	*IT*	*B.A.*	*Engg.*	*IT*	*B.A.*
OA	4.2	4.4	3.7	4.7	4.3	4.2
AUT	3.7	3.5	3.2	4.3	4.2	3.8
CR	2.7	3.2	2.3	3.3	3.7	2.8
EV	3.4	3.7	2.9	4.2	4.4	3.8
TR	2.9	2.7	2.4	3.8	3.6	3.2
INV	4.3	3.9	3.6	4.7	4.3	4.2
PH	3.2	3.3	2.6	4.2	4.5	3.9
COP	3.7	3.9	3.2	4.3	3.8	3.5
EA	3.8	3.5	3.2	4.2	3.7	3.3
ES	3.2	3.5	2.7	4.2	3.8	3.4
as	3.3	3.6	2.7	4.2	3.7	3.2

HRM AND ORGANIZATIONAL HEALTH

When HRM practices are correlated with organizational health perception, it is observed that the relationship is greater for the promoters than the faculties range from .23 to .73); on the other hand, the correlations for faculty member range from .12 to .37 only. Very few correlations are statistically significant. A comparison of the inter□ correlations among the three groups indicate that HRM practices influence organizational health perception more positively among the promoters of engineering colleges than other two groups. Factors such as autonomy, creativity, evaluation and trust have least correlation. HRM practices and strategies in terms of six motivational aspects and ten organizational processes influence organizational awareness, physical health, coping, involvement, environmental awareness, environmental satisfaction and organizational satisfaction to a great extent. Institutions in parting degrees of PGDBM and MBA seem to lack synergy. Both faculty members and promoters of such institutions require training and should undergo more and more management development programmes and could be exposed to organizational development interventions programmes too. HRD audit is also required for these organizations. MAO-B, MAO-C and OCTAPACE analysis could be undertaken to unravel the dynamics of such relationships, so that, appropriate strategies could be devised for improving organizational health, effectiveness, growth and positive thinking. Unless promoters realize the importance of these factors, the organizations will perish in the long run. Future research must focus on maintaining a rhythm among faculties, promoters and students in technical institutions.

REFERENCES

Drucker, P. (1999) *Management Challengers for the 21st Century*. London: Penguin.

AIMA (2007) India's Best B-Schools. September

Sahoo, K.C. (2007) Philosophical Foundation for Creativity and Innovation. *Vishleshak,* Volume 1, January, 2-8.

Saini, D.S. & Khan, S.A. (2000) *Human Resource Management*. Delhi: Response Books.

30

Impact of Work Culture on Employee Health and Well Being

Chapala Mishra*

ABSTRACT

As a result of globalization of the market and liberalization of the economy, there are sea changes in the psychosocial environment of Indian organizations and in the values, attitudes and behaviour of employees in these organizations. The present study's major objectives were to find out and explain the impact of work culture on the occupational stress and psychological well being of employees in two different types of organizations. The sample consisted of 100 bank employees and 100 graduate engineers from a manufacturing industrial unit. Standardized tests measuring work culture and occupational stress and wellbeing were used to collect data. The findings revealed that work culture influences several facets of occupational stress as well as wellbeing status. Proactive work culture reduces occupational stress and enhances psychological wellbeing. Work culture seems to be more positive in banking sector than manufacturing sector. Occupational stress level is higher in the industrial unit compared to bank employees. Occupational stress and psychological wellbeing seem be inversely correlated for both types of organizations. The study implicates certain stress management strategies to reduce specific occupational stress dimensions.

* **Reader & Head, P.G. Department of Psychology, G.M. Autonomous College, Sambalpur – 768 001, Orissa.**

Early Indianization of management started during fiftees and continued up to late seventies. Growth of Indian managers took place in the initiatives of Unilever, Bird & Co., and Imperial Tobacco. In a protected economy, managing the environment was a critical skill. In the era of license Raj, for business group owners and CEOs like Russi Mody, buying into the system was crucial for success (Rao, 2007). Because of the development of public sector management, entrepreneurial skills took a backseat and the bureaucracy gained importance. It was not possible to distance the government in such a way that there was management autonomy in the state enterprises. CEOs like Y.C.Deveshwar of ITC are products of corporate management trainee schemes. SBI created probationary officers. The establishment of the IIMs was a key milestone for the emergence of a new work culture in India. Management graduates from business schools have been the backbone of corp'orate management in modern India. It took time for Indian Companies to build managerial and corporate confidence when the economy opened up in the ninetees. 'Winds of change also influenced professionalization of family/managed businesses. New generation leaders like Anand Mahindra and Aditya Mangalam Birla are the faces of professionals at family business houses. Board structures and top managements have undergone radical changes. The impact of corporate governance is visible in our work culture.

In his book 'Work Culture in the Indian Context', J.B.P.Sinha (1990) observed that our employees live in a soft work culture. In 2007, the key to turning around a successful company is finding the areas of competitive advantage and driving through them. While doing so, occupational stress is generated which affect the psychological wellbeing of employees at work place (Stalk, 2007). In different work cultures, the organizational climate, ethos, atmosphere and work environment is perceived in different ways. Therefore, in-depth analysis is required to explain the relationships and effects in different types of organizations. Of late, banking and insurance sector is booming. Core and manufacturing sector is facing new challenges. Mergers and acquisitions are taking place. As such, work culture is changing its focus and facets. Most Indian studies on organizational culture have included such concepts as values, ethos, ethics, beliefs, climate and environment (Pareek, 1997).

In an autocratic/feudal culture, people are more dependent and affiliated. The ethos of such a culture is closed, mistrusting and self-seeking. A bureaucratic culture is concerned with following proper rules and regulations. Its climate is dominated by control and backed up by dependency. The ethos of a bureaucratic organization is, characterized by playing safe, inertia, lack of collaboration and intimacy. A technocratic culture generally has an apex climate – expert power being dominant, with a back up climate of extension. The ethos is positive - pro-action, initiative, autonomy, collaboration and experimentation. An entrepreneurial culture is primarily concerned with results and customers. Its climate is generally that of achievement, or concern for excellence, and extension, or concern for larger groups and issues. The ethos is positive, and characterized by the eight values of OCTAPACE.

RATIONALE AND OBJECTIVES

Keeping in view the changing work culture and organizational climate, the present study aims at finding out the impact of work culture on occupational stress and psychological wellbeing of employees in two different types of organization, one from the service sector (banking) and the other one from industry (manufacturing).

SAMPLE

The sample consisted of 100 bank employees and 100 graduate engineers from one manufacturing industrial unit.

METHODOLOGY

Standardized tests to measure work culture and occupational stress were used to collect data, and appropriate statistical techniques were applied to interpret the data obtained.

Organizational Culture Profile developed by Pareek (1997) was used. It measures four organizational cultures: autocratic/feudal, bureaucratic, technocratic, and entrepreneurial/organic/democratic. The instrument has eight sets dealing with values, beliefs, primacy, leadership, communication, rituals in meetings, celebrations, and rooms and furniture. The respondent is required to rank the for statements in each set in terms of their applicability to the organization concerned. The total for each cultural type can vary from 8 to 32. The lower the score, the higher is the value given in that culture

Organizational Role Stress scale is used to measure ten role stresses: self-role distance, inter-role distance, role stagnation, role isolation, role ambiguity, role expectation conflict, role overload, role erosion, resource inadequacy, and, personal inadequacy. ORS is a 5-point scale (0-4), containing five items for each role stress and a total of fifty statements.

RESULTS AND DISCUSSION

Table 1

Showing total scores of bank employees and industry employees on four culture types.

Groups	*Autocratic*	*Bureaucratic*	*Technocratic*	*Entrepreneurial*
Banking	30	28	14	08
Manufacturing	23	32	15	10

Both sectors perceive that their organizational culture is dominated by technocratic and entrepreneurial work cultures.

Table 2

Showing ORS scores of employees of both sectors.

Role stress	*Groups*	
	Banking	*Manufacturing*
SRD	08	12
IRD	07	10
RS	12	08
RI	10	12
RA	11	08
REC	12	14
Ro	10	16
RE	06	07
Rln	07	12
PI	10	14

Employees in banking sector seem to perceive less organizational role stress than employees in the manufacturing sector. Role expectation conflict an~ role overload is found to be more in the manufacturing sector than banking sector. Resource inadequacy and personal inadequacy generates greater role stress in the manufacturing sector. But, role ambiguity is little more in banks than industries. Among all the sources of role stress, role erosion seems to be the lowest in both organizations. That is a healthy indication for work culture. Correlations among the four types of organizational cultures and ORS scores reveal that stress is more in autocratic and bureaucratic culture. Stress is lowest in an entrepreneurial work culture.

CONCLUSION

The study implicates that if we take care of the work culture and make it more and more entrepreneurial, we could reduce organizational and occupational stress and bring synergy to the organization.

REFERENCES

Rao, S.L. (2007) Sixty Years of Professional Management. *Indian Management,* 46, 8, 45-52.

Pareek, U. (1997) *Training Instruments for Human Resource Development,* Delhi: Prentice-Hall of India.

Sinha, J.B.P. (1990) *Work Culture in the Indian Context.* Delhi: Sage.

31

Population Education
Perceptions of the Rural Masses

P. Viswanadha Gupta*, B.S.Vasudeva Rao**

ABSTRACT

UNESCO identifies Population Education "as an educational programme to develop in the people (a) understanding of inter-relationships between population and quality of life (b) responsible attitude and behaviour towards population issues (c) skills in making rational decisions about population related matters." In this regard an attempt was made to present the perceptions and knowledge of the rural people in a micro-level situation. This paper contains the population situation in India, population education history and different definitions, nature of population education, need of population education, goals of population education are discussed.

POPULATION SITUATION OF INDIA

India was the first country in the world to formulate a National Family Planning Programme in 1952 with the objective of reducing birth rate to the extent necessary to stabilize the population at level consistent with requirement of national economy. Health care of women and provision of contraceptive services has been the focus of India's Health Programme.

* **Professor, Department of Adult and Continuing Education, Andhra University, Visakhapatnam.**

** **Research Scholar, Department of Adult and Continuing Education, Andhra University, Visakhapatnam.**

The dominant thinking today is that national problems cannot be tacked by concentration of power in Delhi or State capitals nor can bureaucracy or the departments solve them. Decentralization of power and decentralized planning is the only answer to major problems facing the country and motivating and aware the people.

POPULATION EDUCATION: HISTORY AND DEFINITION

The idea of Population Education had its origin in 1941, when Alva Myrdal in her book "Nation and Family" attempted to convince the United States of America that population policy was nothing less than social policy at large. The role of education was seen as that of influencing children through the schools and adults through other educational agencies to appreciate national population goals. It is likely that Myrdal's book provided the inspiration for an article entitled, "A unit on the population of United States" by Kennath Rehange in 1942 in "Social Education". It was followed by an article by Frank Loriner and Frederick Osborn in 1943 setting out the case for the inclusion of population issues in the social studies curriculum of the secondary schools. Nothing of note pertaining to the inclusion of population content in curricula happened during the next two decades.

NATURE OF POPULATION EDUCATION

Common belief in the present day world speaks of population as a problem. Small population hampers growth as the working force is scarce. Large population has surplus working force but resources become scarce as users are much more. The large population, however, would not have posed a concern if the natural resources, employment opportunities, food, housing, health and other social services were expanding at the rates commensurate with population growth. The unplanned population growth tends to pose severe stress on the nation its resources and most of the social and public services. This has been the case in most of the developing countries. Imbalance created by poverty, malnutrition, illiteracy or ill-health persist, social tensions and population pressure disparagingly affects the quality of life. Over-crowding in urban areas leads to increase in crimes, violence, squalor and a life full of dearth and tensions.

NEED FOR POPULATION EDUCATION

The need for the institutionalization of population education arose from the following factors:

1. Population Explosion
2. Age Composition
3. Population and Development
4. Population and Environment
5. Development o New Values

GOALS OF POPULATION EDUCATION

The role of Education is to endow learners with the kinds of tools that will help them understand the various aspects of any given phenomenon. This is precisely the foal that population education sets for itself. It proposes to help the learners to define and understand the nature, causes, and consequences of demographic phenomena and their inter-relationships with the realities of economic, social and cultural development.

POPULATION EDUCATION IN ADULT EDUCATION SECTOR

The National Conference on Population Education conducted by NCERT in 1971 recommended that population education should be integrated into the ongoing programmes of functional literacy and the ideas of population education be systematically incorporated in the literature being produced for neo-literates. Since then, population education has found a place in all the non-formal education (including Adult/Continuing/Social Education) programmes initiated by the Government of India. But the major breakthrough in this regard happened after the launch of the National Adult Education Programme (NAEP) on 2nd October, 1978. The major aim of NAEP was the total development of the individual through education. In this context, population education was recognized as one of its vital components. Having recognized the need of population education in NAEP, a National Seminar on Integration of Population Education in NAEP was organized at Bombay jointly by the Directorate of Adult Education and the Family Planning Association of India on March 3-7, 1979 which recommended the integration of population education in the overall framework of NAEP, including training and material preparation and evaluation, by establishing systematic linkages between population education and NAEP.

The objective of this study are to experiment and determine as to which approach of teaching population education more effective in bringing about the desired changes in the knowledge, attitude and beliefs and the behaviour of our younger generation who would soon occupy our places and will join ranks with the reproductive couples and swell the population of this already over-populated country. The aim is to discover a very effective approach through which knowledge is imparted to bring changes in their beliefs and to create in them a positive attitude towards the necessity of checking the unwanted population growth by all possible means. This approach can then be constantly used to bring about a healthy change in their behaviour which in times to come will help the nation overcome this very serious problem which as endangered the very existence of this beautiful country.

The government of India, organizing many programmes like health and family welfare campaigns, need of small family and incentives to the people of adopted family welfare activities the main aim is to provide better quality of life to people if population is limited, the national reserve will be less utilized and provide better education to the children more ever the family can be able to live in some health and consume better food. All the factors occurred only people must aware about the concept of population education.

India lives in villages our country consists about 8,30,000 villages about 80% people lives in villages it implies if majority people from rural areas well aware about positive and negative effects of over population, than the country will provide better facilities to its people. Under these circumstances the study was taken up to estimate the opinions of people on micro-level may in a rural village of Visakhapatnam district.

SIGNIFICANCE OF THE STUDY

This study is unique in nature because about 80% of the people lives in rural areas and their reflections may be considered. The study finds new insight to understand the thinking of rural people about population and family welfare activity. This study is supposed to break new grounds in what areas counselling and guidance is necessary to change their outlook.

LOCALE AND SAMPLE OF THE STUDY

In order to study the reflection of the rural people towards population education, Thotada village, Munagapaka Mandal of Visakhapatnam district in Andhra Pradesh has been chosen an area of the study. The data was collected from a total sample of 76 members from Thotada village.

COLLECTION OF DATA

The questionnaire for rural people was administered to the sample drawn from the village and also personal observations were also recorded.

ANALYSIS OF THE DATA

The data/information gathered in the present research all under qualitative. Percentages are only calculated for the purpose of data analysis.

FINDINGS OF THE STUDY

Socio-economic variables are considered to be the most important factors influencing the quality of population in a community. The quality of life depends upon the prevailing socio-economic and cultural situation in the community. Some of the variables are examined to know their opinion towards population education.

PROFILE OF THE SAMPLE

The data was collected from Totada village, Munagapaka Mandal of Visakhapatnam District to estimate the attitude or opinion or reflections of the rural people towards population education. The village consist majority of Backward Caste. A total number of 76 members were interviewed. The sex, age, social class, marital status and educational background of the respondents were presented in the following tables.

Table 1
Profile of the Sample Respondents

Sl. No.	*Character*	*Variable*	*Number*	*Percentage*
1.	Gender	Male	27	28.14
		Female	49	71.86
2.	Age	Below 25	8	10.52
		26 – 35	35	46.05
		36 – 45	30	39.47
		46 and Above	3	03.94
3.	Marital Status	Married	45	59.21
		Unmarried	31	40.79
4.	Social Class	O.C.	11	14.47
		B.C.	60	78.94
		S.C. & S.T.	5	06.57
5.	Educational Qualifications	Illiterate	22	28.94
		Below 10th	35	46.05
		Degree	10	13.15
		Post Graduation	9	11.84
6.	Occupation	Employee	12	15.79
		Agriculture	39	51.31
		Business	5	06.57
		House Wife	15	19.78
		Others	5	06.57
7.	Family type	Joint	13	17.11
		Nuclear	63	82.89

From the sample sex-wise male respondents consist 27 (28.14%) and female are 49 (71.86%), 8 (10.52%) respondents are from Below 25 years age group, above 46 years age group the sample consist 3 (03.94%) respondents. There are 35 (46.05%) respondents, 30 (39.47%) respondents under, 26-35, 36-45 age groups respectively. The marital status of the sample respondents are married 45 (59.21%) and unmarried 31 (40.79%). Majority of the respondents

60 (78.94%) are belongs to Backward Caste followed by 11 (14.47%) and 5 (06.57%) from Others Castes community and Scheduled Castes & Scheduled Tribes respectively.

Regarding educational qualifications, figures indicates that 22 (28.94%) are illiterates. A majority of respondents 35 (46.05%) are having below 10th class qualifications. 10 (13.15%) respondents are having the graduates. Only few 9 (11.84%) respondents are post gratuities. Majority 39 (51.31%) respondents were agriculture allied works, 12 (15.79%) respondents were from employees, there were 5 (06.57%) respondents are doing business and 5 (06.57%) are other works means students, unemployed etc., Majority 63 (82.89%) are belong to nucleus family and rest belong to joint family 13 (17.11%).

FAMILY PLANNING

India is the first country to adopt official birth control programme in the world. But the results are not satisfactory. If the desired and the expected family size is in accordance with national norms and is achieved by the adoption of effective contraceptive methods, the birth and growth rate of population can be reduced to a level where the country can assume better standards of living to its citizens. India is the first country in the world to have national population policy and population control programme in the world. This section deals with attitude of family planning methods in the study area.

Table 2 reveals that the majority 58 (76.31%) of the respondents negatively responded towards doing abrasions with medicine is sin; only 6 (07.89%) respondents reported that they do not know about the doing abortion with medicine is sin, due to lack of education they reported in this way. 65 (85.52%) respondents negatively responded towards don't encouragement of family planning methods. 3 (03.94%) members opined positively in this aspect.

Table 2

Perception of the Respondents towards Family Planning

Sl. No.	Statement	Yes	No	Don't Know
1.	Doing abortion with medicine is sin	12 (15.78)	58 (76.31)	6 (07.89)
2.	Don't encourage family planning methods	3 (03.94)	65 (85.52)	8 (10.52)
3.	Approaching hospital for Birth control is shame	12 (15.78)	60 (78.94)	4 (05.26)
4.	Family planning is a sin because it is a disposal of god	8 (10.52)	62 (81.57)	6 (07.89)
5.	Family planning is not good for health	6 (07.89)	60 (78.94)	10 (13.15)

(Percentages are indicated in parentheses).

12 (15.78%) members responded towards approaching hospital for birth control is shame and 60 (78.94%) responded negatively towards this statement. 62 (81.57%) responded negatively towards family planning is a sin because it is a disposal of god. 8 (10.52%) responded positively towards this item. 6 (78.94%) respondents responded towards family planning is not good for health. 60 (78.94%) people negatively responded towards in this aspect.

POPULATION

In social sciences population is a demographic variable which affects on the one hand, the size of the family and on the other hand, the development of economy of a Nation. It plays an important role in formulating economic and social plan of a country or a state. Although, minimum change in size of population is helpful in production and development, yet its rapid change may staginess or hinder growth rate of development. So, rapid rate of population increase is not good for the welfare of human being as well as for the welfare of the economy and society.

Population dynamics is a branch of knowledge which includes all aspects of population change and regulation of human fertility. In population dynamics, we study the components of population change, namely fertility, mortality, health and migration where special importance is given to the regulation of human fertility. The main objective of the present study is to analysis the attitude of the rural people towards the over population.

Table 3

Perception of the Respondents towards Over Population

Sl. No.	*Statement*	*Yes*	*No*	*Don't Know*
1.	More population leads to environment problems	50 (65.78)	6 (07.89)	20 (26.31)
2.	Illiteracy is not having connection with population	22 (28.94)	40 (52.63)	24 (31.57)

(Percentages are indicated in parentheses).

Table 3 reveals that the 50 (65.78%) people responded positively that more population leads to environment problems and 6 (07.89) negatively responded. 22 (28.94%) sample reported that illiteracy is not having connection with population and 40 (52.63%) members negatively opined on this issues.

POPULATION EDUCATION

Explosive growth of population is the most significant terrestrial event of the past million. Three and a half billion people now inhabit the earth and every year this number increases by 70 million. No geological event in a billion years has posed a threat to terrestrial life comparable to that of human overpopulation. The most striking feature of world's population growth in the 1970s is that "the annual rate of increase decreased from an all time high of about two per cent in the late 1950s and early 1960s to about 1.8 percent in the 1970s. Although the slow-down is not, yet, very pronounced, it represents a significant turn from the previous trend of growth at a progressively accelerating rate, whereby the number of the earth's human inhabitants doubled and more than redoubled during the past two centuries. The climax in speed of multiplication seems now to have passed and the rate is expected to go on abating gradually in the future.

Table 4

Attitude of the Respondents towards Population Education

Sl. No.	Statement	Yes	No	Don't Know
1.	Due to more population low feeding and wrong feeding occur	35 (46.05)	25 (32.89)	16 (21.05)
2.	Education is useful to explain population literacy to the volunteers	62 (81.57)	10 (13.15)	4 (05.26)
3.	Primary Education onwards should taught about population education	70 (92.11)	0 (00.00)	6 (07.89)

(Percentages are indicated in parentheses).

From the Table 4, 35 (46.05%) members responded positively that due to more population low feeding and wrong feeding occurs and 16 (21.05%) members have no idea about this statement. 62 (81.57%) responded positively towards that education is useful to explain population literate to the volunteers and 10 (13.15%) members negatively responded towards this issue. 70 (92.11%) sample population responded positively that primary education onwards should taught about population education and 6 (07.89%) members told that they don't know about this issue.

SUPERSTITIONS

The term "Superstition" refers to the thinking of a person, which is permanent in nature and is affected by social, religious as well as economic conditions. Person presents his thoughts and behaviour in the society on the basis of his beliefs. Dictionary of Education defines the term superstition as under:

- The acceptance of a proposition as true or of a situation or object as actually existent
- The object of superstition, or the things believe in and
- Escape from doubt to the settlement of opinion, not an individual matter only but one that occurs in the community.

Table 5

Attitude of the Respondents towards Superstitions

Sl. No.	*Statement*	*Yes*	*No*	*Don't Know*
1.	Is god will decide number of children for family	5 (06.57)	70 (92.11)	1 (01.31)
2.	It is can to have two or three children without having disparities	59 (77.63)	4 (05.26)	13 (17.11)
3.	Due to population control joint families are decreased	42 (55.26)	24 (31.57)	10 (13.15)
4.	Religion is not a problem to maintain Birth control	30 (39.47)	40 (52.63)	6 (07.89)

(Percentages are indicated in parentheses).

The above Table-5 informs that 5 (06.57 %) members responded positively that god will decide number of children for family. 70 (92.11 %) people responded negatively. 59 (77.63 %) sample members positive responded that it is can to have two or three children without having disparities and 4 (05.26 %) members are negatively reported. Majority 42 (55.26 %) of the members reported positively that due to population control joint families are decreased and 24 (31.57 %) are negatively noticed. 30 (39.47 %) members positively said that towards religion is not a problem to maintain birth control and 6 (07.89 %) members they have no idea about this aspect.

RESOURCES

Table 6

Opinion of the Respondents towards Resources

Sl. No.	*Statement*	*Yes*	*No*	*Don't Know*
1.	Population of India having sufficient human resources	35 (46.05)	35 (46.05)	6 (07.89)
2.	To give better feature to India give importance to family planning	49 (64.47)	11 (14.47)	16 (21.05)
3.	The restricted age limit towards child marriage is good	70 (92.11)	3 (03.94)	3 (03.94)

(Percentages are indicated in parentheses).

Above Table 6 reported that 35 (46.05%) members agreed that population of India having sufficient human resources. To give better feature to India give importance to family planning, 49 (64.47%) are positively opined and 11 (14.47%) are negatively reported. 70 (92.11%) members are responded positively and 3 (03.94%) inclined towards the statement "The restricted age limit towards child marriage is good.

The government of India through its agencies and support of NGO's doing meticulous efforts to bring positive change among people towards negative effects of over population. In spite of gigantic efforts from the study it was observed still nearly 20 to 30 percent of people are not in a position to change their mind, may be due to ignorance, dogmatism, traditions and beliefs. In this regard, it is necessary to introduce constant persuasion and counselling to create positive mind set.

AREAS TO BE STRENGTHENING

From the study area it was observed though about 60 to 70 percent people have positive opinion in the village situation towards population education. But about 20 to 30 percent has either negative opinion or no knowledge.

MAJOR FINDINGS

1. About 23.17% people felt that abortions by using medicine are not advisable.
2. 85% has positive opinion towards Family Planning and population control.
3. Approaching to hospitals for delivery is not accepted by 21% of people.
4. Adoption of the Family Planning is against the wishes of the god according to 18.51% of people.
5. Family Planning leads to ill health viewed by 22% of the respondents.
6. Though 65.75% of the respondents agreed that more population leads to environmental problems, but 34.22% disagreed with the statement.

7. Respondents have mixed opinion about relation between education and population.
8. Majority (92.00%) agreed the population education to be imparted from primary level.
9. The respondents' has opinioned about 53.95%, more population is not resulting low feeding of children.
10. Majority (92.11%) agreed that it has to be decided by individual, about number of children to his family.
11. About 60% opinioned that religion has a role on birth control.
12. The adoption of population control can brighten the India's future accepted by 64.47% but 35.53% not agreed with the statement.

The study is taken up in a micro-level situation and confined to a rural village. From the study it was observed that 20 to 30 percent of people need counselling, guidance and persuasion to change their opinion towards population, population education and family planning. At present, the presences of 36.54% f illiterates are in India and among them 45.84% are women. Education has an impact on the behavioral and thinking capacity of human being. It is time to formulate appropriate strategies to educate the rural masses.

REFERENCES

Commission of the status of women in India (1974) "Towards Equality" department of social welfare, government of India, New Delhi.

Reproductive and Child health project rapid household survey report (2001) conducted by Population Research Centre, Andhra University, Visakhapatnam.

Vasudeva Rao. B.S. (1988) "National Adult Education Programme in Visakhapatnam District" Himalaya Publishing House, New Delhi

Vasudeva Rao B.S et. al. (2006) "Knowledge and Practices of the Rural Women towards adoption of Family Planning Methods" *Journal of Adult and Extension*, Vol.2, No.2, July-December

Vasudeva Rao B.s. et. al. (2006) "Integration of Population and Sex Education in Adult and Continuing Education Curriculum" *Journal Adult Education and Development*, Vol. 19, No.3-4, May-August.

SECTION—4
DISABILITY

32

Intellectual Disabilities and Intellectual Impairment in Switzerland

Varisco S.*, Legay Y.**, Galli-Carminati G.***

The first collaboration between our Psychiatric Unit of Mental Development (UPDM) in Switzerland and an Indian institution called Lebenshilfe began in 2004 with a research project (HUG THEM TIGHT) that gave way to an intercultural reflexion. Our common interest: persons with Intellectual Disabilities (ID). Lebenshilfe is an educational institution in Vizag, Andhra Pradesh, India that daily greets more than 400 persons with ID (aged from 2 to 50 years) and offers them adapted and diverse educational care. UPDM is a unit of the division of adult psychiatry that belongs to the University Hospital of Geneva. Within the UPDM framework there is an ambulatory, a day hospital, two hospital units and a mobile team (see figure I).

We provide care to adult persons (i.e. older than 16 years) presenting ID and one (or more) psychiatric comorbidities (G. Galli Carminati, 1999; G. Galli Carminati 2002; Galli Carminati et al.,

* Psychiatric Unit of Mental Development (UPDM), University Hospital of Geneva (HUG), Switzerland.

** Psychiatric Unit of Mental Development (UPDM), University Hospital of Geneva (HUG), Switzerland.

*** Psychiatric Unit of Mental Development (UPDM), University Hospital of Geneva (HUG), Switzerland.

2003; Lehotkay et al., 2008). It is important to underline that providing care to this population is complex and implies a pluriprofessional and a multidisciplinary approach. All the patient's caregivers have to join their effort to function as a network: every change in patient care has to be pointed out and discussed (Galli Carminati, 2007). This is the fundament of the UPDM partnership work (Galli Carminati, 2003; Guerdan & Galli Carminati, 2006). Every unit belonging to UPDM functions according to specific rules and all interventions are adapted to the specific needs of the patient with ID.

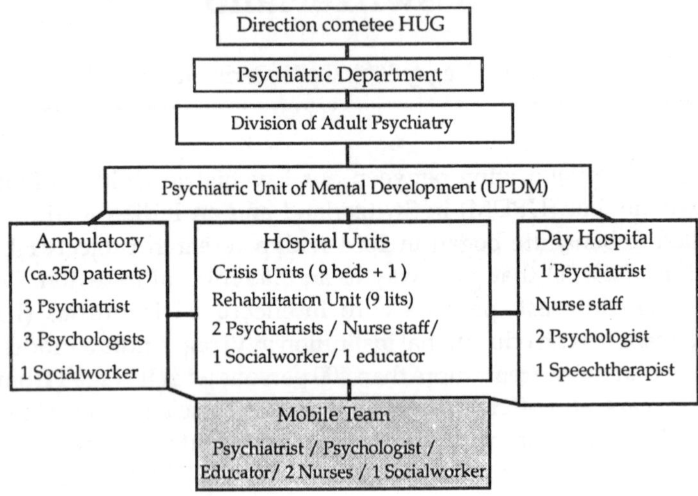

The **ambulatory** offers, among other services, psychiatric, psychological and social assessment and support, the elaboration and coordination of a care project (which includes pertinence or the type of living environment, educational care and activities proposed to every patient with ID, and the assessment of specific medical investigations or treatment), as well as the setting-up and monitoring of drug treatment (Galli Carminati et al., 2005; Galli Carminati et al., 2006a; Galli Carminati et al., 2006b). The family of the patient with ID can also benefit from psychological support. Psycho-educational support is also provided to the educational staff (i.e. in order to develop other educational strategies for the treatment of these type of patient). In short, the principal aim of the ambulatory is to assure a regular contact with the patient and his environment, in order to function as a secure therapeutic landmark where caregivers know the patient's history, centralise multidisciplinary interventions and are warrant of therapeutic goals. When the patient with ID presents unmanageable problems that require hospitalization, very often it is the ambulatory psychiatrist that prescribes it.

A **crisis unit** and a **rehabilitation unit** compose the two psychiatric hospital units, where a specific program is established for each patient. But every hospitalization is often experimented by the patient as a severe rupture with the daily familiar environment. In order to avoid rupture and consequently limit hospitalizations, the **mobile team** was created which allows the crisis intervention to be directly done in the realm of the patient's life environment, as shown in figure II (Galli Carminati & Legay, 2003; Legay & Galli Carminati, 2006□; Galli Carminati & Legay, 2007).

Figure II: Mobile Team Crisis Intervention Scheme

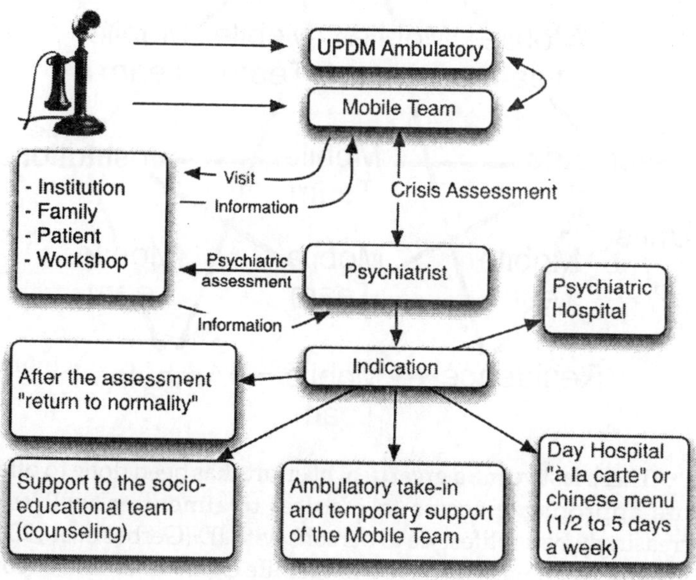

The **day hospital** care program is essentially based on group therapy (Galli Carminati, 1998a; Galli Carminati, 1998b; Schaya & Galli Carminati, 2000; Galli Carminati 2002; Schaya & Galli Carminati 2002; Galli Carminati et al., 2003a; Galli Carminati, 2003b; Schaya & Galli Carminati, 2003; Galli Carminati & Méndez 2003; Galli Carminati, et al., 2004a; Galli Carminati et al., 2004b; Galli Carminati et al., 2005; Douibi et al., (2006); Galli Carminati et al., 2007). The patient attends the day hospital during the day and returns to his home in the evening: the patient is in touch with his familiar environment, which is particularly important for persons with ID. In fact, for these persons it is very difficult to manage changes in daily routine and they feel quickly distressed. During crisis periods, the mobile team can be seen as the warrant of the partnership and collaboration between all patients' network caregivers (see figure III).

Figure III: Role of the UPDM Mobile Team

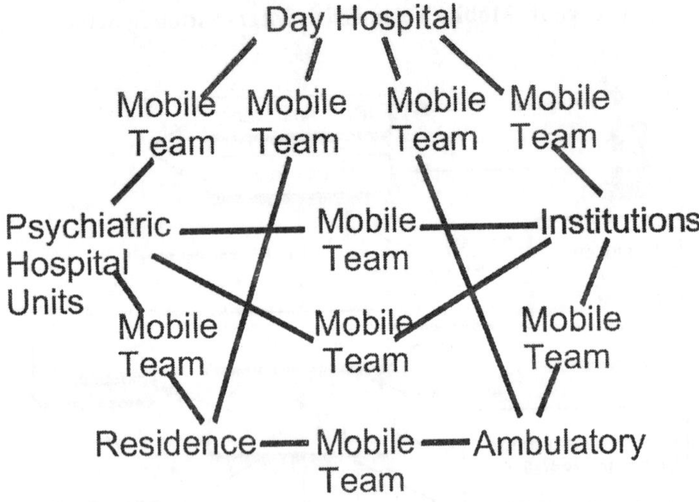

These last years, a great deal of efforts has been done to offer a more appropriate access to medical treatment as well as an increasingly better lifestyle to persons with ID (Gerber et al., 2008). Today, persons with ID have a longer life expectancy and become elderly. Thus, in our daily practise, we are more and more faced with ageing persons with ID.

We are gradually realizing that their psychological and medical cares have to be modified, because on the one hand their needs evolve and may differ from conventional treatment and on the other hand, as elderly persons in the general population, persons with ID may additionally present intellectual impairment. The big problem with this population is that it is very hard to distinguish the signs of intellectual impairment and moreover to measure decline in cognitive functioning. In fact, persons with ID are mostly unable to answer questions involving memory or higher cognitive function even when they don't have intellectual impairment. If we have a look at the diagnostic and statistical manual of mental disorder (DMS-IV-TR), we immediately realize that many diagnostic criteria for intellectual impairment depend on observational data from the patient's environment, and we can suppose that frequently they are readily applied to persons with ID.

A recent textbook of the Diagnosis of Mental disorders in persons with Intellectual Disabilities (DM-ID) published by the National Association for the Dually Diagnosed (NADD) in collaboration with the American Psychiatric Association (APA), underlines the limitations of applying DSM-IV-TR criteria to persons with ID. The mains problem of intellectual impairment is the recent memory disturbance. Other non-cognitive behaviors classified in DSM-IV-TR are violence, insomnia, wandering, dependency and incontinence. But all these elements are also part of the diagnosis observed in the etiology and pathogenesis of ID, as mentioned by the MD-ID. This underlines that the prevalence of intellectual impairment in persons with ID correlates with the general population: 5% in persons aged ≥65 years. Unfortunately, the diagnosis of intellectual impairment (especially at early stages) is difficult to make, due to the lack of reliable and standardized criteria and diagnostic procedures. Some factors predisposing intellectual impairment in persons with ID are increasing age, a positive history of intellectual impairment, or having the Down syndrome. In fact, adults with ID and Down syndrome seem to be especially vulnerable to developing intellectual impairment (25% in persons ≥40 years, and 65% in persons aged ≥60 years). It is also interesting to note that 31% to 78.5% of persons aged ≥65 years with ID (without Down syndrome) show Alzheimer neuropathology. The MD-ID gives some other interesting information concerning Intellectual impairment in persons with ID. For example, in adults with mild to moderate ID (I.Q. range of 50–69 and of 35–49), first noticed are changes in activities of daily living and work habits. In addition, epileptic seizures may occur at earlier or later stages. At earlier stages of disease, memory loss is not always noticed, even if cognitive changes are frequently present. Unfortunately it is difficult to evaluate them, because of cognitive limitations and the absence of tests adapted to ID persons showing deterioration in memory functions. In fact, standard tests applied to the general population are inappropriate for ID. In adults with severe to profound ID (I.Q. range of 20–34 an I.Q. <20), who already have significant cognitive deficits, neither memory loss nor disorientation would be recognized if measured with standard tests. However, some non-cognitive behaviors may be observed, such as irritability or apathy and the loss of the ability to use eating tools. Non-verbal tests may be used. One method is showing something the patient might value, hiding it, and asking the patient to find it after a few minutes. The MD-ID shows that a research of different criteria allowing the detection of Intellectual Impairment in ID persons as early as possible has to be continued.

And what about the management of care of elderly persons without ID in Geneva?

The widespread philosophy to provide care for the outpatients of the geriatrics clinic is to improve the quality of life of the elderly. More and more associations to protect elderly persons are created. Some studies show that living in one's home as long as possible gives a higher life expectancy. To make this possible, multidisciplinary staffs are on call 24h/24 for home care (physician/nurse/auxiliary nurse) and a pluridisciplinary mobile team already exists. The mobile team is called by the general practitioner or by the patient's family or neighbors. A physician evaluates the case in situ, and if necessary, a psychologist is consulted for a psychological and neuro-psychological assessment. Afterwards, on the basis of these collected elements, some suggestions are formulated: home care (intervention of a nurse, a physio-or an ergo-therapist, a social worker, the lunch-service or one of the different associations for elderly); the day hospital (where some group activities are proposed, i.e. mobility exercises, principle alimentation courses and cooking workshops, memory training for early intellectual impairment or for advanced intellectual impairment difficulties, relaxation and an alcohol group talk); a short hospitalization (in order to solve the crisis and allow the patient to return to his own home, or also to give the patient's family members some time to regenerate themselves) (see figure IV).

Figure IV: Mobile Team for elderly people

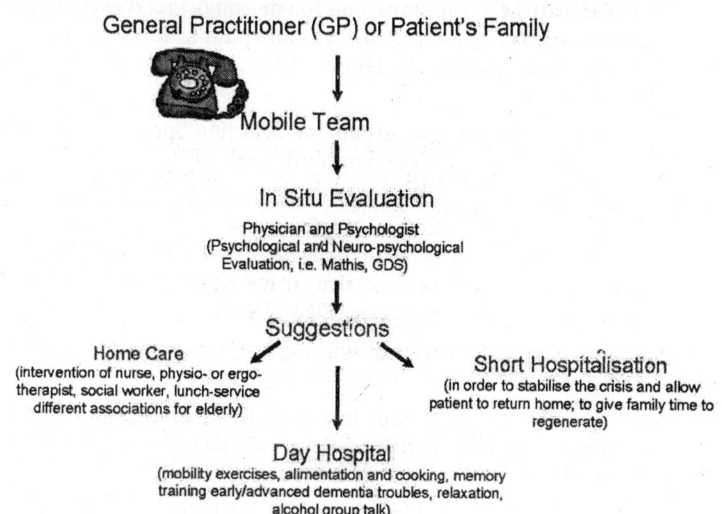

Since 2007, an ambulatory service in collaboration with the geriatric units provides support to the patient's family at the crucial moment of intellectual impairment diagnosis. More precisely: they assist the family by providing more information about intellectual impairment and helping them to better understand some "strange" behaviors dictated by intellectual impairment; they support and guide family members in elaborating and shaping their relationship with the patient; they coach on how to deal with and manage the patient, step by step. This is highly important because the patient's personality changes, as well as his manner to interact and behave with other family members. These transformations are also recognized in ID patient's behaviors with their environment.

The big challenge for caregivers next year will be to detect as early as possible the different signs of intellectual impairment in persons with ID, as well as to develop more adapted tools and interventions for specifically this population.

REFERENCES

H. Douibi, F. Gerber, M. Géoui, D. Nsonde, P. Claus, G. Galli Carminati (2006). Le groupe « BdBd ». *Revue Francophone de la déficience intellectuelle,* vol. 16, 129-136.

G. Galli Carminati: Le groupe sans mots (ou presque), Prix d'encouragement décerné par la Fondation P. B. Schneider pour le développement de la Psychothérapie Médicale, février 1998a, *Psychothérapies*, Vol. XVIII, N° 3, 159 169.

G. Galli Carminati: Approches groupales. Sélection Spécial, Psychiatrie et Handicaps HUG, Genève, mars avril 1998b, N° 167, 24-26.

G. Galli Carminati, M. Gex Fabry Pun, M. F. Kummer, M. Pilar Blanco & A. M. Van der Schueren: Etude Epidémiologique sur la prévalence des troubles psychiatriques dans la populations des Etablissements Publics Socio-Educatifs pour personnes mentalement handicapées, *Médecine et Hygiène,* 22 septembre 1999, 57e année, 1763-1766.

G. Galli Carminati: Le double diagnostic, *Pages Romandes* "Déficience mentale, Déficience psychique" février 2002, N° 1, 11 14.

G. Galli Carminati: Group therapy in a mentally disabled population: from contraindication to specificity. *Funzione Gamma Journal (WEB Journal: http://www.funzionegamma.edu/),* February 2002, N°8.

G. Galli-Carminati, Y. Legay, L'équipe mobile: intervention de crise et soutien aux sorties des unités hospitalières, *Pages Romandes,* février 2003.

G. Galli Carminati, M. Gex-Fabry-Pun, M. F. Kummer, A. Mendez, O. Baud, P. Blanco & A. M. Van der Schueren: Epidemiological study on prevalence of psychiatric disorders amongst the population of Public Socio-Educational Institutions for Intellectually disabled people, *European Journal of Mental Disability*, N°25, mars en 2003, version en français, 34-56 (version en anglais, 32-47).

G Galli Carminati, Y. Legay, B. Tschopp, L. Zid, A. Hermet, P. Thibault, P. Gorianz, M. Schaya, M. Gex-Fabry-Pun, Le groupe «Sonar», *Avances en salud mental relacional- Advances in relational mental health-Revista Internacional On-line –An International On-line Journal*, Vol. 2, no. 1, March 2003.

G. Galli Carminati, A. Méndez: *Groupes, psychopathologie et retard mental. L'expérience genevoise.* Médecine et Hygiène, Genève, Juin 2003.

G.Galli Carminati, Les Groupes pour la population avec disabilité intellectuelle et troubles psychiques, *Avances en salud mental relacional-Advances in relational mental health-Revista Internacional On-line –An International On-line Journal*, Vol. 2, no. 3, August 2003.

G. Galli Carminati : Les groupes des parents. In : G. Galli Carminati, A. Méndez: *Groupes, psychopathologie et retard mental. L'expérience genevoise.* Médecine et Hygiène, Genève, 2003.

G. Galli Carminati, N. Constantin, M. Schaya, M. Gex-Fabry, M.-F. Kummer, L.Canellas, Evolution, en hôpital de jour, de 30 personnes avec retard mental et trouble psychiatrique. *Archives suisses de neurologie et de psychiatrie* 2004a, 155.1, 24-34.

G. Galli Carminati, N. Constantin, Y Legay, B. Tschopp, L. Zid, A. Hermet, P.Thibault, P.Gorianz, M Schaya, M Levental, C Carrel, S. Ritter : «Sonar Group» Underwater Music Therapy. Evolution of 2 persons with severe disability on a period of 3 years, *European Journal of Psychiatry* 2004b, Vol 18 Supplement, 106-114.

G Galli Carminati, Fabienne Gerber, Nadine Constantin, Day Hospital for Adults with Intellectual Disabilities and Psychiatric Disorders: A Longitudinal Study, *Psychiatric Services*, may 2005, Vol. 56 No. 5, 609.

G. Galli Carminati, Retard Mental et toxicomanie – les limites improbables, *Pages Romandes* "Le cannabis s'arrête-t-il aux portes des institutions?" avril 2005, N° 2, 4 5.

G. Galli Carminati, N. Deriaz, G. Bertschy, Low-dose venlafaxine in three adolescents and young adults with autistic disorder improves self-injurious behavior and ADHD-like symptoms, *Progress in Neuro-Psychopharmacology and Biological Psychiatry* 2006a, 30, 312-315.

G. Galli-Carminati, I. Chauvet, Nicolas Deriaz, Prevalence of gastrointestinal disorders in adult clients with pervasive developmental disorders. *Journal of Intellectual Disability Research*, October 2006b, Vol. 50, 711-718.

G. Galli Carminati, Les réunions tripartites, *Bulletin insieme-Genève*, N°2, 14-16 novembre 2007.

G. Galli-Carminati, Y. Legay, L'équipe mobile□: intervention de crise et soutien aux sorties des unités hospitalières, *Bulletin insieme-Genève*, n°2 , 24-28 novembre 2007.

Galli Carminati G., Schaya, P Gerber F., Carminati Garbino M.V.G., Constantin N, (2007). Prospective Evaluation of a Day Treatment Intervention in Adults with Intellectual Disability and Psychiatric Disorders. *European Journal of Intellectual Disability*, 1 (revue online, September 2007).

F. Gerber, MA.Baud, M.Giroud, G. Galli Carminati, Quality of Life of Adults with Pervasive Developmental Disorders and Intellectual Disabilities. *J Autism Dev Disord.* 2008 Feb 12; [Epub ahead of print] PMID: 18266098.

V. Guerdan, G. Galli Carminati: Le partenariat: confronter ses points de vue pour éviter les abus. In: G. Galli Carminati, A. Méndez: *J'Abuse? La personne avec retard mental et troubles psychiatriques face à l'abus*. Médecine et Hygiène, Genève, 2006.

R. Lehotkay, S. Varisco, N. Deriaz, A. Douibi, G. Galli Carminati : Intellectual disability and psychiatric disorders: More than a dual diagnosis..., Swiss Archives of Neurology and Psychiatry, submitted.

Y. Legay, G. Galli Carminati: Equipe mobile : Intervention de crise et soutien au sortir des unités hospitalières. Dans *Déficience Intellectuelle: Savoirs et perspectives d'action, Tome I,* publié par l'AIRHM, sous la direction de H. Gascon, D. Boisvert, M.-Cl. Haelewyck, J.-R.Poulin et J.-J.Detraux, 2006.

M. Schaya & G.Galli Carminati, Expérience pilote de l'évolution d'un groupe verbal, auprès de huit patients à l'Hôpital de Jour, *Revue Francophone de la Déficience Intellectuelle,* décembre 2000, Vol 11, N°2, 137-147.

M. Schaya & G. Galli Carminati: Coffee & Cookies group. *Funzione Gamma Journal, (WEB Journal: http://www.funzionegamma.edu/),* February 2002, N° 8.

M. Schaya, G. Galli Carminati, , Evolution des patients dans le groupe Homme-Femme, *Revue Francophone de la Déficience Intellectuelle,* juin 2003, Vol 14, N° 1, 49-57.

33

Special Population

Beyond Psychological Perspective

Gautam Gawali*, Janbandhu, S.**

ABSTRACT

In psychology the term "Special Population" generally refers to those having learning disabilities, such as mentally or psychologically challenged and those suffering from Dyslexia, Dysgraphia, Agraphia, Dyscalculia and Alexia. Even the Orthopedically Handicapped, Visually Handicapped, and Speech and Hearing Handicapped are treated as Special Population. It is so because the categories of people to be incorporated in "Special Population" were decided by the psychologists working in developed countries. They had done extensive work, for imparting training to these people, for eradicating the inferiority complex from them, and for rehabilitating them. Also they had worked on racial discrimination, racial prejudices etc. However, they had not worked on caste discrimination, probably because "caste" was either unknown phenomenon or very little known phenomenon for the psychologists of most other countries. Because, the most inhuman caste system was/is predominant in India, those who were deprived of even basic necessities for thousands of years were recognized as "Special Population" by those who framed the "Constitution of

* **Professor, Dept. of Applied Psychology, University of Mumbai, Mumbai.**

** **Professor, Dept. of Applied Psychology, University of Mumbai, Mumbai.**

India". Non – psychological but materialistic facilities were provided to them, such as reservations, scholarships etc. but what about eradicating the stigma of caste, which is inherited, which results mostly in developing inferiority complex among them and wasting energy and time in hiding the caste identity from others. Hardly, a few, even highly educated, members of this "Special Population" can speak their mother tongue in the way the Hindu high caste people speak. This deficiency restricts their interactions with the relatively more developed people. It was revealed in a study that they were doing so for hiding their caste identity. Changing names and surnames is a common practice among them. School dropout is maximum among the children of this special population. Innumerable atrocities, on this special population, are being committed even today. Two or three decades before, this special population was an "anathema" for the psychologists; now a days some of these communities are featuring in some of the psychological studies. Present study intends to seek guidance from the expert psychologists, to frame action plans to bring the special population into the mainstream.

We don't claim that we are correct, but it is commonly observed that, the topics, the problems and the concepts on which extensive research work has been done in the developed countries, are repeated in India. For example, during 1970 to 1980 most of the psychologists in India were working in the field of learning-serial learning, paired associate learning, measuring meaningfulness of learning material etc. Later on most were impressed by the work of Atkinson and McClelland and studies were done on n-Ach; afterwards they started measuring self concept of Indian people etc. Those working in clinical areas, worked on mentally challenged or psychologically challenged population, and a good number of them worked on those having learning disabilities, such as, children having dyslexia, dysgraphia, agraphia, dyscalculia and alexia. In fact, on these problems and topics extensive work had been already done, and there is ample literature available in the libraries and on internet. Experts in their fields have studied all the possible aspects, and suggested training procedures for bringing positive and useful changes among them; even the techniques of rehabilitating them are already given. Still, similar research work is done on the "Special

Population" by the psychologists in India. It definitely helps in improving the CVs of the researchers; but what about its utility? Answers to this question is not at all encouraging.

Second author of this paper was associated with CSD, New Delhi, for a short duration, when Dr Bishwanath Mukherji, was Director of Research. Research work, could be useful to the society was made known to him, during his association with CSD. YMCA, Calcutta, posed a problem to CSD; children from slum areas do not attend the school, suggest the solution, so that the children can attend them regularly. On the spot investigation revealed that, in all the families both mother and father were going out for earning livelihood, there was no one to look after their hutments and younger children in the family. Obviously, the school age children, because they had to take care of their hutments and young siblings, were not going to school. So, the concept of pavement school was introduced. The children were not going to school, the school went to them.

In an another study, socio-economic standard of the tribals of Mehboobnagar was enhanced. Despite language barriers, the psychologists could won the confidence of tribals; taught them stitching and sewing, and first helped them to increase their economic standard, and then gave lessons of formal education. Let us make clear that CSD is not an NGO, in the sense the term NGO is known in our country.

Millions of rupees are being spent on studies of personality, stress, education of school children etc. Most of the factors explored in such studies are more or less similar to those which were already studied by the researchers in developed countries. Let us consider a few examples, how many Indians experience job stress? except those who are in IT industries. People in metro cities experience stress, but their causes are entirely different, than the causes for stress are being studied. In India life stress is much more than occupational stress, but studies on life stress are much less than studies on occupational stress. It appears that the researchers first explore the easy availability of sample, and then the topic for research are finalized. The ultimate result is, utility of such studies is almost nil.

Most studies carried out on personality incorporated mainly those factors, which were studied extensively. These studies included mainly those factors which were studied by the researchers in developed countries. There is hardly any study on personality carried out in India, considered the most important factor which is mainly responsible for the development of personalities of youths. In India every individuals personality is mainly shaped by the CASTE in which he or she is born and brought up. The factor of caste was not considered by the researchers in other countries, because, they never experienced the "LUXURIES" of caste. Rather it was unknown to them. But racial discrimination, they had studied in depth. Unfortunately psychologists in India either failed to recognize the importance of caste in psychological studies, or purposely, they had ignored it.

Caste, if one thinks seriously, then he finds that it is inherent, caste is associated with birth itself, and does' end even after death. Even today the "SANSKARAS" done after childbirth differ from one caste to another caste. In the colonies with whom the child will play depends upon his caste. Informal intercaste interactions are there; and in most cases they are inevitable. But they are just "REMOTE ASSOCIATIONS. "CLOSE ASSOCIATIONS" are encouraged with the same caste children. There is no need to tell the psychologists that these interactions are the foundation stones of future personalities. It is one's caste which determines his identity, self concept and perceptions too.

Among the four major castes the fist three enjoyed the benefits which their religion had given to them. The fourth one had been gifted with the dirtiest possible inhuman atrocities and it continued atleast for three thousand five hundred years directly, and for the last sixty years indirectly. Just imagine, during day the temperature is 45° Celsius, you are thirsty; there is water source, but you can't quench your thirst, unless somebody offers you water, and such possibility is extremely rare. It is because according to your religion you are "UNTOUCHABLE". A dog, a swine are touchable, they are the re-incarnations of the god. It is this population of "UNTOUCHABLES" which is the "SPECIAL POPULATION" of India, which remained beyond the perspective of psychology.

This population was forced to remain illiterate for thousands of years. They were forced to remain popper by their religion. In some parts of this land they had to tie an earthen pot around their neck, and a broom around their waist. They had to spit in the earthen pot and a broom was eradicating their footprints imprinted on the dust. The psychological consequences of untouchability need to be explored. Personality characteristics of the untouchables or the ex-touchables must be measured. What psychological damage the untouchability had done, need to be studied, and then through counseling, guidance, and using psychological techniques efforts must be made to bring this "special population" in the "main stream" of India.

Reports, published in newspapers, telecasted on T V channels, government reports, and speeches of political leaders portrait an excellently attractive scenario about these ex-untouchables. But the ground realities are extremely different than what is being painted. The reasons are simple, newspapers are published in cities, T V reports, like Indian doctors are more interested in cities, reliability of the government and that of politicians is well known, so the unimaginable difference is bound to occur. What is more disheartening that, it is believed that, in urban areas there is no caste discrimination, and even in the rural areas casteism has been eradicated successfully. Reality is that, in India Indians do not observe untouchability, only when, it is impossible to observe (Janbandhu, 1991). In present study, the special population is not the one which is treated as special population by the psychologists, but it is that population which is recognized as "special population" by the constitution of India.

AIM OF STUDY

The aim of study is to search evidences of caste discrimination and untouchability among the educated families living in urban areas, and understand the psychological consequences of untouchibility and caste discrimination on the ex-touchables.

OBJECTIVES OF STUDY

(i) To search the methods and styles of observing untouchability, used by the castes Hindus, in modern times.

(ii) To investigate the manners through which people recognize the caste of colleagues and neighbors and then decide the strategy of interacting with them.

(iii) To find out the psychological consequences of untouchability and caste discrimination on the ex-unouchables.

HYPOTHESES

Indians do observe untouchability whenever it is possible, they do not observe untouchability when it is impossible to observe it.

Sophisticated manners and styles are used to observe caste discrimination, by the caste Hindus.

Psychological consequences of untouchability and caste discrimination results in laying down atrocities on the ex-untouchables, thereby hampering their overall development.

METHODOLOGY

Sample

Sixty eight families living in flats in a MHADA complex in a big city (more than 30 lac population) of Maharashtra, comprised the sample. Of these sixty eight families, nine were ex-untouchable families. These families embraced Buddhism. The remaining 59 families comprised of, four Christians, 3 Muslims, 24 Marathas, 14 Brahmins, 4 North Indian Brahmins, 2 Bengalis, 4 South Indians and 2 each Gujaratis and Punjabis. The MHADA complex is a separate colony having a common open space as community ground. This community ground was used mostly by the children and the senior citizens of the complex.

TOOLS USED FOR DATA COLLECTION

Interview Schedule

The interview schedule was devised specially for the present study. It is consisted of 34 items. The items were related to visits of the Ss to other Ss, names of friends of their children, their group and social activities etc.

A BATTERY OF SCALES

It includes a few scales devised to measure casteism and untouchability. The first scale was "caste awareness scale", it was devised by Janbandhu and Labhane (2003). Test – retest reliability of the scale was .87. Second scale was a Bogardus Type Scale, which consist of seven statements. It's test retest reliability was .83. The third scale was devised to measure the distance from which the S would like to converse with the people of different castes. In this scale there was a drawing room of 20′ x 20′, attached to which there was a veranda where the visitors could sit and wait. For entering the drawing room one has to remove the shoes or chappals. Visitors belonged to four different castes; at what distance each of them would be entertained by the head of the family. In addition to these there was blank space to note down the observations.

MATRIMONIAL ADVERTISEMENTS

Matrimonial advertisement published in leading newspapers were studied for searching the casteism and untouchability.

PROCEDURE OF DATA COLLECTION

Through personal interview and observation the data were collected. The scales were administered individually. The data collection was done by a 50 + Brahmin lady, who has completed her doctorate in psychology, and engaged in psychological research since the last 25 years.

RESULTS AND DISCUSSION

This is a small part of a major research work. Caste awareness was found among 100% respondents, and each one of them was aware of the position of his caste in the caste hierarchy. Not a single Brahmin or Maratha (Kunbi, Patil, Deshmukh etc.) family developed close associations with the family of ex-touchables. Hatred towards ex-untouchables was significantly more among the Marathas than the Brahmins. Favourable attitude towards inter caste marriages was found among Brahmins and ex-touchables, but not a single Maratha family was in favour of intercaste marriages. On Bogardus type scale none of the caste Hindu families preferred to have an ex-untouchable as a life partner. The ex-untouchables did not have any hesitation to accept caste Hindus as life partner.

On festive occasions the frequency of visits was remarkably more among the same caste people. During "Ganeshotsvawa" the whole complex contributes, even the ex-untouchables pay the contributions, but they do not take part in the prayer or "Aarti". Associations of caste Hindus were limited to "Hi", "Hello" with the ex-untouchables, long lasting discussions are avoided. Ex-untouchables argue that the gods and goddesses are imaginary; the concept of soul is also imanagery, all these hurt the faiths of caste Hindus.

Relatively better interactions were observed between Christians, Muslims and ex-untouchables. The south-Indians and Bengalis are more concerned with their family affairs and cultures. Some of them had more interactions with the ex-untouchable families.

Reflections of castes were seen among the children also. On the utility ground, the children of caste Hindus played together, they play mostly cricket. Children of ex-untouchables and others were playing together; they play football, cricket etc. Even the senior citizens had their separate groups, keeping close and frequent interactions with the caste breatherns. Bengali and south-Indian senior citizens were sometimes seen with the group of caste Hindus, and sometimes with that of ex-untouchables. However, they rarely joined these groups.

Most interesting results were observed on the situational test, where there was a 20′ x 20′ drawing room and a veranda. More than 90% caste Hindus, said they will go out of drawing room and talk to the ex-touchables in the veranda. Only six percent allowed then to sit in a chair placed near the entrance. Though very slow but some positive changes in the attitude of caste Hindus were clearly visible. Atleast from the drawing room the untouchability has disappeared.

Regarding marriages, there is rigidity; and negative attitude towards scheduled castes and scheduled tribes is clearly visible. Matrimonial advertisements read as, "CASTE NO BAR, SC/ST SORRY". Every matrimonial having CASTE NO BAR ends with "SC/ST SORRY".

Psychologists in India, knew all these facts about the caste system and untouchability, however, there is hardly any psychological study dealing with these ever present problems. Tall claims are made by the psychologists, with the help of psychological techniques such as BRAIN WASHING, pursuation etc. we can bring in remarkable changes in individuals. Watson is often quoted, "Give me handful of children and my own world ______ ". However, there is hardly any psychologist who had studied this "special population" of India, and came out with remedial measures.

CONCLUSION

Casteism and untouchability still persist in India; the special population of ex-untouchable is still beyond psychological perceptives.

REFERENCE

Janbandhu, D.S. (1991) Evaluation of the Role of Buddhism in Enhancing the Socio-Economic and Psychological Status of Ex-Mahars. Research Project Report. Sponsored by I.C.S.S.R. New Delhi.

34

Psychological Intervention for Developmentally Disabled and Autistic Child Through Computer Aided Instruction

P. Nirmala Devi*, Puja Chandra Verma**

ABSTRACT

The research presents the application of Computer Aided Instruction (CAI) as an intervention program in an attempt to assess its impact on a special child with intellectual and developmental disability. It was demonstrated that CAI was effective in management of the short attention span, restlessness, rocking movement and improved the subject's performance at classroom level resulting in enhancement of self-confidence and improved socialization skills.

INTRODUCTION

Mental retardation is a disability characterized by significant limitations both in intellectual functioning and in adaptive behavior as expressed in conceptual, social and practical adaptive skills. This disability originates before age 18, as described by Luckasson, Borthwick-Duffy, Buntinx, Coulter, Craig and Reeve

* Professor, Department of Psychology & Parapsychology, Andhra University.

** Special Educator, MSc (Computer Science), MA (Psychology), Andhra University.

(2002).According to Allen, Harold and Michael (1994) there are three criteria before a person is considered to have a developmental disability, an IQ below 70, significant limitations in two or more areas of adaptive behavior (i.e., ability to function at age level in an ordinary environment), and evidence that the limitations became apparent in childhood.One common criterion for diagnosis of mental retardation is a tested *intelligence quotient* (IQ) of 70 or below and deficits in adaptive functioning. In early childhood mild disability (IQ 60–70) may not be obvious, and may not be diagnosed until children begin school. Even when poor academic performance is recognized, it may take expert assessment to distinguish mild mental disability from *learning disability* or behavior problems.

As they become adults, many people can live independently and may be considered by others in their community as "slow" rather than retarded. Developmental disability therefore seems to be the most appropriate term in which is recently in use in the place of mental retardation as mentioned in the AAIDD©Journal(2007).

Moderate disability (IQ 50–60) is nearly always obvious within the first years of life. These people encounter difficulty in school, at home, and in the community. In many cases they will need to join special, usually separate, classes in school, but they can still progress to become functioning members of society. As adults they may live with their parents, in a supportive group home, or even semi-independently with significant supportive services to help them, for example, manage their finances. Among people with intellectual disabilities, only about one in eight will score below 50 on IQ tests. A person with a more severe disability will need more intensive support and supervision during his or her entire life. The limitations of cognitive function will cause a child to learn and develop more slowly than a typical child. Children may take longer to learn to speak, walk, and take care of their personal needs such as dressing or eating. Learning will take them longer, require more repetition, and there may be some things they cannot learn. The extent of the limits of learning is a function of the severity of the disability.

Nevertheless, virtually every child is able to learn, develop, and grow to some extent. To facilitate the same to the best of their ability, computers as a medium is well established as a powerful learning tool in an interactive context.Meyers25 was among the first to demonstrate the facilitative effects of using a computer with preschool children with Down syndrome in the early 1980s. It was concluded that severely handicapped children (some of whom had Down syndrome) made improvements in specific fields like that of vocabulary, general language skills, and social skills after an intervention that involved individualized, clinician-facilitated computer training in addition to a classroom communication curriculum.

OBJECTIVE

Mental Retardation or developmental disability represents a widespread and heterogeneous condition, characterized principally by cognitive deficits in relation to the normal population (Zeaman & House, 1963; Ellis, 1963; Milgram, 1982; Anderson, 1986). The nature of this deficit is yet to be described and there is a great deal of debate as to whether persons with MR display slower development of cognitive abilities (Zigler, 1969) or alternatively, develop their cognitive system as the result of different processes, one or more of which may be deficient (Ellis, 1969; Ellis & Cavalier, 1982). More recently Detterman (1987) proposed a possible solution to this historical controversy that MR should be characterised by a deficit of a complex cognitive system of independent but interrelated parts. So, the different theories on MR -delayed versus deviant development- were interpreted as a function of the measurements used (molar versus molecular). Vicari et al. (1992), describing different patterns of cognitive abilities in a neuropsychological test battery from persons with the same IQ and Chronological Age, confirmed Detterman's point of view. According to this conceptual framework, MR would arise not from a homogeneous involvement of mental functions, but rather from a deficit of one or more cognitive abilities.

Thus children with MR of similar significance may show different cognitive profiles. According to Shatin (1982), Psychology Department, the Chinese University of Hong Kong CAI provides educational and rehabilitative supports to improve cognitive development of special children. The principal aim of computer therapy is to increase the eye-hand co-ordination, to enhance the academic course assigned to the students through reinforcements, to impart expertise to students to take up computers as a vocation in accordance with the skills acquired. To these aims specific computer supports are utilized

FORMULATION OF HYPOTHESIS

In management of the child at Sankalp it is suggested that both Pervasive Developmental Disorder PDD (autism) and mild MR be kept in mind and that he would benefit from reduction of rocking movement through psychological intervention. Introduction of dance therapy may help improve smoothness of motor movement and one-on-one instruction focused on socialization and self-management skills may enhance self-confidence.

Specific Interests of the subject were music, playing with toys, puzzles, and watching television. Keen interest and positive response to audio-visual aid was the basis for CAI being used as an intervention program in order to facilitate the academic curriculum by increasing attention span and reducing restlessness and rocking movement.

METHODOLOGY

Research Design

The investigation is based on a longitudinal study as a single subject design which employed a Before-After Experimental Model to assess the impact of Computer Aided Instruction as an intervention program.

SAMPLE

Master NC, aged 14 yrs 6months, is studying in vocational training class at Sankalp. Sankalp is a Special Education and Advisory Center for Children, which was started by the Naval Wives Welfare Association in 1990.Though initially started to serve the Naval Community, the school is now open to children of Armed Forces Personnel as well as the Defense Civilians. The subject was diagnosed with Developmental Disability, Autistic Features and Attention Deficit Hyperactivity Disorder(ADHD) with mild Deystonia which refers to poorly developed muscle tone. Complaints were of short attention span, restlessness, constant rocking movement and general lack of interest in the academic curriculum as noted by behavioral observation before intervention.

TOOLS FOR PSYCHOMETRIC EVALUATION

1. Malins Intelligence Scale For Indian Children(MISIC)
2. Vinelands Social Maturity Scale (VSMS)
3. Childhood Autism Rating Scale (CARS)

TOOLS FOR INTERVENTION

1. Computers
2. Software
   (a) MS Word
   (b) Paintbrush
   (c) Logic Building CD-ROMS (Based on developmental age)
   (d) Schoolroom Educational CD-ROMS (Based on developmental age)

PSYCHOMETRIC EVALUATION

The subject's IQ score was 53.6 (Mild) where PQ was 67 and VQ was 40.2 on Malins Intelligence Scale For Indian Children. On the basis of Vinelands Social Maturity Scale (VSMS),Social Age and Social Quotient were 8 yrs. 3 months and 57.22 respectively while Developmental Age and Developmental Quotient were 8 yrs. 6months and 59.42. With respect to the score on Childhood Autism Rating Scale ,the subject was diagnosed with having Moderate Autism(35).

Having this baseline data , the subject was given CAI as part of the intervention program which was implemented in the following manner.

INTERVENTION PROGRAM

The computer sessions were taken twice a weak for a period of an hour in the form of one-to-one Interactive session for a period of one year during the academic session (2005-2006) and it is an ongoing intervention program.

FIGURE 1

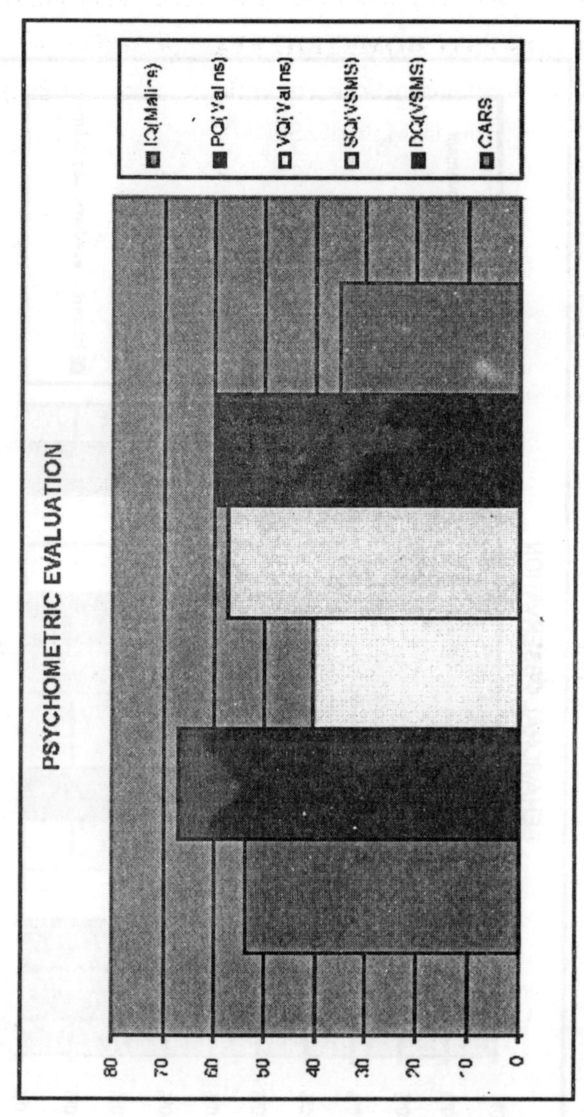
PSYCHOMETRIC EVALUATION
IQ(Mali s)
PQ(Val ns)
VQ(Val ns)
SQ(VSMS)
DQ(VSMS)
CARS
80
70
60
50
40
30
20
0

FIGURE 2

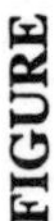
BEHAVIORAL OBSERVATION
100%
90%
80%
70%
60%
50%
40%
30%
20%
10%
0%
Before Intervention
After Intervention
Frequent rocking movement
Restlessness
attention span
eye contact
Interest in academic curriculum

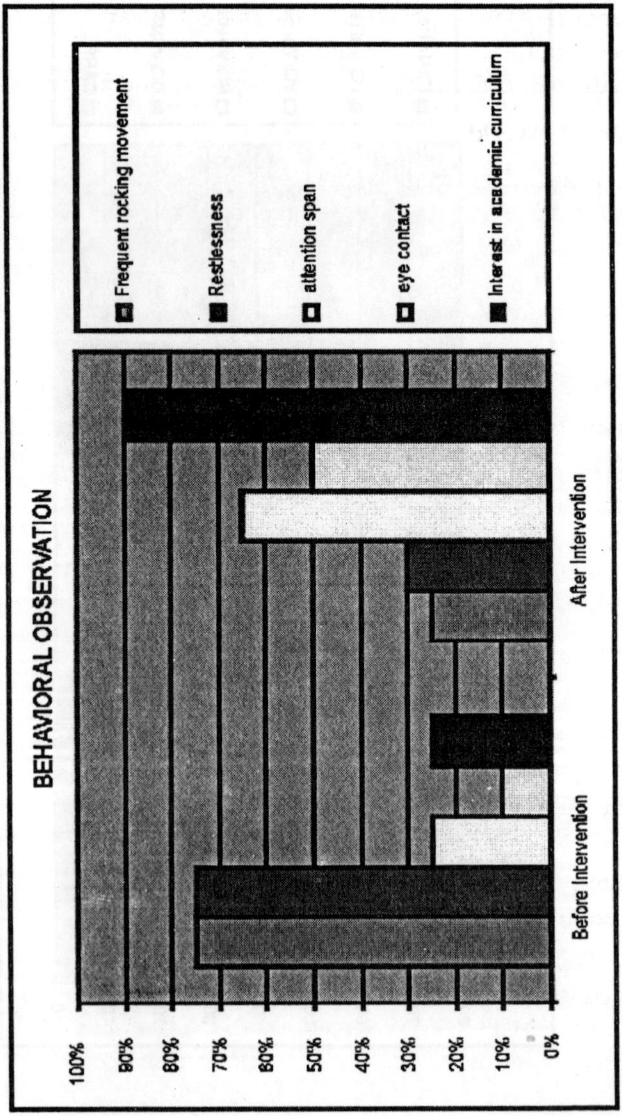

Session 1: Introduction to computers

It involves familiarizing with the different parts of the computer, learning primarily to put on the computer and using the keyboard and mouse. It takes 5-7 classes for the student to learn mouse-control, but eventually depending on their capability they learn to do so with the requisite amount of encouragement and incentives given.

Session 2: Working with the software provided

It includes learning to type numbers and alphabets in MS Word and also learning to access the required software and typing words and sentences (e.g., like the student's name, address, parents and sibling's name, words related to the course material etc). It gives immense amount of satisfaction to the student when they perform the tasks enlisted. In this session spontaneity of both the student and teacher is of utmost importance.

Session 3: Introducing the Usage of Various Options

In this session the subject learns to change the font color, size etc., add clipart and word art and systematic introduction of other options. It was observed that the concentration span of ADHD children increases due to the use of the audio-visual aids and retention of students with mild MR gets enhanced.

Session 4: Reinforcement of class syllabi

After the desired comfort level of the student with the medium of computer was arrived at, class syllabus was reinforced by encouraging the student either to recognize the text or graphics or to type in the keywords. Retention & attention span got enhanced, the result being increase in self-confidence of the child.

Session 5: Introduction to new software and CAI used as a communication tool

Paintbrush was used to help increase eye/hand co-ordination and concentration. New software (Logic Building and Schoolroom Educational CD-ROMS) were introduced intermittently to keep the interest level high. Readymade software in accordance to the student's age and capability was used. Freedom was given to the student to draw whatever he/she desired. While doing these, questions were put forward to the students regarding the drawings to gain insight and promote socialization skills keeping in view the Autistic features of the subject.

Each of these five sessions was repeated minimum five to seven times to get positive results and has to be a one to one session for optimum results. Encouragement and patience are the key elements. The schedule can be altered in accordance to the student's interest & capabilities.

RESULTS AND DISCUSSION

The results pertaining to behavioral observation based on the comparison of pre and post Computer Aided Instruction Program have been presented in Figure 2.

The results reveal that the subject has improved as a result of the intervention program(CAI) with respect to behavioral observations based on feedback reports from the special educator. The improvement is in terms of decreased rocking movements and restlessness along with increase in attention span, eye contact and interest in academic curriculum. Feedback report further revealed that the subject while working on the computer was alert, attentive and showed enthusiasm and willingness to learn and participate through the medium of computer, thereby showing remarkable decrease of restlessness and rocking movements. With increased concentration levels the subject seemed responsive to suggestions by making better eye contact and readily cooperating with the special school staff in fulfilling the tasks and activities given to him as part of school curriculum. CAI classes acted as an incentive for the subject to perform to the best of his capability in the conventional classroom atmosphere by providing self motivation and positive reinforcement.

Thus based on the aforesaid observations, computers seem to act as a foundation for building a sense of achievement resulting in increased self confidence and general well being. Computer Technology having developed into a highly user friendly medium has resulted in facilitating to bring out creativity and originality in an easy, interesting and enjoyable manner. Flexibilty seems to be the guiding feature where the developmentally disabled could take advantage and work effectively both at home and in the office, thus forming a basis for vocational opportunities. In addition parents may be guided with the help of psychologists and special educators to make use of CAI as a via medium to establish greater bonding and enhancing the capabilities of their wards.

CONCLUSION

CAI as an intervention program for a period of one year conducted on the subject with developmental delays and autism is found to be effective in bringing about a positive change with respect to improving attention span, increasing adaptability through better communication skills, reduced restlessness and rocking movements by offering greater flexibility enabling the subject to work at his own pace and preparing him for economic independence in future .From the point of view of the parents , the CAI as a psychological intervention program may probably be of immense benefit as they could be more resourceful by actively participating and interacting with their wards resulting in increased bonding and self acceptance.

REFERENCES

Anderson M (1986). Annotation understanding the cognitive deficit in mental retardation. *Journal of Child Psychology and Psychiatry* 27, 297-306.

Detterman (1987). Theoretical notions of intelligence and mental retardation. *American Journal of Mental Deficiency* 92, 2-11.

Allen F, Harold A P, Michael B F(1994).Diagnostic And Statistical Manual Of Mental Disorders: Fourth Edition. India, Jaypee Brothers.

Ellis NR (1963). The stimulus trace and behavioral inadequacy. In: *Handbook of Mental Deficiency*, N.R. Ellis (ed.), pp.134-58. McGraw-Hill, New York, NY.

Ellis NR (1969). A behavioural research strategy in mental retardation: defence and critique. *American Journal of Mental Deficincy* 73, 557-67.

Ellis NR & Cavalier AR (1982). Research perspectives in Mental Retardation. In: *Mental Retardation: The Development-Difference Controversy*, E. Zigler & D. Balla (eds), pp.121-52. Lawrence Erlbaum Associates, Hillsdale, NJ.

Luckason, Borthwick-Duffy, Buntix, Coulter, Craig (2002) The American Association on Mental Retardation Reference manual on definition and Terminology:10th edition. McGraw-Hill, New York, N.Y.

Milgram N.A. (1982) The rational and irrational in Zigler's motivational approach to mental retardation. In: *Mental Retardation: The developmental Difference Controversy*, E. Zigler & D. Balla (Eds.), pp. 155-62. Lawrence Erlbaum Associates, Hillsdale, NJ.

Shatin, N. T (1982) Introduction: the developmental approach to mental retardation. In: *Mental Retardation: The developmental Difference Controversy*, E. Zigler & D. Balla (Eds.), pp. 3-8. Lawrence Erlbaum Associates, Hillsdale, NJ.

Smith T. (1999). Outcome of early intervention for children with autism. *Clinical Psychology: Research and Practice, 6*, 33-4

Vicari S, Albertini G, Caltagirone C (1992). Cognitive profiles in adolescents with mental retardation. *Journal of Intellectual Disability Research, 36*, 415-423.

Zeaman D. & House B. (1963) The role of attention in retarded discrimination learning. In: *Handbook of Mental Deficiency*, N.R. Ellis (Ed.), pp. 159-223. McGraw-Hill, New York, N.Y.

Zigler E. (1969) Developmental versus difference theories of mental retardation and the problem of motivation. *American Journal of Mental Deficincy* 73, 536-56.

35

Learning Disabilities in Visually Impaired

Some Intervention Strategies for Developmental Dyslexia

K.P. Subba Rao*, D. Lalitha, D.V. Subba Raju*****

ABSTRACT

The paper discusses some of the intervention programmes aimed at teaching linguistic skills and the difficulties encountered by children with Dyslexia—a specific learning disability in visually Impaired. This can provide useful strategies for teachers for improving the academic achievement of learning disabled or dyslexic students in the class. The authors view that a child with dyslexia can be helped by different intervention strategies after conducting some selected cases from a Visually handicapped school.

Children of today are the citizens of tomorrow and they are going to be pillars of the country. Hence, it is essential to ensure that each pillar is strong as the other. Moreover, we cannot think of bringing about optimum human resource development without uplifting all categories of backward students. There is every possibility that each class room has some learning disabled

* **Professor, Department of Education, Andhra University, Visakhapatnam.**

** **Lecturer, Dr. L. Bullayya College of Education, Visakhapatnam.**

*** **Sr. Lecturer, District Institute of Educational Training, Bheemili.**

students. The fact that learning disabled students have near normal, normal or above normal intelligence, envisages that these students should be identified as early as possible, so that required intervention strategies can be planned at the earliest. A sound educational programme for learning disabled students comprises atleast 3 important steps. They are Assessment, Identification and Planning instructional interventions.

In order to read and write, children have to learn how to map the sound of the heard word, the sight of the written word and the articulatory sequence of the spoken word on to each other. Additional codes have to be learned concerning segment of word sounds, word spellings, specific sequences of letters and their relation to speech sound. Thus both whole word and segmented codes are involved in the acquisition of written language and the child needs to learn to relate these codes correctly to each other (Paulesu. Frith. Snowling, Gallagher, Morton, Frackowaik, and Frith. 1996).

Learning Disabilities: Learning disabilities affect the manner in which individuals with average or above average intelligence receive, process, retain and/or organize. The areas of difficulty will vary from one student to another.

Learning disabilities concern a specific group of handicapped children and youth. The Education for all Handicapped children Act, defines "learning disabilities as "specific learning disability means a disorder in one or more of the basic psychological processes evolved in understanding in using language, spoken or written which may mean test themselves in an imperfect ability to listen, think, speak, write, spell or to do mathematical calculations. The term includes such conditions as perceptional handicaps, brain injury, dysfunction, dyslexia and developmental aphasia. The term does not include children who have learning problems, which are primarily the result of visual hearing or motor handicaps, of mental retardation or of environmental, and economic disadvantages".

Definition: The definition of a learning disability is as follows: Learning disability is a persistent condition of presumed neurological dysfunction which may also exist with other disabling conditions. This dysfunction continues despite instruction in standard classroom situations. Learning disabled, a heterogeneous group, have these common attributes: average to above average intellectual ability; severe processing deficit; severe aptitude-achievement discrepancy and measured achievement in an instructional or employment setting.

Characteristics: Students with learning disabilities might exhibit one or more of the following characteristics: Reading confusion of similar words, difficulty in using phoniems, problems in reading multi-syllable words, difficulty in finding important points or main ideas. Slow reading rate and/or difficulty in adjusting speed to the nature of the reading task, difficulty with comprehension and retention of material that is read, but not with materials presented orally. Writing difficulty with sentence structure, poor grammar, omitted words, frequent spelling errors, inconsistent spelling, letter reversals difficulty in copying from chalkboard poorly formed handwriting – might spring instead of using script, writes with an inconsistent slant; have difficulty with certain letters; space words unevenly, compositions lacking organization and development of ideas, listening difficulty, paying attention when spoken to, difficulty listening to a lecture and taking notes at the same time easily distracted by background noise or visual stimulation might appear, to be hurried in one-to-one meetings, Inconsistent concentration, oral language difficulty, expressing ideas orally which the student seems to understand, difficulty in describing events or stories in proper sequence, difficulty with grammar, using a similar sounding word in place of the appropriate one, difficulty in memorizing basic facts of mathes, confusion or reversal of numbers, number sequences or symbols, copying problems, aligning columns difficulty in reading or comprehending work problems, study skills problems, problem with reasoning and abstract concepts, exhibits an inability to stick to simple schedules, repeatedly forgets things, loses or leaves possessions, and generally seems "personally disorganized", difficulty in following directions, poor organization time management and social skills, difficulty in "reading" facial expressions, and body language, problems interpreting subtle messages - such as sarcassam or humour seems disorganized in space – confuses up and down, right and left, gets lost in a building, is disoriented in time, i.e. is often late to class, unusually early for appointments or unable to finish assignments in the standard time period, expresses excessive anxiety, anger, or depression because of the inability to cope with school or social situations.

Reading represents an important area of an integrated programme of language development which includes speaking, pronunciation and spelling. Reading involves three processes i.e. Interpreting symbols, making the correct sound and understanding the sense. So it is defined as a process of sight, sound and sense. Some children, though they have normal intelligence, fail to achieve this basic skill at an expected rate. This may be due to specific learning disability in the area of reading. Learning disability refers to specific retardation or disorder in one or more processes of speech, language perception, reading, spelling or arithmetic.

This does not include learning problems which are due to Sensory handicap, motor problem, mental retardation, emotional disturbance or adverse environmental factors.

The term "Dyslexia" is used to represent the specific learning disability. It is most commonly observed among learning disabled children. It is defined as "the inability to learn to process written language despite adequate intelligence, sensory ability and exposure" (Grubin, D. 2002).

The term "Dyslexia" was coined by Rudolf Berlin of Stuttgart, Germany, in 1887. He used this word to describe reading difficulties that students had with words and letters. The American Heritage Dictionary defines Dyslexia as "a learning disability marked by impairment in the ability to read". More recently, dyslexia has been defined as "the inability to learn to process written language despite adequate intelligence, sensory ability, and exposure" (Grubin 2002). Symptoms of Dyslexia common symptoms of dyslexia include, but are not limited to: problems with spelling; difficulty in recognizing individual sounds in words; reading difficulties; differences between a child's ability and his actual level of achievement; difficulties in naming things; problems with getting things in the right order. Just as every child is different, so are the symptoms of dyslexia. Some dyslexic children may show only one or two of these signs, while others may have more.

CHARACTERISTICS OF CHILDREN WITH DYSLEXIA:

(A) In a Pre-schooler

- Late talking compared to other children.
- Pronunciation problems.
- Slow vocabulary growth, often unable to find the right word.
- Difficulty in rhyming words
- Trouble in learning numbers, the alphabet, days of the week.
- Extremely restless and easily distracted
- Trouble interacting with peers.
- Poor ability to follow directions or routines.

(B) At primary level

- Slow to learn the connection between letters and sounds.
- Confuses basic words.
- Make consistent reading and spelling errors including letter reversals (b/d).
- Inversions (u/w).
- Transpositions (felt/left).
- Substitutions (house/home).
- Slow recall of facts.
- Slow to learn new things.
- Relies heavily on momorization.
- Impulsiveness on slack of planning.
- Unstabled pencil grip.
- Trouble learning about time.
- Poor coordination.
- Unaware of physical surroundings.
- Prone to accidents.

What happens in the brains of dyslexia children, when learning to read?

Many researchers suspect that the brain areas controlling language, particularly the angular gyrus, play a critical role (Ariniello, L. 1999). Research by Pughet al (2001) found that reading – disabled children had dysfunctions in the posterior areas of their left hemispheres. According to Shaywitz, S. (2003) "Good readers have a pattern of activation in the back of the brain – the system that includes the occipital region, which is activated by visual features of the letters: the angular gyrus, where print is transcoded into language; and wernicke's region, the area of the brain that accesses meaning. This posterior area is strongly activated in good readers, but we saw relative under activation in poor readers (O'Arcangeleo 1999).

According to Shaywitz (D. Arcangelo, M. 1999) people with dyslexia do not have problems in copying letters and words. They may make some reversals in writing, but no more so than other children. To use an example given by Shaywitz, a child can copy the letters "w-a-s" correctly, but when asked what was written, a dyslexia child may reply "saw". Problem is not one related to vision, but rather one of perceptual skills of what the child does with a word on a page.

INTERVENTION PROGRAMME FOR VISUALLY IMPAIRED CHILDREN

The school as well as the society have equal responsibility for teaching/remediation/counseling a person with disabilities, basic skills for independence. In schools these skills may be academic (reading, writing, speaking and computing), social (getting along with other children), following instruction, schedules and other daily routines. The underlying assumption of both remedial and habituative programmes is that a person with disabilities needs special help to succeed in the normal settings. Infact, remediation is the central part of intervention which stands for all the efforts on behalf of individuals with disabilities. The other dimensions of intervention are the preventive approaches and the compensatory efforts as well.

The world wide opinion about the remediation was focused after proclamation of PL 94-142 which called as EDUCATION FOR ALL HANDICAPPED CHILDREN ACT. It was proved a block buster legislation and hailed as the law that will probably become known as having the greatest impact on education in history.

Further amendment in PL-94-142 have initiated new chapters not only in remediation but also in the formative dimensions of intervention i.e. prevention. Thus PL-99-457 bring in its sphere the handicapped infants and toddlers from birth through age two, who need early INTERVENTION SERVICES. Similarly PL101-476 the third amendments by U.S congress changed the law which may read now as INDIVIDUALS WITH DISABILITIES EDUCATION ACT. This law has supplemented the schools with TRANSITION SERVICES which means a coordinated set of activities for a student, designed with in an out come oriented process, which promotes movement from school to post school activities, including post secondary education, vocational training, integrated employment, continuing and adult education, independent living or community participation.

INDIVIDUALIZED EDUCATION PROGRAMME: (IEP) BASIC INGREDIENT OF REMEDIATION

An individualized Education programme be developed and maintained for every student with disabilities. Each IEP must be the product of the joint effecter of the members of a child study team, which must include atleast 1. The child's teachers, 2. A representative of the local school district other than child's teacher, 3. The child's parents or guardian and 4. whenever appropriate the child himself. Other professional such as physical educator speech language pathologists and physical therapists, may also be in the IEP conferences.

A continuum of services: Exceptional children their teachers and their families may need a wide range of special education and related services from time to time. The continuum of services is a range of different placement and service opinions to meet students needs. The continuum is often symbiotically depicted as a pyramid, with placements ranging from least restrictive (regular class room placement) at the bottom to most restrictive (special schools or institutions) at the top. The fact that the pyramid is widest at the bottom indicates that the greatest number of exceptional children should be served in regular classrooms, and the number of children who require more restrictive intensive and specialized placements, are smaller as one move upward.

A high school student who can travel independently and succeed academically with only occasional help from the special teacher may do best in an itinerant teacher programme or with the help of a teacher consultant. Young children who are acquiring basic skills will probably require daily contact with a teacher of the visually important and may be best educated under the resource room plan. Children who have severe impairments or handicaps in addition to blindness will probably function best under the special or cooperative class plan. For some students restricted school placement may be most appropriate.

Because children's needs change as they develop it is important to remain flexible determining what programme best fulfils a child's needs. Children should be educated as much as possible in the classes they would be attending, if they were not visually impaired and they should spend as much time as possible in classes with children who have normal vision.

Listening: Visually impaired children both those who are totally blind and those with low vision must obtain an enormous amount of information through the sense o f hearing. A great deal of time in school is devoted to speaking and listening to other visually impaired students, also make frequent use of recorded materials particularly, in high schools. Because many visually impaired students are able to process auditory information at a faster rate than that of average conversational speech, devices are available to increase the play back rate of tapes with out significantly distorting the capacity of the speech.

PRACTICAL LIVING AND SOCIAL SKILLS

Some educators of visually impaired students suggest that academic achievement has traditionally been over emphasized at the expense of important basic living skills. Hatton (1976) calls for giving the most urgent attention to such areas as cooking grooming, shopping, personal hygiene and social behaviour.

Orientation and Mobility: Orientation is defined as the ability to stabilize one's position in relation to the environment through the use of the remaining senses. Mobility is the ability to move safely and effectively from one point to another. Orientation and mobility instruction is a well developed sub specialty who are visually impaired.

CLASS WIDE PEER TUTORING

The regular class room teacher is expected to deliver individualized instruction to the mainstream student, maintained effective programme for the rest of the class and help the main stream child because socially integrated into the class room. In practice 3 different team models have emerged (Giangreco 1989).

1. Multi disciplinary teams are composed of professionals from different disciplines who work independently of one another.
2. Inter-disciplinary team is characterized by formal channels of communication between members which each professional visually conducts discipline specific assessments, to share information and develop intervention plans.
3. Trans disciplinary team is the highest level of team involvement, but the most difficult to accomplish. The members share information and expertise accross discipline boundaries, enabling the selection of goals and primary of services that are discipline free.

CASE STUDIES

Case-1: A 4th class student, Pydithalli, daughter of an agricultural labour from Majjivalasa mandal of Vizianagaram, lost her vision at the age of 3. She belongs to a very poor family hailing from a remote village hence she could not get any sort of counseling or advice to regain the lost vision. Learning disabilities continues to intervene her learning. She lacks memory and wrongly reads and writes words. The dyslexia appears in reading words with different sounds, in writing the words with mistakes like instead of Aavu (Cow) Aava in Telugu. She confuses with the dots in the slate (Briaille) in calculation where she wrongly writes numbers, for example, instead of 36 she writes 63 simply reversing the numbers. It is understood that the girl is too slow in learning, not able to remember the order of the words and has confusion over the series of the numbers.

Case-2: Dalinaidu, a 5th class student from the school for blind, is a son of rikshawpuller. His father is a literate having education upto VII class. He too belongs to a poor family and earns Rs. 1000/- per month. The child commits mistakes in reading, writing and calculating the numbers. For instance, in Telugu he writes Abhyasham in place of Abhyasam the stress 'h' unnecessarily put on Abhyasham. In numbers he usually registers loosely the 'series' that is 1, 2, 3.... He fails to write numbers omitting the next serial number like 1, 2, 3, 6, 5 ... so on. It is considered that the boy could remember 60 percent what he learned and read. He has a lot of confusion over the words which leads to dyslexia.

Case-3: This case about Satyaveni, daughter of Sattibabu from a village from Narasipatnam mandal of Visakhapatnam. Though they belong to upper caste in social status, they also come under below the poverty line. Agriculture is the main occupation in the area. Satyavenis father works as an agricultural labour earning Rs. 6000 per anum. Satyaveni is now studying V class in the blind school. She lacks memory in recognizing the dots on the Braille sheet hence she fails to remember words as well numbers. She writes '*neru*' (water) instead of *neeru* omitting the dypthong '*ee*'. She fails to write numbers serially. She only corrects the wrongly written words when the teacher instructs promptly. It is opened that she has poor memory and confusion over the reading and writing including calculating.

CONCLUSION

Intervention research on dyslexia has clearly demonstrated reading deficits can be effectively remediated. Intervention programmes need to be structured so that inductive interference will occur and through extensive practice in different contexts transfer is possible. Such initiatives will represent progress conceptually and therapeutically for individuals with different profiles of processing defiant and reading disability.

REFERENCES

Barron, R (1996) Word Recognition in Early Reading; A review of the Direct and Indirect Access Hypotheses Cognition, 24, 93-119.

Das, JP., Mishra, RK, Pool, J.E (1995): An experiments on cognitive remediation or word reading difficulty. Journal of learning disabilities 28, 66-79.

Ashum Gupta (2002) Intervention Strategies for developmental Dyslexia. Journal of Indian Education 45-46.

Loweth, M.W., Steinbach, K.A., and Frijters, J.C. (2000): Remedicating the cone, deficits of developmental reading disability: A double deficit perspective. Journal of learning disability, 33, and 334-358.

Ariniello, L. (1999), Dyslexia and language brain areas. Society for Neuroscience Brain Briefings. Retrieved November 17, 2002 from

http://apu.sfn.org/content/Publications/BrainBriefings/dyslecxia.html.

Grubin, D. (Producer), (2002). The secret life of the brain. (Television series). Alexandria, VA: Public Broadcasting Service.

D'Arcangelo, M. (1999). Learning about learning to read: A conversation with Sally Shaywitz. Educational Leadership. 57 (2), 26-31.

Shaywitz, S. (2003). Overcoming dyslexia. New York: Alfred A. Knopf.

Giangreco, MF et al. (1989): "Providing Related Services to Learners with Severe Handicaps in Educational Settings – Pursuing the Least Restrictive Opinion. "Pediatric Physically Therapy, 1 (2): 55-63.

Hatton, Dominey D (1996): Developmental Growth Curves of Young Children Who are Visually Impaired. DAI, 56(7): 2555.

www.sangeeth.com

www.dyslexia.com

Mala Tandon, Learning Disabilities – Role of parents Edutracks, July, 2004.

Shudra Chatuvedi, (2002): *Psychological make up on Visually Impaired children*, Ms. Seema Wasan, Ranjit Publications, New Delhi.

Index

J

K

L

M

□□□